"I considered myself a good listener before reading this book, and was repeatedly surprised when I recognized myself in the examples of what not to do! It helped me immediately with my spouse, giving me tools to really listen and understand, even when we disagree, so we can find our way to a compromise. I love how funny the authors are and the great examples they weave in. I highly recommend this book to anyone!"

—Christina H., Brattleboro, Vermont

"This book delivers countless epiphanies that will help you become a better listener in all of your relationships. The questions in each chapter guide you to actively explore your own communication strengths and blind spots. The genius of this book comes from its well-told, engaging stories and anecdotes, which are wise and never preachy. The third edition has been superbly updated to cover the impact of technology, and offers invaluable advice for talking across our ever-widening political and social divides." —Anne K. Fishel, PhD,
coauthor of *Eat, Laugh, Talk: The Family Dinner Playbook*

"This book could not have come along at a better time. With the bombardment of noise and the narrowing of our screen sizes, everyone needs to read this book to remind us that there is nothing more important than tuning in to one another. *The Lost Art of Listening* should be required reading!" —Tammy Nelson, PhD,
author of *The New Monogamy*

"It will be hard for readers not to see themselves, and everyone they listen to, in this book. Drs. Nichols and Straus offer an insider's look at what can go wrong in the two-sided process of communicating. Whether you want to improve communication with family, colleagues, or friends, you will learn the skills to listen for the meaning behind the message. The book also takes on the other side of conversation—speaking with clarity. Drs. Nichols and Straus masterfully demonstrate how to open conversations that invite the listener to hear."

—Margaret Wehrenberg, PsyD, author of
The 10 Best-Ever Anxiety Management Techniques

THE LOST ART OF LISTENING

Also by the Authors

Stop Arguing with Your Kids: How to Win the Battle of Wills by Making Your Children Feel Heard
Michael P. Nichols

Treating Trauma in Adolescents:
Development, Attachment, and the Therapeutic Relationship
Martha B. Straus

THE LOST ART OF LISTENING

How Learning to Listen Can Improve Relationships

THIRD EDITION

Michael P. Nichols, PhD
Martha B. Straus, PhD

THE GUILFORD PRESS
New York   London

Last digit is print number: 9 8 7 6 5 4 3 2

Library of Congress Cataloging-in-Publication Data

Names: Nichols, Michael P., author. | Straus, Martha B., 1956– author.
Title: The lost art of listening : how learning to listen can improve relationships /
   Michael P. Nichols, Martha B. Straus.
Description: Third Edition. | New York : The Guilford Press, 2021. | Revised
   edition of The lost art of listening, c2009. | Includes bibliographical references
   and index.
Identifiers: LCCN 2020033630 | ISBN 9781462542741 (trade paperback)
   ISBN 9781462545049 (cloth)
Subjects: LCSH: Listening. | Interpersonal relations. | Interpersonal
   communication.
Classification: LCC BF323.L5 N53 2021 | DDC 153.6/8—dc23
LC record available at *https://lccn.loc.gov/2020033630*

Contents

Introduction   1

Part One. The Yearning to Be Understood

1. "Did You Hear What I Said?":   9
   Why Listening Is So Important

2. "Thanks for Listening":   29
   How Listening Shapes Us and Connects Us to Each Other

3. "Why Don't People Listen?":   50
   How Communication Breaks Down

Part Two. The Real Reasons People Don't Listen

4. "When Is It *My* Turn?":   83
   The Heart of Listening: The Struggle to Suspend Our Own Needs

5. "You Hear Only What You Want to Hear":   106
   How Hidden Assumptions Prejudice Listening

6. "Why Do You Always Overreact?!":   123
How Emotionality Makes Us Defensive

Part Three. **Getting Through to Each Other**

7. "Take Your Time—I'm Listening":   151
How to Let Go of Your Own Needs and Listen

8. "I Never Knew You Felt That Way":   176
Empathy Begins with Openness

9. "I Can See This Is Really Upsetting You":   204
How to Defuse Emotional Reactivity

Part Four. **Listening in Context**

10. "It Takes Two to Tango":   235
Listening between Intimate Partners

11. "Nobody Around Here Ever Listens to Me!":   268
How to Listen and Be Heard within the Family

12. "I Knew *You'd* Understand"   291
Being Able to Hear Friends and Colleagues

13. "I'm Not Wasting My Time Talking to *That* Person!":   322
How to Listen to People It's Impossible to Agree With

Epilogue   345

Notes   351

Index   355

About the Authors   368

Introduction

Nothing hurts more than the sense that people we care about aren't really listening. We never outgrow the need to have our feelings known. That's why a sympathetic ear is such a powerful force in human relationships—and why the failure to be understood is so painful.

My ideas about listening have been sharpened by forty-five years as a psychoanalyst and family therapist. Refereeing arguments between intimate partners, coaching parents to communicate with their children, and struggling myself to sustain empathy as my patients faced their demons has led me to the conclusion that much of the conflict in our lives can be explained by one simple fact: People don't really listen to each other.

Talking without listening is like snipping an electrical cord in half and hoping that somehow something will light up. Most of the time, of course, we don't deliberately set out to break the connection. In fact, we're often baffled and dismayed by feeling left in the dark.

Contemporary pressures have, regrettably, shrunk our attention spans and impoverished the quality of listening in our lives. We live in increasingly hurried times, when dinner is something you pick up on your way home from work, when keeping up with the latest music and movies means catching snatches on your commute, and when reading is limited to blog posts and short articles online. That's all we've got time for.

1

Meanwhile we're bombarded with so much competing input vying for our attention—not only from the Internet, TV, and emails but now also from social media posts and Instagram—that our attention is fractionated. We like to think we're good at multitasking. We check our email while talking on the phone. We look for things to buy in catalogues while watching TV. We fool ourselves into thinking that we can do more than one thing at a time. The truth is that we just end up doing one thing after another poorly.

We've gained unparalleled access to information and lost something very important. We've lost the habit of concentrating our attention. These days most people are overwhelmingly busy. From pop music at the gym to commercials on TV and radio, we're bombarded with so much noise that we've become experts at tuning things out. If a television show doesn't grab our attention in the first two minutes, we change the channel; if we're listening to someone who doesn't get right to something we're interested in, we tune out.

In the limited time we still preserve for family and friends, conversation is often preempted by soothing and passive distractions. Too tired to talk and listen, we settle instead for the lulling charms of electronic devices that project pictures, make music, or bleep across display screens. Is it this way of life that's made us forget how to listen? Perhaps. But maybe the modern approach to life is the effect rather than the cause of the decline of meaningful discourse. Maybe we lead this kind of life because we're seeking some sort of solace, something to counteract the dimming of the spirit we feel when no one is listening.

How we lost the art of listening is certainly a matter for debate. What isn't debatable is that the loss leaves us with an ever-widening hole in our lives. It might take the form of a vague sense of discontent or deprivation. We miss the consolation of lending an attentive ear and of receiving the same in return, but we don't know what's wrong or how to fix it. Over time this lack of listening impoverishes our most important relationships.

Conflict doesn't necessarily disappear when we acknowledge each other's point of view, but it's almost certain to get worse if we don't. So why don't we take time to hear each other? Because the simple art of listening isn't so simple.

Often it's a burden. Not, perhaps, the perfunctory attention we grant in the casual interchanges of everyday life. But the sustained attention of careful listening—that takes strenuous and unselfish restraint. To listen well we must forget ourselves and submit to the other person's need for attention.

Most failures of understanding are not due to self-absorption or bad faith, but to our own need to say something. We tend to react to what is said, rather than concentrating on what the other person is trying to express. Emotional reactions make us respond without thinking and crowd out understanding and concern. In these busy times we may think that we're listening, but with obligations and distractions, we often listen only perfunctorily. We get the gist of what someone is saying and restlessly move on. Each of us has characteristic ways of reacting defensively. We don't hear what's said because something in the speaker's message triggers hurt, anger, or impatience.

Unfortunately, all the advice in the world about "active listening" can't overcome the maddening tendency to react defensively to each other. To become better listeners, and to transform our relationships, we must learn to control the emotional triggers that generate anxiety and cause misunderstanding and conflict.

If this task seems too formidable, remember that most of us are more capable than we give ourselves credit for. We concentrate pretty hard at work, and most of us still enjoy earnest, open conversation with a few friends. In fact, talking with friends is a model of what conversation can be: safe enough to talk about what matters, concerned enough to listen, honest enough to tell the truth, and tactful enough to know when not to. More relationships should be like this.

In the process of writing this book, I've tried to become a better listener in my personal as well as professional life, to listen a little harder to my wife's complaints without getting defensive, and to hear my children's opinions before giving my own. However, I've had conversations that left me feeling bruised and defeated. My wife would speak sharply to me about not helping out more around the house or not listening to her, and I'd feel attacked; or I'd call my editor one too many times to complain about the burdens of writing and she'd make *me* feel like a burden for complaining; or my friend Rich would call me the part of the anatomy you sit on for acting like I was entitled to some special consideration. Not only didn't I listen at these times—hear and acknowledge what the other person was saying—but I got hurt and angry, and completely unwilling to talk to that person, *ever again, as long as I live.*

I'm sure you know how painful such misunderstandings can be. When my wife "yelled at me," my editor was "mean to me," and my friend "picked on me," I got hurt and withdrew. But what made these incidents especially painful was that just when I thought I was learning to listen better, these setbacks set me all the way back. Instead of just thinking that things hadn't gone well and needed repair, I felt defeated. How could I, who can't even get along with the people in my own life, have the temerity to write a book about listening?

Maybe you know how that feels. When we try to change something in our lives, whether it's our diet or work habits or listening skills, and we experience a setback, we have a tendency to feel hopeless and give up. Suddenly the progress we thought we were making seems like an illusion. Maybe if I were reading a book about listening and experienced these setbacks, I would have given up. But since I was *writing* this book, after a while of brooding in hurt silence I'd go back and try to talk to the person I'd quarreled with— only this time with the resolve to listen to his or her side before telling mine. In the process, I learned to see how my relationships go through cycles of closeness and distance and, even more important, how I could influence those cycles by the quality of my own listening.

This book is an invitation to think about the ways we talk and listen to each other: why listening is such a powerful force in our lives; how to listen deeply, with sustained immersion in another's experience; and how to prevent good listening from being spoiled by bad habits. There's no question that listening is an even greater challenge than it was when I wrote this book.

Because I (MPN) am an old fossil and don't know much about the digital world, I'm happy to be joined in this edition by Dr. Martha Straus as coauthor. Marti is a clinical psychologist and professor with expertise in the novel challenges of online conversations. She has helped me update this new edition to account for the important ways that the digital devices and social media have transformed the rules for communication and made it even harder for people to get their fair share of nourishing, in-person listening.

In this third edition we also talk about how much tougher it has become to have a meaningful conversation with someone who views the world very differently than we do. Today we comfortably curate our newsfeeds and social lives, hanging out as much as possible with people and ideas that match our own. Knowing it will be upsetting for us, we don't push ourselves to listen to anyone whose perspective is diametrically opposed to our own—and so obviously wrong. Instead of learning to handle our own emotionality to have difficult conversations, we avoid them altogether. Chapter 13 explains how to listen when it feels almost impossible—to relatives and colleagues who make our blood boil or about hot-button topics like politics, culture wars, and painful family disputes.

Among the secrets of successful communication we describe are:

- The difference between real dialogue and just taking turns talking
- Hearing what people mean, not just what they say
- How to reduce arguments
- How to ask for support without getting unwanted advice
- How to get uncommunicative people to open up
- How to share a difference of opinion without making other people feel criticized
- How to make sure both sides get heard in heated discussions
- How speakers undermine their own messages
- How to get people to listen to you
- How to listen when communicating by text, phone, video chat, and social media
- How to converse with difficult people
- How to listen across social and political divides

The Lost Art of Listening is divided into four parts. Part One explains why listening is so important in our lives—far more important than we realize—and how, for many people, it's a lack of sympathetic attention, not stress or overwork, that accounts for the loss of real connection in their relationships. Part Two explores the hidden assumptions and emotional reactions that are the real reasons people don't listen. We'll see what makes listeners too defensive to hear what others are saying, how digital communication can fuel anxiety and misunderstanding, and why you may not get heard even though you have something important to say.

After exploring the major roadblocks to listening, we'll examine in Part Three how you can understand and control emotional reactivity to become a better listener. And we'll explain how you can make yourself heard, even in relationships with deeply entrenched misunderstandings. Finally, in Part

Four, we'll explore how listening breaks down in intimate partnerships, in family relationships, between friends, and at work. We'll explain how listening is complicated by the dynamics of these relationships and how to use this knowledge to break through to each other. And we'll describe how to listen across social, cultural, and political divides, even when such conversations feel deeply personal and threatening, and the other person seems impossibly obtuse.

Throughout this book we've added invitations to reflect on how the legacy of our past affects our listening in the present, because the way we listen now has been shaped by how we've been listened to from the beginning of our lives. We've also scattered in the book discussions of common struggles parents have with listening to their children and teens. And at the end of each chapter, you'll find a set of exercises designed to help you become a better listener. Actually doing these exercises may help transform the passive experience of reading into an active process of improving your ability to listen.

Regardless of how much we take it for granted, the importance of listening cannot be overestimated. The gift of our attention and understanding makes other people feel validated and valued. Our ability to listen, and listen well, creates goodwill that comes back to us. But effective listening is also the best way to enjoy others, to learn from them, and to make them interesting to be with. We hope that this book can help take us a step in the direction of showing more of the concern we feel for each other.

PART ONE

The Yearning to Be Understood

1

"Did You Hear What I Said?"

WHY LISTENING IS SO IMPORTANT

Sometimes it seems that we're all so preoccupied that nobody listens anymore.

"He expects me to listen to his problems, but he never asks about mine."

"She can't remember what I've told her because she's always busy with something else."

"She often doesn't answer my texts, but she gets upset when she doesn't get an immediate response from me."

"The only time I find out what's going on in his life is when I overhear him telling someone else. Why doesn't he tell *me* these things?"

"I can't talk to her because she's so critical."

Wives complain that their husbands take them for granted. Husbands complain that their wives take forever to get to the point.

She feels a violation of their connection. He doesn't trust the connection.

Few motives in human experience are as powerful as the yearning to be understood. Being listened to means that we are taken seriously, that our feelings are recognized, and, ultimately, that what we have to say matters.

The urge to be heard is a longing to escape our isolation and bridge the space that separates us. We reach out and try to overcome that separateness by revealing what's on our minds and in our hearts, hoping for understanding. Getting that understanding should be simple, but it isn't.

Joan saw a suit she'd like to buy for work, but wasn't sure she should spend the money. "Honey," she said, "I saw a really nice suit at the outlet store."
"That's nice," Henry said, and went back to his iPad.

Sanjay was upset about having had a fender bender, but he was afraid that if he said anything Denise would get on his case about it. So he kept quiet and worried about how he was going to get it fixed. Denise felt Sanjay's distance and assumed that he was angry at her for something. She didn't feel like having an argument, so she didn't say anything either.

The essence of good listening is empathy, which can only be achieved by suspending our preoccupation with ourselves and entering into the experience of the other person. Part intuition and part effort, it's the stuff of human connection. And, maybe paradoxically, these days it seems that the more ways we have to communicate, the less we seem able to find the time for conversation.

A listener's empathy—grasping what we're trying to say *and showing it*—builds a bond of understanding, linking us to someone who hears us and cares, and thus confirms that our feelings are legitimate and comprehensible. The power of empathic listening is the power to transform relationships. When deeply felt but unexpressed feelings take shape in words that are voiced and come back clarified, the result is a reassuring sense of being understood and a grateful feeling of shared humanness.

· · · · · · · · · · · · · ·

The art of listening is critical to successful relationships.

· · · · · · · · · · · · ·

If listening strengthens our relationships by cementing our connection with one another, it also fortifies our sense of self. In the presence of a receptive listener, we are able to clarify what we think and discover what we feel. Thus, in giving an account of our experience to someone who listens, we are better able to listen to ourselves. Our lives are defined in dialogue.

It Hurts Not to Be Listened To

The need to be taken seriously and understood is frustrated every day. Adults complain that their children and partners don't listen. Children complain that their parents are too busy scolding them to hear their side of things. Even friends, usually a reliable source of shared understanding, are often too busy to listen to one another these days. And if we sometimes feel cut off from sympathy and understanding in the private sphere, we've grown not even to expect courtesy and attention in public settings.

Our right to be heard is violated in countless ways that we don't always remember, by others who don't always realize. That doesn't make it any less frustrating.

When I told a psychiatrist friend that I was collecting experiences on the theme "It hurts not to be listened to," he sent me this example:

"I called a friend and left a message asking if we could meet at a particular time. He didn't answer, and I felt a little anxious and confused. Should I call again to remind him? After all, I know he's busy. Should I wait another day or two and hope he'll answer? Should I not have asked him in the first place? All this leaves me uneasy."

The first thing that struck me about this example was how even a little thing like an unanswered phone message can leave someone feeling unresponded to—and troubled. Then I was really struck—like a slap in the face—by the realization that my friend was talking about me! Suddenly I was embarrassed, and then defensive. The reason I hadn't returned his call—doesn't matter. (We always have reasons for not responding.) What matters is how my failure to respond hurt and confused my friend and that I never had any inkling of it.

If an oversight like that can hurt, how much more painful is it when the subject is of urgent importance to the speaker?

. . . .

Listening is so basic that we take it for granted.
Unfortunately, most of us think of ourselves
as better listeners than we really are.

. . . .

When you come home from a business trip, eager to tell your partner how it went, and he listens but after a minute or two something in his eyes goes to sleep, you feel hurt and betrayed. When you call your parents to share a triumph and they don't seem really interested, you feel deflated and perhaps foolish for having allowed yourself to even hope for appreciation.

Just as it hurts not to be listened to when you're excited about something special, it's painful not to feel listened to by some*one* special, someone you expect to care about you.

Jalen's best friend in college was Derek. They were both political science majors and shared a passion for politics. Together they followed every revelation of congressional dysfunction, relishing unfolding news items as though they were a series of deliciously wicked Charles Addams cartoons. But as much as they took cynical delight in examples of hypocrisy and folly in Washington, their friendship went beyond politics.

Jalen remembered the wonderful feeling of talking to Derek for hours, impelled by the momentum of some deep and inexplicable sympathy. There was the pleasure of being able to say anything he wanted, and the pleasure of hearing Derek say everything he'd always thought but never expressed. Unlike Jalen's other friends, Derek wasn't a competitive conversationalist. He really listened.

When they went to graduate schools in different cities, they kept up their friendship. Jalen would visit Derek, or Derek would visit Jalen, at least once a month. They'd play pool or see a movie and go out for Chinese food; and then afterward, no matter how late it got, they'd stay up talking.

Then Derek got married, and things changed. Derek didn't become distant the way some friends do after marriage, nor did Derek's wife dislike Jalen. The distance Jalen felt was subtle, but it made a big difference.

"It's difficult to describe exactly, but I often end up feeling awkward and disappointed when I speak with Derek. He listens . . . but somehow he doesn't seem really interested anymore. He doesn't ask questions. He used to be so involved. It makes me sad. I still feel excited about the things going on in my life, but telling Derek just makes me feel unconnected and alone with them."

Jalen's lament says something important about listening. It isn't just not being interrupted that we want. Sometimes people appear to be listening but aren't really hearing. Some people are good at being silent when we talk. Sometimes they betray their lack of interest by glancing around, checking their phones, and shifting their weight back and forth. At other times, however, listeners show no sign of inattention, but still we know they aren't really hearing what we have to say. It feels like they don't care.

Derek's passive interest was especially painful to Jalen because of the closeness they'd shared. The friends had reached an impasse; Jalen couldn't open himself to his friend the way he'd done in the past, and Derek was mystified by the distance that had grown between them.

Friendship is voluntary, and so talking about it is optional. Jalen didn't want to complain to Derek or make demands. Besides, how does one guy tell another that he feels no longer cared about? And so Jalen never did talk to Derek about feeling estranged. Too bad, because when a relationship goes sour, talking about it may be the only way to make things right again.

> It's especially hurtful not to be listened to
> in those relationships we count on for understanding.

After a while most of us learn to do a pretty good imitation of being grownups and shrug off a lot of slights and misunderstandings. If, in the process, we become a little calloused, well maybe that's the price you pay for getting along in the world. But sometimes not being responded to leaves us feeling so hurt and angry that it can make us retreat from relationships, even for years.

When a woman discovered that her husband was having an affair, she felt as if someone had kicked her in the gut. In her grief and anger, she turned to the person she was closest to—her sister-in-law, whom she considered her best friend. The sister-in-law tried to be understanding and supportive, but it was, after all, hard to listen to the bitter statements about her brother. Still, she tried. Apparently, however, the support she offered wasn't enough. Eventually the crisis passed and the couple reconciled, but the woman, feeling that her sister-in-law hadn't been there when she needed her, never spoke to her again.

The sister-in-law in this sad story was baffled by her friend's stubborn silence. Other people's reactions often seem unreasonable to us. What makes their reactions reasonable *to them* is feeling wounded by a lack of responsiveness.

To listen is to pay attention, take an interest, care about, take to heart, validate, acknowledge, be moved . . . appreciate. Listening is so central to human existence as to often escape notice; or, rather, it appears in so many guises that it's seldom recognized as the overarching need that it is. Sometimes, as Jalen, the estranged sister-in-law, and so many others have discovered, we don't realize how important being listened to is until we feel cheated out of it.

Once in a while, however, we become aware of how much it means to be listened to. You can't decide whether or not to take a new job, and so you call an old friend to talk it over. She doesn't tell you what to do, but the fact that she listens, really listens, helps you see things more clearly. Another time you're just getting to know someone, but you like him so much that after a wonderful dinner in a restaurant you take a risk and ask him over for coffee. When he says, "No thanks, I've got to get up early," you feel rejected. Convinced that he doesn't like you, you start avoiding him. After a few days, however, he asks you what's wrong, and once again you take a risk and tell him that your feelings were hurt. To your great relief, instead of arguing, he listens and accepts what you have to say. "I can see how you might have felt that way, but actually I would like to see you again."

Why can't it always be that way? I speak, you listen. It's that simple, isn't it? Unfortunately, no. Talking and listening create a unique relationship in which speaker and listener are constantly switching roles, both jockeying for position, each one's needs competing with the other's. If you doubt this, try telling someone about a problem you're having and see how long it takes before he interrupts to describe a similar experience of his own or to offer advice—advice that may suit him more than it does you.

A man in therapy was exploring his relationship with his distant father when he suddenly remembered the happy times they'd spent together playing with his electric trains. It was a Lionel set that had been his father's and grandfather's before him. Caught up in the memory, the man grew increasingly excited as he recalled the pride he'd felt in sharing this family tradition with his father. As the man's enthusiasm mounted, the therapist launched into a long story about *his* train set and how he had gotten the other kids in the neighborhood to bring over their tracks and train cars to build a huge neighborhood setup in his basement. After the therapist had gone on at some length, the patient could no longer contain his anger about being cut off. "Why are you telling me about *your* trains?!" he demanded. The therapist hesitated; then, with that level, impersonal voice we reserve for confiding something intimate, he said lamely, "I was just trying to be friendly."

. . . .

It takes two people to share a feeling—
one to talk and one to listen.

. . . .

The therapist had made an all-too-common mistake (actually he'd made several, but this is Be Kind to Therapists Week). He assumed that sharing his own experience was the equivalent of empathy. In fact, though, he switched the focus to himself, making his patient feel discounted, misunderstood, unappreciated. That's what hurt. It might have even been more distressing because therapists are paid to listen empathically; however, the experience of invalidation is awful no matter who is co-opting the conversation.

As is often the way with words that become familiar, *empathy* may not adequately convey the power of appreciating the inner experience of another person. Empathic listening is like the close reading of a poem; it takes in the words and gets to what's behind them. The difference is that while empathy is actively imaginative, it is fundamentally receptive rather than creative. When we attend to a work of art, our idiosyncratic response has its own validity, but when we attend to someone who's trying to tell us something, it's understanding their feelings, not creativity, that counts.

Bearing Witness

Listening has not one but two purposes: taking in information and bearing witness to another's experience. When people tell you about their lives, it is reasonable to assume that they expect you to pay attention and perhaps offer a supportive response. Of course, this seemingly simple personal exchange still poses plenty of challenges. But now we are also asking people to listen to us through a variety of social media—texts, images, posts, blogs, tweets, and shares—offering so many more ways to bear witness to the experiences of others but also to let each other down by not responding sufficiently, if we respond at all.

Indeed, the act of posting a comment or picture can be a way of casting a wide net to friends and followers to ask them to bear witness to our experience. Getting comments and "likes" on social media might be a less direct strategy for seeking support; yet our hurt and disappointment when no one responds may feel much the same as if we had asked in person. Whether we speak face-to-face or through electronic communication, we are still giving voice to our need to be heard. By momentarily stepping out of his or her own frame of reference and into ours, the person who really listens acknowledges and affirms us. That validation is essential for sustaining the confirmation known as self-respect. Without feeling listened to, we are shut up in the solitude of our own hearts.

A thirty-six-year-old woman was so unnerved by an upsetting incident that she wondered if she needed psychotherapy. Estela, the executive vice-president of a public policy institute, had arranged a meeting with the lieutenant governor to present a proposal she'd developed involving the regulation of a large state industry. Of necessity she'd invited her boss to the meeting, although she would have been able to make a more effective presentation without him. The boss, in turn, had invited the institute's chief lobbyist, who would later have to convince legislators of the need for the proposed regulation. The meeting began, as Estela expected, with her boss rambling on in a loose philosophical discussion that circled but never quite got to the point. When he finished, he turned not to Estela but to the lobbyist to present the proposal. Estela was stunned. The lobbyist began to speak, and fifteen minutes later the meeting ended without Estela's ever having gotten to say a word—about *her* proposal. In her male-dominated workplace, this was not the first time that Estela had had the experience of being disregarded, but, of course, it still rankled. Yet, in hindsight, that wasn't even what was most upsetting for her.

Estela couldn't wait to tell her husband what had happened. Unfortunately, he was traveling for work and wouldn't be back for three days. She was used to her husband's business trips; what she wasn't used to was how cut off she felt. She really needed to talk to him. As the evening wore on, Estela's disappointment grew and then changed character. Instead of simply feeling frustrated, she began to feel inadequate. Why was she so dependent on her husband? Why couldn't she handle her own emotions?

Estela decided that her problem was insecurity. If she were more secure, she wouldn't need anyone this much. She wouldn't be so vulnerable; she'd be self-sufficient. It wouldn't bother her so intensely that she was overlooked at work and lonely at home.

Estela's complaint—the unexpected urgency to be heard—and her conclusion, that if she had more self-confidence she wouldn't need to depend so much on other people's attention and responsiveness, is a common one. Needing someone to respond to us tempts us to believe that if we were stronger we wouldn't need other people so much. That way they wouldn't be able to disappoint us like this.

Being listened to does help us grow up feeling secure; but, contrary to what some people would like to believe, we never become whole and complete, finished products, like a statue or a monument. On the contrary, like any living thing, human beings require nourishment not only to grow up strong, but also to maintain their strength and vitality. Listening nourishes our sense of worth.

The more insecure we are, the more reassurance we need. But all of us, no matter how secure and well adjusted, need attention to sustain us. In case this isn't immediately evident, all you need to do is notice how we all have our own preferred ways of announcing our news. If my wife has news, for example, she's likely to call me at work or tell me as soon as she gets home. If she has something to say, she says it. Not me. If I have good news, I hoard it, save it up to announce with a fanfare—dying to be made a fuss over.

I once worked for months trying to land a book contract. My wife knew I was working on the book, but I didn't let her know that a contract was imminent. Waiting and hoping, and trying not to let myself hope for too much, I had extravagant fantasies about getting good news—no, about sharing it. Telling my wife would be the payoff. What I didn't want to do was simply tell her; I wanted—I needed—my announcement to be a big deal. The day the contract finally arrived I was ecstatic. But the best part was looking forward to telling my wife. So I called her at work and told her I had a surprise for her: I was taking her out for a fancy dinner. She said fine and didn't ask any questions. (She's only known me for forty years.)

By the time I got home, my wife had changed into a silk dress and was ready to go out. She could tell I was excited, but she waited patiently to find out why. At the restaurant, I ordered a bottle of champagne, and when it came she asked, still patient, "Do you have something to tell me?" I pulled out my contract and presented it with all the savoir faire of a ten-year-old showing off his report card. She saw what it was and her face lit up with a huge grin. That look—her love and pride—was indescribably sweet. My own smile was wet with tears.

What elaborate lengths some of us go to for such moments! Those of us who feel the need to arrange special occasions for our announcements share a good deal with those who don't need to calculate so. The period of time during which we're waiting to tell our news is charged with anxious anticipation. We can feel the tension building. The tension has to do with an aroused impulse—to confess or confront or show off or propose—to make an impact on another person and be responded to. The excitement comes from hope for a positive response; the anxiety comes from fear of rejection or indifference.

One of the diabolically clever features of the iPhone is the display of thought bubbles—the "typing awareness indicator" that flashes rhythmically when someone (hooray!) is texting back to us after we have sent a message. We await the reply with heightened anticipation: the other person heard us and we are connecting! If he or she gets distracted and the bubbles disappear for a few seconds, or if the response appears as a cutesy emoji instead of a thoughtful sentence, we are apt to deflate a bit. And just as in person, we may feel even more disappointed when we get no response at all.

Whom you choose to tell what says something about your relationship to yourself—and to the other people in your life. Your presentation of self involves pride and shame—and whom you choose to share them with. With whom do you feel safe to cry? To complain? To rage? To brag? To confess something truly shameful?

> A good listener is a witness,
> not a judge of your experience.

As soon as you're able to say what's on your mind—and be heard and acknowledged—you are unburdened. It's like having an ache suddenly relieved. If this completion comes quickly, as it often does in day-to-day conversations, you may hardly be aware of your need for understanding. But the disappointment you feel when you're not heard and the tension you feel waiting and hoping to be heard are signs of how important being listened to is. There are times when all that can be thought must be spoken and heard, communicated and shared, when ignorance and silence are pain, and to speak is to try to alleviate that pain.

> **"Guess What!"**
>
> Remember the last time something really wonderful happened to you. Do you remember waiting to tell someone? Whom did you choose, and how did it work out?

Being Heard Means Being Taken Seriously

The need to be heard, which is something we ordinarily take for granted, turns out to be one of the most powerful motives in human nature. Being listened to is the medium through which we discover ourselves as understandable and acceptable—or not. We care about the people who listen to us. We may even love them. But, for a time at least, we use them.

When we're activated by the need for appreciation, we relate to others as *selfobjects*, psychoanalyst Heinz Kohut's telling expression for a responsive other, someone we relate to, not as an independent person with his or her own agenda, but as someone-there-for-us.

Perhaps the idea of using listeners as selfobjects reminds you of those bores who are always talking about themselves and don't seem to care about what you have to say. When they listen, their hearts aren't in it. They're only waiting to change the subject back to themselves.

This lack of appreciation can be especially painful when it occurs between us and our parents. It's maddening when they can't seem to let us be people in our own right, individuals with legitimate ideas and aspirations. Watching our parents listen to other people right in front of us can be especially aggravating. Why don't they show *us* a little of that attention? Here's the writer Harold Brodkey in *The Runaway Soul* dramatizing this irritating experience through the conversation of a young woman and her boyfriend (the boyfriend speaks first):

"Does your dad ever listen, or does he just do monologues?"

"He just does monologues. Doesn't he let you talk?"

"Only if I insist on it. Then we do alternate monologues."

"Well, that's it, then. He talks to you more than he does to me now."

Of course the woman's father talks to her boyfriend more than he does to her. The boyfriend is a fresh audience, new blood.

The people who hurt us most are invariably the ones with whom we think we have a special relationship, who make us feel that our attention and understanding are particularly important to them—until we see how easily they shift their interest to someone else or notice them checking their phones. Right in the middle of confiding in us, they'll catch someone else's eye and break off to talk to that person; they might be seeking virtual feedback from an online "friend" even though we actually made the effort to show up in person for them. We discover that what we thought was an understanding shared only with us is something they've told a dozen people. So much for our special status as confidants! What's so hurtful about these promiscuous "intimates" isn't that they use us, but that they rob us of the feeling that we're important to them, that we're special.

Although none of us likes to see (especially in ourselves) the kind of blatant narcissism that disregards the feelings of others, the truth is, much of the time we're all hopelessly absorbed with our own concerns. The subject of narcissism turns out to be crucial in exploring the art of listening, especially today, when we add social media to the mix. It's a whole new level of narcissism out there with people jostling for the limelight, carefully curating their preferred identities to maximize attention, and grabbing a few extra crumbs of recognition by counting their virtual "likes." It's a fact that one aspect of our need for other people—in person and online too—is entirely selfish. Being listened to maintains our narcissistic equilibrium—or, to put it more simply, it helps us feel good about ourselves.

When Briana and her parents finished unloading the car, she felt a sinking sensation and was conscious for the first time of all the things she didn't have. Anxiously she watched as the other students and their families trooped into the dormitory, loaded down with beautiful pillows and down comforters, expensive AirPods, HDTVs, tennis rackets, road bikes, and lacrosse sticks. Briana had never even seen a lacrosse stick. By the time her parents drove off, leaving her standing alone in front of South Hall, her excitement about starting college had given way to dread.

Briana never did get over her sense of isolation that first year. Everyone else seemed to make friends so easily. Not her. She felt she didn't belong there. She called home a lot and tried to tell her parents how awful it was. But they said, "Don't worry, honey; everybody's a little lonesome at first," and "You should make more friends," and "Maybe you just have to study a little harder." If only it were that easy!

. . . .

Reassuring someone isn't the same as listening.

. . . .

By the first of December Briana was skipping classes, missing meals, and crying herself to sleep. When she couldn't stand it anymore, she made an appointment at the counseling center.

Briana was pleased when the therapist smiled and said to call her Noreen, then attended closely to what she had to say. She wasn't used to that kind of warmth and interest from adults. Noreen turned out to be the most sympathetic person Briana had ever met. She didn't tell Briana what to do or analyze her feelings; she just listened. For Briana, it was a new experience.

With Noreen's help, Briana was able to get through that first year and the three years that followed. Noreen helped her discover that her feelings of insecurity stemmed from never feeling really listened to by her parents. Briana had always thought that they were pretty good parents, but she could see now that they never actually took the time to get to know her very well. Her father was remote and often too busy to talk with her, and her mother seldom took her seriously as a person.

Eventually Noreen convinced Briana that she would never be free of her anger—and vulnerability to depression—until she worked things out with her parents. When Briana agreed, Noreen suggested that she get in touch with me for a few family therapy sessions.

Briana and her parents arrived separately for our first meeting, and although they were all smiling, the three of them seemed as wary as cats circling a snake. I had suggested to Briana over the phone that we go slow in this first meeting, that she try not to unload the full weight of her anger on her parents but rather search for some common ground. But that wasn't the truth about what she was feeling, and the truth was what she was after. She started in on her father. When she was little, she'd loved him, she said, but as she got older she increasingly saw him as ridiculous and irrelevant. He worked hard, was a patriot, and almost nothing in his life caused him second thoughts. He had toiled long hours to be able to send her to this fine college and, to him, she must have seemed entirely ungrateful. After listening to his daughter's ungenerous assessment, Briana's father said, "So that's how you see me?" and then retreated into silence, his brand of armor. He disengaged so completely that it was no surprise when he didn't return for a subsequent session.

Then Briana turned to her mother. She called her "shallow," "phony," and—one of the cruelest things a child can say to a mother—"interested only in yourself." Briana's mother tried to listen but couldn't. "That's not true!" she protested. "Why do you have to exaggerate everything?" This only infuriated Briana more, and the two of them lashed out at each with escalating rage and intensity.

I tried to calm them down but wasn't very successful. Briana was hell-bent on communicating—not talking, that old-fashioned process of give-and-take, but *communicating*—that important development where one insistent family member imparts some critical information to the others, confronting the person with "the truth" whether she wants to hear it or not. Briana's mother left the session in tears.

The following week I met with Briana alone. She was sorry the meeting hadn't gone better but was glad to have gotten her feelings out. She thought her mother had shown herself to be the unaccepting person Briana knew her to be. They weren't on speaking terms for a while and that was just fine with Briana.

Six months later, much to my surprise, Briana called to say that she and her mother wanted to come for another meeting. This time the conversation began superficially. Briana complimented her mother on her shoes and asked about her younger sister. Her mother asked Briana how she was doing. Had she gotten over all that bitterness? Briana, feeling once again patronized and dismissed, tried to avoid reacting but couldn't. Furiously, she accused her mother of not really being interested in how she was feeling and caring only about polite formalities. My heart sank. But this time Briana's mother didn't react angrily or cut her daughter off. She didn't say much, but she didn't interrupt to defend herself either. What enabled her to listen to her daughter's angry accusations this time? I don't really know. Perhaps she didn't want to be estranged any longer; she really did try harder to listen.

One of a mother's heaviest burdens is being the target of her children's primitive swings between need and rage. The rage is directed at the hand that rocks the cradle no matter how loving its care. With daughters, it's often part of breaking away *and* staying connected at the same time. Briana's mother seemed to sense this, seemed to remember that her daughter was still her feisty little girl in some ways.

Briana may have expected retaliation from her mother. But when it wasn't forthcoming, she calmed down considerably. She had wanted, it seemed, only to be heard.

After that, Briana's relationship with her mother changed dramatically. Previously limited to monologues or muteness, they entered into dialogue. Briana phoned and wrote. She shared confidences with her mother. Not always, of course, and not always successfully, but Briana had become more open to her mother as a person, rather than perceiving her simply as a mother who was somehow supposed to selflessly make everything right. She, in turn, became less a child and more a young woman, ready for life on her own.

Briana's unmet need to be listened to had cut her off from other people and filled her with resentment. Unburdening herself was like breaking down a wall that had kept her from feeling connected to other people. That she expressed her feelings in such an infantile emotional flood says only that they were a long time unspoken. Talking to Noreen, who didn't have a stake in defending herself, helped Briana find her voice and express her feelings in ways that others might be better able to hear.

That second meeting with Briana and her mother had produced one of those moments that happen once in a while in families, when someone says something and everything begins to shift. Only it wasn't what Briana said that caused the shift; she'd said it all before. It was that, this time, her mother put aside her own claims to being right and just listened.

When we learn to hear the unspoken feelings beneath someone's anger or impatience, we discover the power to release the bitterness that keeps people apart. With a little effort, we can hear the hurt behind expressions of hostility, the resentment behind avoidance, and the vulnerability that makes people afraid to speak or truly listen. When we understand the healing power of listening, we can even begin to listen to things that make us uncomfortable.

Digital Communication: The Struggle to Feel Heard When You Can't Be Seen

When you speak with someone you care about who is upset—especially if it's with you—your empathy for the distress can get all mixed up with your own reactions of defensiveness or anger. It's likely, for example, that Briana's rage in that first meeting was overwhelming for her parents; their emotional reactivity meant they couldn't really listen to her.

But what about when we communicate online—how do you really listen to a disembodied someone out there in cyberspace? These days, we are spending significant amounts of time in virtual conversations with people we can't see; arguably, the whole culture of listening has changed as the balance tips away from actual human contact. Now, we often have to make do without that extra information we get about someone by actually being there—tone of voice, facial expression, body language, eye contact, our knowledge of what is happening for the other person when she chews her lip like that. Our strategies for listening in the digital world are compromised by the lack of social cues; perhaps not surprisingly, in the land of texting, many of our most important emotional exchanges are rife with a whole new level of misunderstanding.

Of course, there are many trade-offs with online communication; we are discovering more about both the opportunities and challenges as time goes on. In any event, 96% of Americans have cell phones, so we do well to think about how digital communication affects us and the people we are listening and speaking to.

On the positive side, maybe you like having the luxury to read a text or email carefully and edit your response so that you say what you really intend, instead of feeling on the spot and making a regrettable retort. If you are upset or preoccupied, you can wait to write back at a time when you can pay fuller attention and a situation doesn't get out of control as it might have in person. Or if you've been unwell and can't go out, it can be a wonderful diversion to keep up with a group of friends and let them know how you're doing. Studies suggest, overwhelmingly too, that parents are enthusiastic about the increased digital communication with their teens and young adults; they really like staying connected in this extra way.

On the other hand, without seeing the impact of your words register on someone's face, you might react with unnecessary cruelty or disregard for someone's feelings. Cyber bullying isn't just for teens; adults of all ages engage in it too. Comments scrawled in a harsh impulse on social media can be devastating. For example, I know a young mother, Renata, who'd posted on Facebook about her whiny toddler's ear infection, simply seeking sympathy. Minutes later, she instead found herself in the middle of a full-throttle debate about the evils of antibiotics and reading insinuations about the negligent quality of her mothering. Instead of feeling heard—as might have happened if people had just been able to listen to her exhausted voice—Renata reported that she'd been completely misunderstood; she was only looking to commiserate about how hard it was to console a sick baby.

And there is a growing body of evidence that we are actually becoming poorer listeners: all this reliance on virtual communication is directly implicated in this problem. Recent research suggests that some kids who are using social media to navigate relationships seem to be more self-involved and less self-reflective than their age-mates from past generations; it's possible they might be so busy with presenting a particular image—seeing themselves from the outside—that they aren't exerting as much effort getting to know themselves from the inside.

Some studies suggest that the digital experience may be making all of us less empathic, more impatient, and, maybe because our inboxes are flooded, more selective about what we even bother to pay close attention to. Because we can text (or "ghost"—simply disappearing from a text conversation) instead of having a difficult face-to-face dialogue, we might not be working as hard as we once did on developing those skills to navigate the hard patches, to find the courage to ask for forgiveness, and to offer it in return.

The desire to go online to announce an accomplishment, post a picture of an exciting vacation, or otherwise present an amazing version of our real life is perfectly understandable; it's basically the same need we have to share our joy in person with our parents, partners, and friends—and it's probably easier to do. Out of the same need for empathy, some might post a photo of a beloved dog who died or share the news of a bad diagnosis with all their friends on social media. Our yearning to connect with others about things that matter to us is hardwired. Yet the result will never be quite as satisfying as a real conversation. All the "likes" and hearts and sad emojis you can receive from a post probably won't ever amount to one nourishing listen.

Being heard means being taken seriously. It satisfies our need for self-expression and our wish to feel connected to others. The receptive listener allows us to express what we think and feel. Being heard and acknowledged helps us clarify both the thoughts and the feelings, in the process firming our sense of ourselves. By affirming that we are understandable, the listener helps confirm our common humanity. Not being listened to makes us feel ignored and unappreciated, cut off and alone. The need to be known, to have our experience understood and accepted by someone who listens, is food and drink to the human heart.

Without a sufficient amount of sympathetic understanding in our lives, we're haunted by an amorphous unease that leaves us anxious and lonely. Such feelings are hard to tolerate, and so we seek solace in passive escapism; we snap on the TV, shop online, watch porn, play Fortnite, scroll through Facebook, binge Netflix, treat ourselves to Ben and Jerry's, or escape into popular fiction about people whose imaginary lives are more exciting than our real ones. There is, of course, nothing wrong with relaxing. But why can't we stand in line in the grocery store without checking our phones? Why do we turn on the TV even when there's nothing to watch? And why do we feel restless without the car radio playing, even when it's just noise?

We usually associate escapism with release from stress. While it's true that many of us feel used up at the end of the day, it may not be overwork that wears us down, but a lack of understanding in our lives. Chief among the missing elements is the attention and appreciation of responsive people who care and listen to us with interest. When the quality of our relationships isn't sufficient to maintain our equilibrium and enthusiasm—or when we're not up to making them so—we seek escape from morbid self-consciousness. We seek stimulation, excitement, responsiveness, gratification, all seemingly available in the virtual world at the click of a button. How sad for us that we have come to depend so much on devices that only *almost* work to make us less lonely. But really, these are the kinds of feelings that can best be satisfied by a heart-to-heart talk with someone we care about. And without the consolation of someone to talk to, some of us will continue to drown out the silence, imagining that the next screen we look at might actually distract us from those low rumblings of despair and disconnection.

EXERCISES

1. Who is the best listener you know? What makes that person a good listener? (Not interrupting? Asking interested questions? Acknowledging what you've said?) What is being with that person like? What can you learn from that person that would make you a better listener?

2. What do you hesitate to talk to your partner about? Why? What happens to those withheld thoughts and feelings? What are the consequences of that withholding for you? For the relationship?

3. If you improved the way you listen, who would you want to notice? What conversations would you like to go differently?

4. If people think you aren't listening to them, what will they assume it means? What will this lead to?

5. If people think you are listening to them, what will they assume it means? What will this lead to?

6. The next time something is really bothering you, notice how you feel about wanting to talk with someone. Does something hold you back? What do you worry about? If you do share your feelings with someone, what happens?

7. What are some differences for you in how you communicate in person compared with texting? What kinds of conversations would you rather have in person? By text?

8. Have you ever spoken to people on a dating or social networking site and then met them in person? How were they different than when they presented themselves in writing?

9. Are there times when you have an emotional exchange on text that you realize would go better in person or on the phone?

2

"Thanks for Listening"

HOW LISTENING SHAPES US
AND CONNECTS US TO EACH OTHER

We define and sustain ourselves in conversation with others. Recognition—being listened to—is the response from another person that makes our experience meaningful. It allows us to realize our own agency and authorship in a tangible way. But, as we saw in Chapter 1, the expression and recognition so fundamental to our well-being is a mutual, reciprocal process. Our lives are coauthored in conversation. So, if being recognized through listening is to define and sustain us, it must come from someone whom we in turn recognize. Striking a balance between expression (talking) and recognition (listening) is what allows us and the people we care about to interact as sovereign equals.

If your life, or even a key relationship in it, is unbalanced—if it doesn't allow you sufficient self-expression and mutual recognition—you will be the poorer for it. Listening and being listened to are critical to the formation of a strong and healthy self *and* to the formation of strong and healthy relationships.

What makes listening such a force in shaping character is the power of words to match and share experience—or contradict and falsify it. What is understood and accepted—"Yes, isn't that wonderful!"—becomes part of the social self, the self you own and share. What doesn't get appreciated—"You shouldn't be feeling that way in the first place"—becomes part of the

29

private self, known but not shared, or disowned, kept secret, sometimes even from yourself. Ominously, much of what fails to find acceptance becomes part of the disavowed self, what psychoanalyst Harry Stack Sullivan called the "not me."

Of course, your parents may have had burdens of their own, and it's likely they did the best they could. Maybe, on balance, they provided you with much that you value today, listened as best they were able, supported you to be successful. And now, as an adult, you have some perspective and are ready to learn more about the parts you have buried to stay safe—that you may have sensed or known your parents would not be able to help you manage or approve of. Or perhaps you find yourself in a relationship with someone now, and you would like to be able to hear that person's secrets without judgment, but you are finding that curiously hard to do. How did this happen?

Some parents may be too anxious to tolerate a child's anger; others may be too embarrassed to tolerate their children's sexual feelings. Perhaps your parents were dealing with the legacy of their own struggles as kids; no one listened to them either. Each of us grows up with some experiences of self so poisoned with anxiety and shame that they aren't assimilated into the rest of our personality. Listening shapes us; not feeling heard twists us.

A young mother in the toy aisle was berating her little girl for wanting a Barbie doll. It was a *stupid* thing to want; the child *should be ashamed of herself*; she *should have more self-respect*. It was painful to hear. The sad irony of a mother hammering away at a little girl's pride to teach her self-respect was hard to escape. Should a mother let her daughter have a Barbie, like all the other kids? That's up to her; but she should respect her daughter's right to have opinions of her own.

Gradually, with cooperation between parent and child, a self is formed, organized by language and listening, holding and consistency, opportunities to reconnect after inevitable ruptures, and sufficient acceptance and understanding over time. A vast body of clinical and research findings concur that the secure self develops in relationships; how we learn to love and feel lovable is based on our early and ongoing experiences with our parents—in their responsiveness to us beginning long before we have language, in the goodness of fit between our temperaments, and along with their particular needs, values, and resources.

The listened-to child feels effective in relationships and has a better chance of growing up whole and secure. The unlistened-to child lacks the understanding that firms self-acceptance and is "bent out of shape" by the wishes and anxieties of others. Children exert significant energy trying to get needs met by caregivers who aren't paying enough attention. They may survive by going to the extremes of defensive detachment or desperate acting out to get an adult to notice them. Neither strategy allows them the emotional security required to develop with the confidence that they are important and will be heard.

Notably, though, babies are astonishingly adaptable, and they somehow learn how to attach to the caregivers they get, even those who are poorly attuned. If you felt insecure about whether your parents would be there for you when you needed them, it's still likely that you figured out how to get some of those needs met—perhaps by anxiously intensifying the demand until you got a response. Alternatively, and even when still very young, you might have determined that you simply wouldn't be able to depend on them (or anyone) and became very self-reliant. These less secure strategies probably helped you get through childhood, but they are likely to make it quite a bit harder for you in relationships now.

If you had the great good fortune to have safe and reliable caregivers, your capacity to listen and expect others to hear you is greatly expanded. It's much easier to listen when you know what it feels like to be listened to. Most of us have had some experience—with someone we know a little or even a complete stranger— and are amazed by the person's capacity to listen. We not only feel heard; we feel felt. There's a high probability that this attentive person has grown up knowing secure love—lucky enough to have had that experience of being listened to with respect and compassion and acceptance from the very beginning of life.

The seeds of listening are sown in childhood, in the quality of the relationship between parent and child. Parents who listen make their children feel worthwhile and appreciated. Being listened to helps build a secure self, endowing a child with sufficient self-respect to develop his or her own unique talents and ideals and to approach relationships with confidence.

That understanding builds self-assurance is hardly news. Most of us can picture a mother with smiling eyes listening enthusiastically to a child eagerly describing some triumph or a father comforting a sad-faced toddler weeping over some minor tragedy. And we all know how bad it feels to watch a parent reduce a child to tears of humiliation for making a mistake. Of course such scenes, repeated over and over, have an impact on a child.

What may not be so obvious is how early or how profoundly the quality of listening begins to shape character.

How Listening Shapes Self-Respect

To begin with, the self is not a given, like having red hair or being tall, but a perspective on awareness, and an interpersonal one at that. The self is how we personify what we are, as shaped by our experience of being responded to by others. Character is formed in relationships, and the vitality of the self depends on the quality of listening we receive.

Among scientific findings with the most profound implications for understanding the importance of listening is the work of infant researcher Daniel Stern. Stern's most radical discovery was that the infant is never totally undifferentiated from the mother—they are not one symbiotic fused unit as was once believed.

And once we accept the idea that we don't begin life as part of an undifferentiated unity, the question isn't how we separate from our parents but how we learn to connect. The challenge isn't to become free of people, but, from the very start, to make ourselves understood in relationship to them. In the early dance of attachment between mother and infant, both are at work to understand the other, listening with their bodies as well as their ears to the sounds, rhythms, and feelings in the presence of the other one. Over time, when things go well enough, they gradually figure each other out, beginning with this earliest kind of listening and attuning.

This view of the self as having a fundamental need for expression and recognition emerged not only from the observation of infants, but also in consulting rooms, where psychotherapists hear the child's cry in the adult voice. The anguish of those who feel empty and alone, unable to connect to other people, leads to the question "What does it take to make us feel whole?" A large part of the answer is being listened to.

In charting the development of children, Stern identified four progressively more complex senses of self, each defining a different domain of self-experience and social relatedness. Second only to the need for food and shelter is the need for understanding. Even infants need listening to thrive. "Listening" to an infant—the quality of parental attunement and responsiveness—plays a decisive role in making us who we are.

The benefit of loving and responsive attention for healthy development has been studied widely. Stern builds on this burgeoning literature by including a useful description of how listening shapes character during infancy and through childhood and adolescence.

"Here I Am": The Sense of an Emerging Self (Birth to Two Months)

The infant's need for listening is simple but imperative. With the sudden pressure of physical need, life goes from lovely to all wrong. Hunger breaks over the body like an angry storm. It starts slowly; the baby has a sense of something going awry. Then fussing turns to full-throated crying as the baby tries to hurl the pain sensations out and away. This crying serves as a distress signal, like a siren, to alert the parents and demand a response from them.

Being a parent at this stage is simple. As I recall, my wife and I, our empathic sensitivities honed to razor sharpness by months of sleep deprivation, were flung into action by the slightest peep. Blessed with a disposition as placid as a howler monkey, our first little darling would ever so gently summon us for her nightly lactose intolerance test. I, never the insensitive father, was usually first to respond. "Honey," I'd coo, grinding my teeth to keep them warm, "do something!" At which my mate, ever appreciative of my support, would hasten to the little one's side to administer whatever first aid was required. Ah, parenthood.

Babies are cute and seem so helpless, but their smiling, fretting, and crying are commanding messages; they must be listened to. At this stage parents, thinking primarily about satisfying the baby's needs, may not recognize the extent of the social interaction involved in the process. Almost automatically, parents are making little adjustments each time they pick her up, figure out what her different cries mean, and adjust as she develops new skills and needs. Well before the baby achieves self-consciousness, parents invest her with their expectations and aspirations. From day one, they both see the baby as who she is and begin to imagine the person she is becoming.

In turn, the baby is also shaping the parents. For example, a "good" baby who sleeps well and is soothed easily helps parents feel competent. They become less anxious and more confident about their ability to listen to him. A fussy, restless baby is harder to read; perhaps despite their best efforts, some parents can feel inadequate and overwhelmed if they can't figure out what he's trying to tell them. This early miscommunication can take on lifelong meaning for parent and child and for their relationship. A baby who is seen as "hard to soothe," "oversensitive," or "rejecting" may have the experience of not being heard from the start. Sometimes the steps to learning the graceful dance between parent and infant require great effort involving trial and error, and love.

Our impulse toward understanding is irresistible. Developmental psychologist Aidan Macfarlane's observations of new mothers talking to their infants for the first time after delivery show that the mothers attribute meaning to each sign and sound. "What's that frown for? The world's a little scary, huh?" Mothers don't really believe the infant understands, but they assign meaning to what their infants are doing and respond accordingly. This maternal mirroring of feeling and compassionate naming provide coregulation of overwhelming feelings and are the baby's entry into the world of empathic listening and acceptance. In time, together they create little formats of interaction, jointly constructed little worlds. This attachment relationship is the child's first culture; it serves as a kind of template for what kind of relationships the child will expect to have in the future and provides a key to the world the child has entered. Most of all, it lets the child know if what she is "saying" matters to someone.

Parents immediately ascribe intentions to their babies ("Oh, you want that"), motives ("You're doing that so Mommy will hurry up and feed you"), and authorship of action ("You did that on purpose, didn't you?"). In so doing, parents are responding to and helping create an emergent self that is learning how to be in a relationship. We are storytelling creatures by nature; attuned parents tend to ascribe motivation whether or not the infant is intending to communicate much at all. These early narratives help caregivers make sense of their infants as understandable beings—supporting them both in their current state of utter dependence and as the people they are to become (just so long as they become the people their parents want them to become).

Who we are and what we say triggers other people's response
to us. That response and our connection to others remain vital
to our psychological well-being.

When babies are too young to talk, their parents have to understand what they feel but cannot say. When a baby cries, the parents must figure out what's wrong. Does he want to be fed? Does she need a diaper change? Does he want to be held? (Imagine the baby's feelings. What a chasm separates her from these giant, nervous creatures nature has assigned as her waitpersons. Would they ever catch on?) When the baby grows up and learns to talk, she becomes better at putting her needs and feelings into words. Better, not perfect. Sometimes we all need a little help making ourselves understood. And, truth be told, no matter what age we are, there are times when *we* might not exactly know why we're feeling so off-kilter ourselves.

Infants are helplessly dependent on their parents. When the parents are absent, angry, or otherwise unresponsive, the child is alone and terrified; he feels the bottom dropping out of his world. Whether a caregiver is physically or emotionally unavailable actually makes little difference to the baby: infants register this as an existential danger either way. Utterly unable to soothe themselves, they urgently need to be held and comforted. It's important to understand, then, that infants only learn how to calm down if and when someone takes the time—over and over again—to offer them comfort when they are distressed. There is actually no other way to find out what that feels like. But here's the thing: Even if you got picked up and held a lot as a baby, in times of great stress, you will still need someone to talk to now. And even if you have become an A-plus self-soother in ordinary life, there will always be periods when you become so upset that you can't feel better on your own. The attention of someone who responds to you with compassion will feel much the way a mother's arms feel to her distressed baby.

Over time, if we've had good enough care and attention, we learn about what works for us when we are lonely or upset. Sometimes we feel better after we curl up with a book, take the dog out for a walk, or watch a movie. At other times, we need to talk it out with someone; our misery is too much to carry alone.

Our adult self-awareness distinguishes us in obvious ways from the infants we once were. And while our yearning for comfort might bear some resemblance to our baby selves—who among us hasn't needed to wail loudly, to be held, to eat comfort food, or to be tucked under a cozy blanket?—over the years our connections gain in depth and dimensionality as we experience the give-and-take of adult relationships.

What listening provides for us as adults is an opportunity to articulate and integrate deeper layers of ourselves. Attention and appreciation on the part of a caring listener create a feeling of safety and witnessing that we might not ever have had before. Our shameful, hidden, or exiled parts might even find their way into the conversation. In this relationship, feeling accepted as we are, we may have the transformative experience of becoming a fuller, more integrated, version of ourselves.

Being listened to promotes an unfolding of aspects of experience that may have been closed off because they were never vitalized by being shared and acknowledged—or worse, were denied and rejected. For an infant, being listened to helps confirm that he or she is a self. For an adult, being listened to helps that developmental process to continue—enabling us to get to know and accept more fully our multidimensional selves.

Adrienne had been going out with Phillip for three years when she met Cliff. She hadn't made any promises to Phillip, but they'd been together so long that she didn't really feel okay about seeing another guy. After about a month of wondering what to do, she finally talked to her friend Judy.

Judy had been married long enough to know that you never know how relationships are going to turn out. So when Adrienne told her about Cliff, she just listened. She asked a few questions, like what did Adrienne want, what was she afraid of, and what did she hope would happen, but mostly she just allowed Adrienne to talk.

Adrienne didn't make any final decisions as a result of that conversation, but she did get a lot clearer about what she wanted. She knew she didn't want to be alone, but she wasn't ready to get tied down, either. Phillip was a genuinely nice guy, but she wasn't really in love with him. Cliff was more exciting, but she wasn't sure he was the kind of person she could count on. She was happy to have Phillip in her life, but since she didn't think she wanted to spend the rest of her life with him, she wasn't willing to close off other options. If she saw Cliff occasionally without breaking up with Phillip, there might be complications, but she was willing to risk them.

Sometimes in injury or illness, confusion or stress, we may realize that no one fully leaves behind those childhood feelings of dependency. At times like these our lifelong need for other people is self-evident; their response to us either validates our experience or not.

When Valerie got one of those migraines that struck without warning, she told her husband that she couldn't go out to dinner because she had a headache. He said he was sorry she didn't feel well and suggested that she take some aspirin and lie down. She was disappointed in his response. Aspirin didn't work for her, and she'd rather stay downstairs and put an ice pack on her forehead. Shouldn't he know that by now? Valerie was glad not to have to go out, but she felt that her husband's suggestion to go upstairs and lie down was just pushing her away. He liked going out to dinner with her, liked having her go to the gym with him, liked having her listen to his problems and accomplishments; but it didn't seem to her like he was willing to be with her when she didn't feel well.

Most of us eventually grow up, but we never outgrow the need to be taken seriously—to have our feelings recognized and to hope for the comfort of others.

"Hey, Look at Me!": The Sense of a Core Self (Two to Seven Months)

Between eight and twelve weeks, infants become gregarious. The social smile emerges; they begin to vocalize and make eye contact. When the baby looks up and smiles and coos, or splashes in the bath, or giggles with delight, how could you *not* love her? Surely, we would like to think, all parents respond intuitively, right away, to such communications. Unfortunately, that isn't so. There is ample evidence to suggest that no parents are perfectly attuned; one study concludes that the most successful mothers—with securely attached babies—still get it wrong 70% of the time on the first try. The important element here is not that they are so well attuned from the start, but that they are willing to try and try again until they've listened successfully.

Of course, it can be hard to persevere if you are exhausted or don't know what to do. Some parents are so overwhelmed, preoccupied, depressed, or otherwise distracted that they haven't been able to really figure out what their babies need. Many parents who struggle this way have few resources, insufficient social support, and problems from the past that they haven't been able to resolve. If they don't have the ability to soothe themselves, they'll find it more difficult to offer such comfort to a wailing infant. Some might even struggle to see their babies as little people with their own rhythms and moods and instead look to the infant to be a comfort to them.

Every infant has an optimal level of excitement. Activity beyond that level constitutes overstimulation, and the experience becomes upsetting; activity below that level is, well, unstimulating. Parents must learn to read their babies. By taking their infants seriously as persons, responding to the infants' feelings rather than imposing their own, parents convey acceptance that children take in and transform into self-respect.

The next time you see an adult interacting with a baby, notice the difference between responding in tune with the child's level of excitement and imposing the adult's emotions on the child. When you see a parent with blunted emotions ignoring a bright-eyed baby, you're witnessing the beginning of a long, sad process by which unresponsive parents wither the enthusiasm of their children like unwatered flowers.

Having quite enough unwatered flowers at the office, thank you, I wasn't about to have any around my house. I remember tiptoeing into the baby's room at eventide, right about the time she was dozing—or pretending to. What my masculine intuition told me she really wanted was not to rest but to be hurled violently up to the ceiling and then come crashing toward the floor—like a skydiver without a parachute—only to be plucked from the jaws of death by Daddy. Whee!

Too choked with joy to speak, the little mite showed her pleasure by widening her eyes like saucers while her face turned a lovely shade of blue.

Excessive enthusiasm may be less depressing, but it isn't necessarily more responsive. We've all seen grownups at it—"baby love"—the fulsome tone of voice, the honeyed words, the endless marveling and exclaiming. When babies are little, it's almost automatic; babies are so animated themselves that they drive up the intensity of our response. But when this adult enthusiasm exceeds the baby's own, the result is a jarring discontinuity. Loving parents share the moods of their children and show it. And when they get it wrong, they try again.

. . . .

It isn't exuberance or any other emotion
that conveys loving appreciation,
it's being understood, and taken seriously.

. . . .

The baby whose parents tickle and poke and jiggle and shake her when she's not in the mood is as alone with her real self as the baby whose parents ignore her. Not being understood and taken seriously as a person in your own right—even at this early age—is the root of aloneness and insecurity.

Eleanor appreciates getting flowers from her adult children on Mother's Day but wishes they'd find time to call more often.

Ted tells Katie that he's worn out and wants to stay home and watch a movie on TV. Katie says that maybe he'd feel better if they went out for a walk.

Nikki tells her father about an older colleague at work who often interrupts her at staff meetings. She doesn't want to make a fuss, but she wants to be able to finish saying what's on her mind. Her father tells her that the next time he does that, she should tell him to shut up, she's not finished. Nikki thanks him and changes the subject.

What these examples have in common is that when people respond to us in terms of their own preferences rather than tuning in to ours, it feels like they don't really know us, don't really get who we are—aren't really listening.

"Honey, I'm Cold. Don't You Want a Sweater?": The Sense of a Personal Self (Seven to Fifteen Months)

By about one year of age the baby realizes that she has an inner, private mental world, with desires, feelings, thoughts, and memories, which are invisible to others unless she makes an attempt to reveal them. The possibility of sharing these invisible contents of the mind is the source of the greatest human happiness and frustration.

Imagine for a moment that you're a baby who hasn't yet learned to talk, and you want a cookie. What do you do if you see the cookie but it's out of reach? Simple. You get your mother to read your mind.

Mind reading may sound extravagant, but isn't that what communication boils down to? The baby must gain his mother's attention, express what's on his mind, and do so in a way that she receives and understands the message.

"I want a cookie" is a simple message, easily sent and easily received, even without words. When it comes to more complicated messages, babies (like you and me) may have to work harder to express themselves—and hope their listeners will work hard enough to understand.

The possibility of sharing experience creates the possibility for confirmation of the self as understandable and acceptable; it also creates the possibility of intimacy, fulfilling the desire to know and be known. What's at stake is discovering which inner experiences we can share and which we can't.

. . . .

Being listened to spells the difference
between feeling accepted and feeling isolated.

. . . .

The possibility of sharing mental states between people also raises the possibility of misunderstanding. For example, babies are remarkably eager explorers. Sitting on Mommy's or Daddy's lap, a baby may probe the parent's mouth or nose with a finger or tug at a strand of hair to see if it will come loose. The parent who takes this exploration as an act of aggression may get annoyed and attribute hostility to the baby. If so, the parent may follow up this feeling with a rebuke, a slap, or some rejection of the baby, who had only been doing what comes naturally at this age.

The misunderstood baby is confused by the parent's lack of understanding, upset and frightened by the rebuke. *Maybe it was a mistake,* the baby may think. So then the baby—who is a kind of tiny scientist exploring the world—pulls at the strand of his mother's hair another time, maybe to clarify the confusion or to try to evoke a different response. He may even give it a real yank, with a more energetic assertiveness, to see what happens. Now, if his mother has no alternative narrative available, she's likely to assume that her original misunderstanding was confirmed: the baby *is* being aggressive.

If this interpretation is repeated over many such "experiments," the parent's incorrect understanding may become the infant's (and later the child's) official and accepted one: exploration is aggression, and it's bad. The baby may come to see himself as aggressive, even hostile. Someone else's reality has become his. Misunderstanding undermines not only our trust in others, but also our trust in our own perceptions.

The word for sharing experience is *intersubjectivity*. The reason for this fancy term, where an ordinary word like *communication* might do, is to keep us from forgetting that understanding is a joint achievement: one person trying to express what's on his or her mind, the other trying to read it, and it goes both ways. Reading a child's mind begins with *attunement*.

Attunement, a parent's ability to share the child's affective state, is a pervasive feature of parent–child interactions with profound consequences. It's the forerunner of empathy and the essence of human understanding. Attunement begins with the intuitive parental response of sharing the baby's mood and showing it. The baby reaches out excitedly and grabs a toy. When the toy is in her grasp, she lets out an exuberant "aah!" and looks at her mother. The mother responds in kind, sharing the baby's exhilaration and showing it by smiling and nodding and saying "Yes!" The mother has understood and shared the child's mood. That's attunement.

One demonstration of the baby's need for an attuned response is the *still-face response*. If a mother (or father) goes still faced—impassive and expressionless—in the middle of an interaction, the baby will become upset and withdraw. Infants after about two-and-a-half months of age react strongly to this still face. They look about. Their smile dies away and they frown. They make repeated attempts to reignite the mother by smiling and gesturing and calling her. If they don't succeed, they finally turn away, looking unhappy and confused. It hurts to reach out to someone who doesn't respond.

"No, I Don't Want a Nap! I Want to Play": The Sense of a Verbal Self (Fifteen to Eighteen Months)

Learning to speak creates a new type of connection between parent and child. The acquisition of language has traditionally been seen as a major step in the achievement of a separate identity, next only to locomotion. But it's more complicated than that: the acquisition of language is also a potent force for interaction and intimacy.

Language increases the child's ability to make herself heard and understood, and it increases the parent's ability to understand. Talking helps children clarify what they want—"Wanna cookie"; "Swing me higher!"—and so cuts down on parents' misreading their child's intentions, if they are responsive to what the child is trying to say.

Emotional unresponsiveness produces a child with a restricted range of emotional expressiveness, fewer attempts to communicate, and a tendency to avoid interactions with others. In other words, a child whose words aren't appreciated and responded to eventually gives up and turns inward or tries to communicate instead with challenging behaviors that require a physical reaction as much as—or more than—a verbal response from an adult.

When we see sadness or depression in someone, we tend to
assume that something's wrong, that something's happened.
Maybe that something is that nobody's listening.

When children learn to talk, some become little chatterboxes. At first, it's cute. One reason little ones prattle on so is that they're delighted with the magic of this wonderful new skill. They can speak their thoughts out loud! Another reason children talk so much is that this talking game is usually played by two people. They talk and someone responds. And they keep talking *until* someone responds.

The name for the ability to accurately hear what your child is saying— actually, *trying to* say—is *empathy*. Empathy means understanding—not just what the other person says, but what the other person feels. You put yourself in someone's shoes and consider his experience—not what you might feel in a similar situation. Empathy is achieved through open and receptive listening with both your heart and your mind. But even if you are able to feel others' pain or joy, you may still have to work to understand why *they* feel that way. As any parent whose kid comes home from school crying knows all too well, empathic feelings can really take over; you do feel the child's misery as if it were your own. But even the most attentive parents will still need to make an effort to try to understand not only the reasons their child is upset but, but also how that experience affects him.

Empathy is conveyed by putting what you understand into words—and it's a good idea to be open to elaboration or corrections. Because we filter empathic understanding through our own thoughts and feelings, we can sometimes get confused—if it's an experience we can relate to, we really might not be clear: is this how I would feel, or is this how you feel? When I'm sitting with a distressed patient, I might wonder, for example, "Are you feeling sad as well as angry about this? I'm feeling a little sad hearing it." Even if I get it wrong, the clarification request means I'm really trying to listen and to understand the person.

The Listened-To Child Is a Confident Child

By the time children get to be four or five, empathy or its absence has molded their personalities in recognizable ways. The securely understood child grows up to expect others to be available and receptive. This is demonstrated by a tendency to draw effectively on preschool teachers as resources. The listened-to child who has a problem at school will confidently turn to a teacher for support. In contrast, it's particularly at such times that insecure children fail to seek contact. Someone hurts a boy's feelings, and he folds his arms and pouts. A girl falls down and skins her knee, and she goes off to be alone. A child feels sad before summer vacation, and he sits motionless and expressionless on a bean bag chair. Such reactions are typical—and, without extra support, might not change much as the unlistened-to child gets older.

Preschoolers with a history of empathic listening are usually securely attached. As such, they are more engaged and more at ease with their peers. They expect interactions to be positive and thus are more eager for them. They are able to make more friends and are happier. They are also good listeners. Already by four or five, empathic failure—not necessarily abuse or cruelty, but simple, everyday lack of emotional understanding—results in a self that is isolated and insecure, vulnerable to rejection and therefore fearful of new people and experience.

"He Never Talks to Me."

The reticence of some men may have as much to do with a history of not being empathically responded to as to anything inherent about gender. Getting uncommunicative people to open up requires an extra effort to demonstrate acceptance of their feelings—including feeling like not talking about something right now. Patient listening can help someone who hasn't had much practice developing the skill to put shut-away feelings into words.

Imagine five-year-old Tammy, weaned on understanding, telling her playmate about a bully in kindergarten. "And then he pushed me and hogged all the crayons!"

A tiny cloud momentarily overshadowed her friend Ryan's even tinier face. Bullies were not his favorite people. But listening sympathetically, he knew, was for sissies. Confident that if his own ire were sufficiently aroused, he could demolish a grape with a single blow of his fist, Ryan counseled war. "You should put paint in his hair and give him a karate chop when he does that."

Here were two kindred spirits, meeting at last on a plane of perfect understanding. "Thanks," said Tammy gratefully, "but I think I hear my mother calling. Nice talking to you."

Calling attention to the formative influence of listening on building secure and confident personalities might lead to the assumption that by adulthood our emotional security is a finished product. But just as children need to be heard and understood to develop a secure sense of self, so do we as adults need understanding to sustain our sense of emotional security.

This need is based partly on a deep desire to sustain our sense of significance. The listener's understanding presence serves to satisfy our need for attention and appreciation. But the idea that listening is something one person *gives* to the other is only part of the story. Another vital aspect of listening is mutuality.

Listening Bridges the Space Between Us

Mutuality is a sense not merely of being understood but also of sharing—of being with another person. Here it isn't just *I* but *we* that is important. Our experience is made fuller by sharing it with another person.

Social networking sites owe no small part of their success to their commitment to giving us a platform on which to share. We share not only important events like births and deaths, but also political rants, pictures of snowy days, comical videos featuring the antics of a beloved pet, candid shots of friends lolling on the beach, or even just an announcement about how we feel at this moment. My friend Ghita, a real foodie, often posts her status update on Facebook as "feeling blessed," along with a picture of a lavish meal.

Those who have never been inclined to share on social media—or have given it up to get more of their free time back—have good reasons, of course; however, for those who post, tweet, blog, put up snapchat story, and so forth, the yearning to tell others about their lives is another kind of bridge, this one connecting them in cyberspace with friends and followers. The satisfaction may be less than a face-to-face encounter, but the underlying impulse is the same.

When I want to share a thought or feeling that means a lot to me, what I want is to be understood, taken seriously, and appreciated. (Calling this "sharing" is an unctuous affectation made even more insipid by social media; what we really want is to express ourselves and be heard.) It is I who wants to be validated. But if I see an especially funny cartoon in *The New Yorker,* I immediately think of someone to share it with. (Here, "sharing" is appropriate, because the experience sought is mutual, communal.) In this instance I don't want to be admired or valued; I just want to share the laughter.

Mutuality is a powerful but neglected aspect of human experience. When we're young and alive, before life blunts our naked nerve endings, the yearning for mutuality takes its most intense form in the hungering for a soul mate. We find or invent a special someone with whom we can share light moments and deep thoughts.

Mutuality is also the stuff of everyday human exchange. We swap knowing comments about the president's latest gaffe, complain about the weather, and chat idly about the events of the day. Nothing important is happening, just life and shared humanity. My grown daughter texts me a picture of her puppy peeking out from under the covers because she's thinking of me and knows I'll enjoy it. A client explains mutuality this way: "That's why when I'm away on business I call my husband at the end of the day—to tell him that the meeting went okay or it's raining or I forgot to pack my good shoes." My daughter and this woman don't *need* anything; they are just sharing the everyday observations, joys, opinions, and complaints that otherwise back up and burden us in isolation.

Most theories of human relationship emphasize one or another aspect of connection, whether it's mutual sharing, having someone there for us, feeling held, being attached, or caring. All these modes of relatedness are ways of reaching through the space that separates us. Underlying all our agendas, however, is the fact that speech is the primary mode of relating, and being listened to is the primary means of being understood and appreciated. By "appreciated" I don't mean admired, but rather perceived and accepted as we feel ourselves to be. When we talk about being down in the dumps, it doesn't help to be told how wonderful we are; we want our discontent recognized. We want to be known, to feel felt.

As we're reminded from time to time when we're misjudged or hurt more than anyone realizes, no one can really see our selves. They see what they can and are willing to see, and they know what we tell them. The rest is private, mystery.

The way we become known is through empathic responsiveness, when through expression, tone, or some expansion of phrasing, the listener accurately mirrors what we are trying to communicate. The good listener appreciates us as we are, accepting the feelings and ideas that we express as they are. In the process, we feel understood, acknowledged, and accepted.

Empathy—the human echo—is the indispensable stuff of emotional well-being. What is adequately mirrored becomes, in time, part of the true and lived self. The child who is heard and appreciated has a better chance to grow up whole. The adult who is heard and appreciated is more likely to continue to feel that way and be more able to listen in turn.

Unshared Thoughts Diminish Us

Some people are good at getting appreciated, but they work too hard at it. They aren't open to all of themselves, and so what gets appreciated is only the face they show to the world. Reassurance isn't very reassuring to the person with too many secrets.

Why, then, do some people say so little about themselves?

The answer is, life teaches them to hold back. The innocent eagerness for appreciation we bring to our earliest relationships exposes us to consequences. Some people are lucky. They get the attention they need and thereafter approach life with relative confidence. Others aren't so lucky. They don't get listened to, and as a consequence they avoid opening up. What might appear to be modesty in some cases may have more to do with the reluctance to expose old wounds. Many people learn instead to channel their need for appreciation into personal ambition or doing things for other people.

> Not being listened to is hard on the heart, and so,
> to varying degrees, we cover our need for understanding
> with mechanisms of defense.

Some people become experts at avoidance and cultivate the capacity to be alone. The charm of solitude is that it provides space for repose and reflection, time for looking within the self, time for creative endeavor. Solitude offers respite from the noisy claims of everyday social living. I'll discuss later how solitude can give us a chance to listen to our own thoughts. But some of the penchant for being alone is defensive—a response to being hurt by not being heard. The defenses that form the solitary person's character support a grand illusion: the illusion of self-reliance. If we could only examine the contemplation of one's own feelings that passes for introspection, we'd discover that the silence of the solitary is often filled with imagined conversations.

Social media offers avoidant people additional distractions from their loneliness. If someone is uneasy with intimacy, it can feel safer to have Internet "friends" than actual in-person friends, to foster the illusion of being in relationships with less risk, to keep one's vulnerable self protected and present a careful image to others who may also be doing the same.

But people who try to substitute an online social life for the real thing may not be protecting themselves as well as they'd hoped. Recent research suggests that feelings of loneliness and inadequacy are actually exacerbated by this strategy. If real relationships have disappointed and hurt you, it's unlikely that an increased investment of time on social media will give you that longed-for chance to be seen and heard. It may seem paradoxical, but the more you reveal yourself in this "safe" way, the more isolated you may end up feeling.

One of the reasons Sharon found Don so appealing was that he always seemed cool and self-contained. While other people at the office always seemed to be complaining or arguing, Don went about his business with quiet assurance. He never seemed to get into arguments with anyone.

But one morning Sharon couldn't help overhearing a junior colleague come into Don's office and ask if he was annoyed at her for something. In a barely controlled voice, Don said that he didn't care for Ellen's arguing with everything he said in staff meetings. "Oh," she said, sarcastically, "what do you want me to do, agree with everything you say?" At that, Don lost it. He said that she hadn't shown him any respect since she came into the firm; he was sick and tired of her disagreeing with everything he said. She never really considered his ideas, he said in an increasingly shrill voice, she was just being disagreeable. At that point Ellen walked out.

Well, Sharon thought, *I guess Don isn't so self-composed after all. He's just one of those people who stay calm only by avoiding confrontations.*

Unshared thoughts diminish us, not only by making us less authentic and less whole, as we've discussed, but also by eating at us. Repression is not like putting something away in the closet and forgetting about it; repression takes a constant expenditure of energy that slowly wears us down.

The feeling of not being understood is one of the most painful in human experience. Not being appreciated and responded to depletes our vitality and makes us feel less alive. When we're with someone who doesn't listen, we shut down. When we're with someone who's interested and responsive—a good listener—we perk up and come alive. Being listened to is as vital to our enthusiasm for life as love and work. So is being a good listener. Understanding the dynamics of listening enables us to deepen and enrich our relationships. It involves learning how to suspend our own emotional agenda and then realizing the rewards of genuine empathy. When our own listening becomes blocked by the emotions that others arouse in us, we conspire to produce our own isolation. It doesn't have to be that way.

EXERCISES

1. Is there someone who would love to have you listen more attentively? What gets in the way? If you were to listen more closely to that person, how would it affect your relationship? How would your listening affect how the person feels about you? How would your ability to empathize affect that person's feeling of well-being?

2. Make a list of things that might be worth *not* listening to. These might include always turning the radio on in the car, spending time with people

you don't like, answering the phone when you'd rather not, snapping on the TV instead of looking out the window, watching one YouTube video after another, compulsively listening to music rather than to your own thoughts.

3. Think of someone you avoid telling certain things because of the way that person typically responds to you. Plan in advance to make a gentle comment about that tendency the next time he or she does it. Note: Be prepared to respond without emotionality if the other person takes umbrage at your comment. The purpose of this exercise is to get you to practice calling people on their annoying listening habits without turning it into a big confrontation. In commenting on their response to you, focus not on what they are doing wrong but on how you prefer to be responded to.

4. What did you learn about listening while growing up at home, in school, and other places outside of the home? Was listening different for men? For women? For children? If so, in what ways? Who do you think was most listened to in your family? Least listened to? What is your explanation for this?

5. When have you felt really listened to? What elements contributed to that sense of being really heard? When did you *not* feel listened to? What contributed to that feeling?

6. Describe a time when you did some of your best listening. What helped and/or supported you in doing that? When have you done some of your worst listening? What would have helped you listen better in that situation?

7. When do you hesitate to say what's on your mind? What in your upbringing might have contributed to this reticence?

3

"Why Don't People Listen?"

HOW COMMUNICATION BREAKS DOWN

Keisha was finding it more difficult than she'd imagined to stay home all day with two small children. She had planned to go back to work after the children were born, but decided that it was more important to be at home with them until they started school. What she missed most about working was having people to talk with. Listening to who wanted a cookie and who had to go to the potty got pretty tedious by the end of the day. Keisha's husband was surprisingly unsympathetic. He helped put the kids to bed and spent time with them on weekends, but when he came home after work he didn't even pretend to be interested in Keisha's account of her day. She was hurt, and she was angry.

"I know Lamar works hard and wants to rest. But I work hard too. All I want is a few minutes of adult conversation. But if I dare to interrupt his precious six o'clock news to try to talk to him, he just gets mad. It isn't worth it, and I've had just about all I can take." Her eyes were full of tears.

"Did You Hear What I Said?"

Why don't people listen? There's no shortage of easy answers to that question. Most focus on the listener. (Husbands can be notoriously unsympathetic listeners.) Keisha's explanation for Lamar's unavailability wasn't completely critical—"I know he needs time to unwind"—but it was, after all, focused entirely on him. His lack of listening was *his* doing.

In fact, listening (or the lack of it) is a two-person process. According to Lamar, it was frustrating to talk with Keisha about the kids. "She's always complaining. She says they won't leave her alone, even when she goes to the bathroom. But she encourages it! She won't let them alone to play by themselves, and she refuses to take any time for herself. And the thing that really bothers me is the way she always sides with the little one. Everything Terri does is cute; everything Jamal does is wrong. If I try to say anything, even very nicely, she starts crying and says I'm picking on her. So I've learned to keep my mouth shut."

Keisha felt neglected because Lamar wouldn't listen to her or help out much. He seemed to her to just be giving advice. Her contribution to the problem was not being open to his point of view. The fact that Lamar's position differed from hers, and may even be critical, made it hard to hear. Unfortunately, when two people are in conflict about something important, unless each is able to at least acknowledge the other's point of view, the result is likely to be an emotional cutoff.

> Do you have an important relationship with someone in which you often don't feel listened to?
> Can you imagine how you might change your approach to that person to make it easier for him or her to hear what you're trying to say?

Lamar felt discounted because Keisha complained about a problem of her own making (as he saw it) and wouldn't listen to his opinion. And yet Lamar managed neither to listen nor to get his point of view across. If he could separate listening from advising, perhaps Keisha would get some sympathy for her feelings, and then he might be able to communicate his perspective more effectively. Of course it's difficult for him to set aside his own feelings long enough to listen to his wife's, especially on a subject that he feels so strongly about. But maybe that's not a good enough excuse for a husband and father's retreat.

When people don't listen to us, we can't help feeling that it's their fault: they're selfish or inconsiderate. (When *we* don't listen, it's because we're bored or tired or don't like being talked down to.) The truth is, listening is a complex process. Even though failures of listening all end in the same painful experience of not being heard, there are many reasons people don't listen.

Several years ago, a young couple came to me complaining of difficulties in communicating. When I asked what the problem was, the husband said, "It's my wife; she's boring." (Who says men are reticent with their feelings?) Restraining my urge to react to this nasty crack, I asked him to explain. The man was a lawyer, working as a campaign advisor in a gubernatorial election campaign. His days were filled with strategy sessions, speechwriting conferences, meetings with the candidate, television interviews, arranging appearances across the state, defending attacks from the opposition, and planning counterattacks. When he came home at night, his head spinning from the excitement and frustration of the crusade, he mumbled a greeting to his wife and collapsed onto the couch with a drink and the news.

When I asked why he wasn't more eager to talk over the events of the day, he said his wife wasn't interested. She was a graphic design artist and not at all, he contended, concerned about politics.

She protested that although she might not know a lot about the details of the governor's race, she *was* interested in him and what he was doing. He wasn't convinced.

I asked him to think of someone who he *knew* was interested in the campaign, someone with whom he could talk enthusiastically. Imagine, I told him, how different you are with that person. He allowed as that might be true. Then I asked him—just for an experiment—to come home for one week and pretend that his wife was that interested person, the person he found it so exciting to talk to. He agreed to try it.

The next week they returned beaming. "Guess what?" he said. "She's not boring anymore."

When people don't say much, it's less likely that they have nothing on their minds than that they don't trust the other person to be willing to hear it. My suggestion to this man—that he pretend his wife *was* interested—encouraged him to break his silence. But it was his approaching her with enthusiasm, taking an interest in talking to her, that broke the pattern of avoidance. The truth is that we become more interesting when we assume interest on the part of our listeners. And, as this example shows, our listeners become more interesting when we discover they are interested in us.

Why Someone Doesn't Hear What You Think You Said

Sometimes people don't hear us because they've had a bad day. They may be preoccupied with the angry things someone said or with all the extra work they have to do. Or they may be turned off to us by any number of things— they assume that we're talking to them only because we want something or that we're going to give them a lecture or that we don't really care about them. Listeners often don't hear because they have a preconceived notion of what we're going to say. Or they can't hear us because they can't suspend their own needs or because what we say makes them anxious. In short, although hurt feelings may tempt us to blame failures of listening on other people's recalcitrance, the reasons for not listening are many and complex.

When the communicative process breaks down, we—who are doing our best—tend to assume that the other person didn't say what he meant or didn't hear what we were saying. Usually, both parties to misunderstanding feel that way. But it may be helpful to realize that, as relationship expert John Gottman has said, between speaker and listener are two filters to meaning.

The speaker, who has an *intention* of what he or she wants to communicate, sends a *message*, and that message has an *impact* on the listener. Good communication means having the impact you meant to have— that is, *intent* equals *impact*. But every message must pass first through the filter of the speaker's clarity of expression and second through the listener's ability to hear what was said. Unfortunately, there are many times when intent doesn't equal impact and many reasons why this is the case.

Some of the reasons for misunderstanding are simple and can be improved, like learning a skill. For example, by giving feedback, listeners tell speakers about the impact of their messages and give them a chance to clarify their intentions. But many reasons for misunderstanding are less straightforward and not amenable to simple formulas for improvement. Our young lawyer's assumption that his wife wasn't interested in his work is just one example of the psychological complications of listening.

> Have you had trouble understanding what someone is trying to say to you?
>   When and where have you heard something like "That's not what I said! Weren't you listening?"

When We Hear What We Expect to Hear

This dynamic, the speaker's tendency to impose certain expectations on the listener, is what, in the psychoanalytic situation, is called *transference*. For simplicity's sake, the idea of transference is often reduced to the notion that the patient assumes that the silent analyst is a carbon copy of one of his or her parents, judging her harshly just like her father did or enthralled with his accomplishments the way his mother was. In fact, transference refers to all the ways in which a person's experience of a relationship is shaped by subjectivity—past experience, expectations, sensitivities, hopes, and fears. Transference isn't limited to the therapeutic situation—and it isn't only distortion.

Every close relationship we have includes both actual experiences *and* an internal model of how relationships work, dating back to our first days in the world. These models are useful for helping us understand relationships in some ways, but they also serve as self-fulfilling prophesies. For example, if we have a history of being invalidated when we speak, we are likely to take that expectation into our adult relationships. Perhaps unintentionally then, we filter how we understand interactions, paying particular attention to the times that fit our model, when we feel unheard and put down.

Chris grew up with a jealous and competitive older sister who was always proving him wrong. Chris's sister would ask innocent-sounding questions that always led to the same conclusion: Chris was wrong or dumb, or both. Now whenever Chris's girlfriend asked him a question about something he was explaining, he felt attacked.

. . . .

Transference: the way in which a speaker's experience
of a listener is unconsciously organized
according to preestablished expectations.

. . . .

Hector hated his wife's constant criticism. She challenged almost everything he said. Consequently, he didn't say much. According to Julia, Hector was overly sensitive. While he admitted that there might be some truth to that, he insisted that she was critical and controlling. "She's always telling me what to do," he said. "She won't leave me alone." If these protests remind you of a teenager complaining about his mother, you're on to something about transference.

Whenever Hector's wife asked him to do something for her, he felt like she was bossing him around. The burden of being cast in the role of a controlling mother is familiar to many women. What to do? This is a tough one. One solution is for the woman to take into account her man's tendency to overreact by carefully avoiding anything that might sound like a complaint. In fact, Hector's wife tried to do just that. Knowing how sensitive he was, she'd refrain from asking him for anything for weeks at a time. But eventually taking care of the house and yard would get too much for her, and she'd complain that she needed him to take some responsibility for the chores. Having waited so long made it hard to keep the annoyance out of her voice. He'd feel scolded and resentful, and the cycle would start all over again.

Another approach would be to reassure your listener that you are not playing the role ascribed to you. Obviously, for Julia this would not mean saying "I'm not your mother!" in a scolding voice. She might, however, attempt to talk from the heart about her feeling overwhelmed and ask how she might help Hector remember she's his partner even when his reactions to her suggest otherwise.

Transference is usually thought of as distortion. But maybe the way we impose our expectations on others also has to do with what the speaker needs from the listener at that moment. Thus, for example, a woman chatting about a video she saw on YouTube may not impose any particular pressure on the person listening to her. On the other hand, if the same woman has just been in an auto accident, she might project onto the listener her need for an empathic response. In the first instance, she might enjoy the listener's sharing a similar experience, whereas in the second she may not want to be interrupted except to have her feelings acknowledged.

Countertransference, the psychoanalytic term for the complexity introduced by the listener, refers to how the listener's subjectivity distorts his or her experience of the conversation. But like transference, countertransference isn't simply distortion, because our expectations actually shape and reshape our relationships. The woman who expects men to talk only about themselves may inquire more than she discloses, thereby helping to confirm her expectations. The man who expects to find his wife's account of the day uninteresting may fail to ask the questions that might make it interesting to him; as a result, he gets out of the conversation pretty much what he puts into it.

> In what situations do you find yourself hearing the voice of someone from the past?

Dorothy suggested to her brother that they should ask their mother what kind of funeral arrangements she wanted for their father. Ron responded angrily, "Well, I can't just drop everything and fly across the country. I certainly can't stay for a week to sit shiva. I have things to do here and people are counting on me." Dorothy had had no such expectations of her brother and wondered why he had to get so angry at her.

· · · · · · · · · · ·

Countertransference: The listener has an emotional reaction
that interferes with hearing what's being said.
When listeners are in the grip of countertransference,
mature responses, like empathy, perspective, humor, wisdom,
and concern for the other person, are distorted
through the prism of the listener's emotionality.

· · · · · · · · · · · · ·

Although the terms transference and countertransference may not really tell you anything you don't already know, they may remind you that listening can be disrupted by the expectations of either the speaker or the listener. Actually, distinguishing between the two (unless *you* misunderstand something *I've* said) is somewhat arbitrary. The communicative process reflects the actions and interactions of both parties' subjective realities. In other words, when I talk about speaking and listening as separate matters for convenience here, the truth is that, in a relationship, a conversation is dynamically shaped by both participants.

The principal forces contributing to the listener's filter are the listener's own agenda, preconceived notions and expectations, and defensive emotional reactions.

The Listener's Own Agenda

To listen well, it's necessary to let go of what's on your mind long enough to hear what's on the other person's. Feigned attentiveness doesn't work.

Remember Jalen, whose friend Derek grew distant after he got married? Jalen might have been able to talk to Derek if he'd concentrated on saying how he felt, without blaming Derek or forcing him to explain himself. If you can express your feelings without trying to compel anything from the other person, you're more likely to get heard—and more likely to hear what the other person is feeling.

For years, Wayne had trouble listening to Janice's requests for change in their relationship. To his way of thinking, she was always unhappy about something; like many men in this situation, he felt that she expected him to do something about it, to fix it. Therefore, because he felt threatened by her complaints, Wayne listened only reluctantly. In fact, when Janice really did want Wayne to do something, she would make that perfectly clear. The rest of the time she just had the sense that he wasn't interested in her feelings.

When Janice's mother developed Parkinson's, something shifted in the couple's relationship. Now when Janice talked about the problems she was worried about, Wayne could sympathize because it was clear that he wasn't responsible. He could sense her vulnerability and he felt good about being able to listen and comfort her.

What shifted wasn't the result of anything either of them did deliberately. Wayne became a better listener once he realized he wasn't responsible for doing anything about Janice's feelings, and she became easier to listen to when she expressed her feelings of vulnerability even more directly. Too bad it took a crisis to make clear what had always been the case. Wayne wasn't responsible for Janice's feelings, and when she spoke about her worries about her mother, he was able to listen.

> When people are upset, sometimes they just need to talk; they might not be asking for a solution and usually don't want to be told what to do. To listen more clearly, you might ask: "Do you just need to talk, or do you want some advice . . . , or to talk and *then* get some advice?" The answer can guide how you listen effectively to what they say next.

Preconceived Notions

By the time we emerge from adolescence, most of us have become self-protective. We know where our naked nerve endings are and don't often expose them. We open ourselves selectively and, like any creature with a soft underbelly, retreat from unfriendly encounters. Sometimes, however, it's too late to pull back inside our shells. When the pressure of emotion makes us open ourselves to someone we think we can trust, failed understanding can be as bruising as a mugging.

When his son told him he was dropping out of college, Seth did his best to hide his disappointment. Still, he was upset and needed someone to talk to. Hoping that his brother would understand, Seth gave him a call. It wasn't easy for Seth to talk about his feelings, so he started out making small talk. After a few minutes, Seth told his brother that Justin had dropped out of school and that he was very disappointed. There was a pause, and then his brother went on to talk about something else. Seth was stunned. How could his brother be so unsympathetic? With great effort, he confronted his brother, saying "Didn't you hear what I said?" His brother replied that he had never thought of Seth as someone who needed emotional support.

Here was a chance for the brothers to share a deeper understanding; if they would only open up and listen to one another they could reestablish the closeness they'd had so many years ago. But it didn't happen.

The expectations with which we approach others are, as we shall see, just one of many ways we create the listening we get. Nor can the process be reduced simply to the behavior of the participants—the words—and therefore always be improved by "skills training" or pretending to take an interest or other calculated strategies. (Conversation can, of course, be reduced to a behavioral analysis, but only by trivializing the feelings of the people involved and overlooking the dynamic exchange taking place below the surface.) Dialogue takes place between two people with not just ears and tongues but hearts and minds—and all the famous complications therein.

> Having an understanding attitude doesn't mean
> presuming to know a person's thoughts and feelings.
> It means being open to listening and discovering.

Emotional Reactivity

As I mentioned in the Introduction, we all have ways of reacting emotionally within particular relationships. The closer the relationship, the more vulnerable we are to hearing something said as rejection or attack, even if it wasn't meant that way. Because of the dynamics of the relationship or what we've learned to expect, we get defensive, which makes it impossible to listen to and understand what the speaker meant to say.

A simple "Have you taken the garbage out yet?" might be taken as a rebuke by someone whose parents never expected him to do anything right. His response might be an overreactive "Can't you leave me alone for one second!"

It's not always the listener's defensiveness, of course, that gives rise to heated reactions. Sometimes it's the speaker's provocation.

"Why do I always have to ask you three times before you do anything?" when it really means "Would you please take the garbage out?" will almost inevitably trigger a defensive reaction. For that matter, even "Haven't you taken the garbage out *yet?*" could also provoke an emotional response. If you don't watch how you say things as well as what you say, it's easy to provoke those you love.

It's important to note too that the speaker making such demands may well have her own anxiety and frustration, planted long ago when she wasn't listened to as a child. Her distress at having to repeat a request may well be intensified by early experiences of feeling that her needs didn't matter to her parents, and so she had to keep insisting on them to get heard.

Then there are those touchy subjects that can almost be counted on to set off an explosion. As I explain in Chapters 6 and 9, the topics likely to be toxic among couples are money, children, power, in-laws, and sex. To have a constructive discussion about any of these requires special effort. You might have to watch not only what you say and how you say it, but also where, when, and why.

This is not to imply that we need to spend our lives tiptoeing around each other. What it does mean is that we may need to step back and calm down, being aware of what sets us off, where such big reactions come from in our lives, and what sets off those we want to communicate with, if we are to get through to each other.

When we don't, many exchanges degenerate to such clever repartee as "You're such a bitch!" and "Oh, grow up!" before falling apart altogether as someone storms out of the room.

Understanding the Rules of the Listening Game: Beyond Linear Thinking

We don't usually stop to examine patterns of misunderstanding in our lives because we're stuck in our own point of view. Misunderstanding hurts, and when we're hurt we tend to look outside ourselves for explanations. But the problem isn't just that when something goes wrong we look for someone to blame. The problem is also linear cause-and-effect thinking. We reduce human interactions to a matter of personalities. "He doesn't listen because he's too self-absorbed." "She's hard to listen to because she goes on and on about everything." Some people blame themselves ("Maybe I'm not that interesting"), but it's usually easier to recognize the other person's contribution.

Attributing other people's lack of understanding to character is armor for ignorance and insensitivity. That some people repeat their annoying ways with most people they come in contact with doesn't prove that lack of responsiveness is fixed in character; it only proves that these individuals trigger many people to play out the reciprocal role in their dramas.

The fixed-character position assumes that it's hard, if not impossible, for people to change and that they will act the way they do no matter the situation. But you don't change relationships by changing other people. You change patterns of relationship by changing yourself in relation to them. Personality is dynamic, not fixed. How we see ourselves and understand our relationships changes when we discover we can change our responses to each other. We are not victims—we are participants, in a real way, and the consequences of our participation are profound.

To participate effectively, you have to know something about the rules of the game.

I remember how confused I was the first time I saw a lacrosse game. From where I sat, it looked as if some kids were standing around while the rest raced up and down the field, using their sticks to pass the ball back and forth, club each other, or both. I got the gist of it—it was like soccer played by Road Warriors—but a lot of it was hard to follow. Why, for instance, did the team that lost the ball out of bounds sometimes get it back and sometimes not? And why sometimes when one kid whacked another with his stick did everybody cheer, while at other times the referee called a foul? The problem was that I couldn't see the whole field and didn't know the rules of the game.

The same disadvantages—not seeing the whole field and not knowing the rules of the game—keep us from understanding our successes and failures at communicating with one another.

Earlier I said that listening is a two-person process, but even that is oversimplified. Actually, even an uncomplicated communication has several components: the listener, the speaker, the message, various implicit messages, the context, the relationship, and, because the process doesn't flow one way from speaker to listener, the listener's response. Even a brief consideration of these elements in the listening process reveals more reasons for misunderstanding than simply bad faith on the part of the listener.

"What Are You Trying to Say?"

The message is the point of what a speaker says. But the message sent isn't always the one intended.

A family of four is invited to spend Sunday afternoon at the lake house of friends of the father. When the teenage daughter asks if she can bring along a friend, her father says, "I don't think we should bring extra guests when we're invited to dinner." The daughter looks hurt, and the man's wife says, "You're being silly; they never mind extra company." The man gets angry and withdraws, brooding over his feeling that his wife always takes the children's side and never listens to him.

The problem here is a common one: the message sent wasn't the one intended. One of the unfortunate things we learn along with being "polite" and not being "selfish" is not to say directly what we want. Instead of saying, "I want . . . ," we say, "Maybe we should . . ." or "Do you want . . . ?" When we're taking a trip in the car and we get hungry, we say, "Isn't it getting late?"

When I was growing up, I learned that guests weren't supposed to put people to any trouble. If you went to someone's house and wanted a glass of water, you didn't ask; you looked thirsty. If they offered you something, you politely declined. Only if they insisted was it okay to accept. (A really good boy waited until a glass of water was offered at least twice before accepting.)

If you grew up with this convention of indirectness as many people do, it doesn't usually cause problems. If the other person in the room says, "Are you cold?", you can assume he means "Can we turn up the heat?" But indirectness can cause problems when stronger feelings are involved. The father in our example didn't want his daughter to bring a friend. Perhaps he was right; it would be rude to bring guests. Or maybe his wife was right; the people who invited them wouldn't mind. But somehow, *he* minded. Maybe he wanted his daughter to remain more a part of the family and less an independent person with friends of her own. Or maybe he wanted her to be part of the grownups' conversation, instead of off with her friend, because he found it easier to talk about the children's doings than his own. That's the trouble with indirectness: there are always a lot of *maybes*.

When we're conflicted over certain of our own needs, we may infer (rightly or wrongly) that others would object to even hearing our wishes, much less acceding to them. Because indirectness leads to so much misunderstanding, it does more harm than good. Two people can't have an honest disagreement about whether or not they want to move to another city as long as they engage in diversionary arguments about whether going or staying would be better for the children.[1]

One reason others argue with us in a way that seems to negate our feelings is that we blur the distinction between our feelings and the facts. Instead of saying, "I don't want her to bring a friend," the father tries to cloud his motives and bolster his argument by appealing to *shoulds*. When his wife argues with what he says instead of what he means, he feels rejected.

> Like every listener, he measured the intentions of other speakers by what they said—or what he heard—and asked that they measure him by what he meant to say.

As speakers we want to be heard—not merely listened to—we want to be understood, heard for what we think we're saying, for what we know we meant. Similar impasses occur when we insist that we said one thing and our listener heard another. Instead of saying, "What I meant to say was . . . ," we go on insisting what we *did* say.

"Why Don't You Say What You Mean?"

Implicit messages tell us more than what's being said; they tell us how we're meant to receive what's being said. Depending on the situation, "Let's have lunch" could mean "I'm hungry," "I'd like to see you again," "No, I don't want to go to dinner with you," or "Please leave now; I'm busy." The statements "I love you" and "I'm sorry" are notorious for having multiple meanings. Knowing the other person can make it easier to decode implicit messages; speculating about his or her motives can make it harder.

---

[1] There are times, however, when the most effective statement of what you want is less than completely candid. For people who have trouble saying no, rather than trying to explain why they don't want to do something, it may be easier to say, "I'd love to, but I can't."

According to Gregory Bateson, one of the founders of family therapy, all communications have two levels of meaning: *report* and *command*. The report (or message) is the information conveyed by the words. The second or command level (which Bateson called *metacommunication*) conveys information about how the report is to be taken and a statement of the nature of the relationship.

Mara scolds her roommate for running the dishwasher when it's only half full. Hilary says, "Okay," but turns around and does the same thing two days later. Mara may be annoyed that Hilary doesn't listen to her. She means the message. But maybe Hilary didn't like the metamessage. Maybe she doesn't like being told what to do as though Mara were her mother.

In attempting to define the nature of our relationships, we qualify our messages by posture, facial expression, and tone of voice. For example, a rising inflection on the last two words turns "You did that on purpose?" from an accusation to a question. The whole impact of a statement may change, depending on which words are emphasized. Consider the difference between "Are *you* telling me it isn't true?" and "Are you telling me it *isn't* true?" Pauses, gestures, and gaze also tell us how to interpret what's being said. Although we may not need the ponderous term *metacommunication*, misunderstandings about how messages should be taken are a major reason for problems in listening.

> It's hard to metacommunicate by text; without hearing the tone of a voice, people may struggle to read worlds of meaning into individual words, relying on how a single word or short phrase is punctuated and edited, wondering whether autocorrect changed anything, figuring out what that tiny emoji is supposed to convey, and grappling with whatever else our overwrought minds might believe is intended by a communication as cryptic as "Hey."

One winter when I was working hard and feeling sorry for myself, I wrote to a sympathetic friend and said jokingly that I was running away to spend two weeks on the white beaches of a deserted Caribbean island. The only trouble was that I didn't *say* it, I *wrote* it, and she missed the irony I intended. The medium didn't carry my tone of voice or the facial expression that modified the message. Instead of getting the sympathy I was (indirectly) asking for, I got back a rather testy note saying that it's nice to know that some people have the time and money to indulge themselves.

We know what we mean; problems arise when we expect others to. How is our communication to be taken? Is it chat? A confession? An outpouring of emotion? When our listeners fail to grasp that we're upset and need to have our feelings listened to, who's to blame?

A woman told her boyfriend that something her boss said made her afraid she might be in for trouble at work. The boyfriend responded by saying no, he didn't think so; it didn't sound that way. When she replied that he didn't listen to her, both of them got upset. She was annoyed because he didn't listen to her feelings. He was hurt because he *was* listening. He just didn't realize how upset she was. He may even have been trying to reassure her it wasn't as big a deal as she believed.

Perhaps to some people this woman's upset would have been apparent. Maybe a friend would have realized that she needed to have her feelings acknowledged, not disagreed with. But she wasn't living with that friend. She was living with a man who didn't automatically understand how she wanted to be listened to. (Some people are careful to make that clear: "I'm worried about something, and I need to talk about it." "I need some advice." "I just need you to listen.")

Texting makes correspondence so easy that people often send messages in a personal frame of mind that get read by someone in a business frame of mind.

A long-distance boyfriend texts his girlfriend in the morning, saying, "Good morning." She's at work and doesn't respond. He later sends another text with a specific question, and she replies with an answer to the question. He responds with a hurt message about how she couldn't bother to take the time to say good morning. What their cryptic texts didn't convey was "I'm at home, feeling lonely, and I miss you" and "I'm busy at work, and I know that I'll see you this weekend."

Occasionally—but not as often as most people think—the implicit message in a communication is a request for the speaker to do something. The teenage boy who says, "I'm hungry" isn't just making small talk. (A teenager's appetite is not an idle thing.) Usually, however, the most important implicit message in what people say is the feeling behind the content.

When we're little, before we learn to act grown up by masking our feelings, our communications are full of ill-disguised emotion. You don't have to be a linguistics expert to figure out what a child is feeling when she says, "There's monsters under my bed!" or "Nobody wants to play with me!"; it's also clearer how you might need to respond. The same emotions may be implicit, if less obviously stated, when an adult says, "I've got that big meeting coming up tomorrow" or "I called to see if Fred wanted to go to the movies, but he didn't call back." One of the most effective ways to improve understanding is to listen for the implicit feelings in what people say.

Much of communication is implicit and—when people are on the same wavelength—decoded automatically. Often, however, what seems implicit—what we take for granted—isn't obvious to someone else. Much misunderstanding could be cleared up if we learned to do two things: appreciate the other person's perspective and clarify what remains unspoken.

"Is This a Good Time?"

The context of communication is the setting: the time, the place, who else is present, and, because communication can't be reduced to the obvious, people's expectations. We ordinarily accommodate our talking and listening to the context without thinking about it. We don't spring bad news on people the minute they walk in the door, we don't talk loudly on cell phones in public, and we don't argue in front of the kids. (As you can't see by the twinkle in my eye, I'm being ironic.)

But even if we try to choose the right time, there are times when people don't have the patience to listen. If a husband calls his wife at work and starts to talk at length about something that doesn't seem terribly important, she may get impatient sooner than she would if the same conversation occurred at home. By contrast, even though her husband usually retreats to his iPad at the end of the day, a wife may succeed in getting his attention by signaling her need for it. "Honey, I need to talk to you about something."

Unfortunately, in many relationships people have different preferred times to talk. He likes to talk when he comes home at the end of the day. She prefers to talk later, when they're watching Netflix or getting ready for bed. Fishing for understanding at the wrong time is like trying to catch a trout in the noonday sun.

* * * * * * * * * * * *

When to talk:
not when your partner needs some space or time to be alone.

* * * * * * * * * *

That timing affects the listening we get may be painfully obvious; unfortunately, when needs collide the resulting failures of understanding are obviously painful. The end of the day can be especially difficult. Partners may be frazzled. Dinner has to be prepared. Kids need baths, there's homework to supervise, things to do to get ready for tomorrow. Worn out from running around all day, trying to make other people happy, attending mind-deadening meetings, fighting traffic, or chasing after children and answering endless questions, most family members have little energy left over for hearing each other.

The unhappy irony is that the domestic conversation people are too tired to engage in might provide just the emotional refueling they need. Talking and listening reinvigorate us. If we take listening for granted, we may assume that the people we care about will listen to us whenever we feel like talking. But good listening doesn't happen automatically. You have to find the right time to approach people.

Setting has an obvious effect on listening—in terms of privacy and noise level, for example—and an equally powerful effect in terms of conditioned cues. Familiar settings, like a therapist's office or a friend's kitchen, can be reassuring places in which to open up. Other familiar settings, like your own kitchen or bedroom, may be anything but conducive to conversation. Memories of misunderstanding and distraction cling to some places like the smell of wet dog.

Conversation in various settings is governed by unwritten rules, some of which are obvious (to most people). At cocktail parties, for example, where conversational subgroups constantly shift, conversations may be warm, candid, even intimate, but they are also brief (which may explain the warmth and candor). Anyone who tries to talk too long in a such a setting may strain a listener's sense of decorum.

Before the advent of the smartphone, rules of decorum were based on a shared sense of what's appropriate and probably originated from practical considerations, like noninterference with others and respect for special places. Distinctions between public and private places were clearly demarcated. Thus, talking loudly in a cathedral, on the train, or at the movies was frowned on.[2] Because rules of decorum were implicit and widely shared, we took them for granted. But now people walk down the street engaging in full-throttle domestic phone quarrels—you need to look closely to see that they are not talking to themselves but via Bluetooth; people banter through movies and discuss their colonoscopy on speaker phone on the train. It doesn't make all the noise more tolerable, but it's interesting to note that the advent of personal devices, cable, and streaming services has effectively blurred the distinction between public spaces and private spaces.

In addition to general rules of propriety, most of us have personal preferences for settings in which we're comfortable talking. Some people like to talk on the telephone or by video chat, for example. (Why, I have no idea—but of course the COVID-19 pandemic in 2020 reduced the number of other options we had.) Some people like to talk when they go for a ride in the car; others prefer to read or look out the window. And, of course, we may be in the mood for conversation in a particular setting at one time and not another. Some children like to talk after they are tucked in bed, with the lights out. Others become chatterboxes while tossing a ball back and forth. Often the best way to get someone's attention is to invite him or her away from familiar surroundings—by taking a walk, say, or going out to a restaurant. Many of these preferences are sufficiently obvious that we adjust to them automatically. We know not to call certain people at home in the evening or too early in the morning, and we learn the most promising times

---

[2] People who get annoyed at those who talk in the movies forget that the advent of DVDs, cable, and streaming services has blurred the distinction between movie theater and living room. They also fail to consider situational priorities that might make theater conversation understandable. Yes, even people who talk in the movies deserve consideration, and so they should be strangled as painlessly as possible.

and places to get the listening we need. When we don't, feelings get hurt. We blame others for not hearing us, or we feel put upon by their lack of consideration in imposing on us at the wrong time.

Whenever conversation takes place in the presence of others, some aspects of listening are accentuated while others are suppressed. If a couple goes out to dinner and a man talks about problems at work, his partner will probably listen more intently than she does at home because the setting suggests intimacy. If they take along the children, however, they are both less likely to be attentive to each other or to talk about their own concerns. Sometimes that's *why* people take the children. Togetherness is a hedge against intimacy as well as loneliness.

Most of us have had the disconcerting experience of talking to someone who seems to be interested until someone else appears or her cell phone dings. "Just a second," she says. "I need to answer this." Sometimes this interruption is unavoidable. Parents of roving teens or people with a friend in crisis, for example, may need to respond to texts or calls. But many people seem not to be aware of the frequency of their distractions and the extent to which their attention is divided.

If two people are having lunch and a third person joins them, it's not reasonable to expect to continue a private conversation. But in other instances, the person talking about something important might expect the listener not to permit an interruption—to turn off the cell or answer it only to say, "Sorry, I can't talk now; I'm busy." Or if two people are having a confidential conversation in a public place, one might expect the other to greet a casual acquaintance who happens by, but not to break off the conversation or encourage the third person to join in.

Third parties are to intimate conversation
what rain is to picnics.

Sometimes the effect of third parties works the other way. An adult may show more animated interest in a child's conversation when other adults are watching. Similarly, a man who often interrupts his wife at home may show more respect when they're out with another couple. Or a disengaged teenager who sits bored and mute at the dinner table with her mother may become engaged and animated when her beloved uncle shows up.

I remember once when I was being interviewed on a morning television show how the host, an attractive woman in her early forties, was intrigued by the book I'd written. She sat very close, kept her eyes on mine, and asked all the right questions. Here was this radiant woman, totally engrossed in what I had to say. It was very flattering. Then a commercial break came up, and the light in her face went out like the light on the camera. I ceased to exist. After the break the interview resumed, and so did my interviewer's show of interest. Her pretense, in the face of a whole audience of third parties (and my susceptibility), was disconcerting; but after all, it was her job to show interest.

Why Some People Are So Hard to Listen To

Even when you play by the rules, some people are hard to listen to. In some cases, that's because their accounts run on to Homeric length. They're generous with details. You ask about their vacation, and they tell you about packing the car, getting lost on the way, and all the various wrong turns. They tell you about the weather and who said what and where they ate lunch and what they had for dinner, and they keep telling you until something other than tact stops them. Others may not talk at all about themselves but instead go on at great windy length about everyone else, all those inconsiderate others who are such problems in their lives. Some people talk on and on about their view of politics, a Netflix series, a book only they have read, the origins of Bitcoin, a historical event on which they have become expert—seemingly anything that could be interesting only to them.

It's also hard to listen to people who talk incessantly about their preoccupations—a mother with a difficult child who talks of little else, a dieter talking about calories, a struggling drummer who talks constantly about being broke, a man who's always complaining about his sciatica. One person's headache can become another's if she has to hear about it all the time. It isn't just the repetition that we tire of; it's being cast in the helpless role of one who is importuned about a problem with no solution, or at least no solution the complainer is willing to consider.

Some people who talk too much are like that with everybody, but often, whether we appreciate it or not, some of them talk at such length with us because they talk so little with anyone else. Who, other than his partner, does the man with no friends talk to? Who, other than the friend who seems to have her life together, does the overburdened wife talk to? A sister with few friends may call her brother almost every day, just to "check in." Some people need our attention, but if the conversation is consistently one-sided, maybe part of the reason is that we respond too passively.

Sometimes speakers are hard to listen to because they're unaware of what they've said—or of its infuriating implications. When the listener reacts to what is implied, the speaker responds with righteous indignation, wounded by the listener's "overreaction." If a mother says to her teenage daughter "Is that what you're wearing to school?", and the daughter bursts into tears and says, "You're always criticizing me!" the mother might protest that the daughter is reacting unreasonably. "All I said was 'Is that what you're wearing to school?' How come you get so upset about a simple question?" Such questions are as simple as parents are free of judgment and children are free of sensitivity to it.

My father has a way of packing what feels like a whole lot of belittling into one little innocent statement that drives me crazy. If I tell him that something is so, even when it's not something particularly unusual or controversial, he'll often say "It could be." Arghh!! I think he does this because he can't tolerate overt conflict. So if you tell him something he didn't know or isn't convinced is the case, he says, "It could be." To me, this feels worse than an argument. An argument, you can argue with. "It could be" makes you feel discounted. One consequence of these interchanges is that I have become stubborn in my opinions. Having had my fill of being doubted, I can't stand not to be believed when I'm stating a fact. Like the fact that Lake Champlain is one of the five Great Lakes.

In case you think I've slid from talking about speakers to complaining about listeners, you're right. While it's possible in the abstract to separate speakers and listeners, in practice they are inextricably intertwined. Listening is codetermined.

Some people are hard to listen to because they say so little, or at least little of a personal nature. If the urge to voice true feelings to sympathetic ears is such a basic human motive, why are so many people numb and silent?

Because life happens to them—slights, hurts, cruelty, mockery, shame. These things are hard on the heart.

We come to relationships wounded. Longing for attention, we don't always get it. Expecting to be taken seriously, we get argued with or ignored. Needing to share our feelings, we run into criticism or unwanted advice. Opening up and getting no response, or worse, judgment, is like walking into a wall in the dark. If this happens often enough, we shut down and erect our own walls.

Although a speaker's reticence may be seen as a personality trait, like introversion, such tendencies are more often habits based on expectations formed from past relationships.

> People who don't talk to us
> are people who don't expect us to listen.

Analytic therapists who encounter resistance to speaking freely engage in what is called *defense analysis*—pointing out to the patient *that* he is holding back, *how* he is holding back (perhaps by talking about trivia), and speculating about *what* might be on his mind and *why* he might hesitate to bring it up. Therapists have license that the average person lacks to ask such probing questions, but it's not against the law to inquire if a friend is finding it difficult to open up for some reason or to point out that she doesn't seem to talk much about herself. We shape our relationships by our response.

"No, Everything's Fine . . ."

When you ask someone if something is wrong, and the answer is a not-very-convincing "No," how do you respond? One common response is to say, "You don't look fine." This may be intended as an invitation, but it doesn't come across that way. Pressing a reticent person to open up or getting annoyed at the person for not doing so presumes that he or she has no good reason for not telling you what's wrong. People don't do anything for no reason.

When someone seems reluctant to tell you what's bothering him, you might make an informed guess about why the person is reluctant to say what's on his mind: "Are you afraid of how I might respond?" "Is it something you're hesitant to talk about?"

Does the person who isn't very forthcoming with you have reason to believe that you're interested in what he thinks and feels? That you'll listen without interrupting? That you can tolerate disagreement? Anger? Openness is a product of interaction.

Men Are from Mars?

As we head further into the twenty-first century, the social construction of gender—men do this, women do that—continues to polarize relations between the sexes in needless ways. As the old complementarity gives way to a new symmetry, growing pains abound. Most women are working; most men are more engaged in life at home. As old rules cease to apply and couples struggle to figure out who does what, increased conflict seems to be inevitable.

Several books in the 1970s and 1980s gained enormous popularity by telling us that men and women communicate differently and then explaining what those differences are. Among the most popular was John Gray's *Men Are from Mars, Women Are from Venus,* in which the author argues that men need space while women crave company. If we learn to respect the inevitable differences that crop up between two people who live together by attributing such differences to gender rather than to stubbornness or ill will, maybe that's a good thing. And if we learn to react sympathetically to what our partners say, that's certainly an improvement. But perhaps the most important thing is not so much learning *how* to react to these other, supposedly alien creatures, but learning not to overreact: learning instead to listen. Perhaps the best response to Freud's famous question "What do women want?" might have been "Why don't you ask?"

Once, differences between men and women were thought to be bred in the bone, and this biological determinism was used to justify all manner of inequity. After years of effort to break down these separate but unequal categories, an early wave of feminist scholars reasserted what they once fought: gender differences. Jean Baker Miller emphasized responsiveness and mutuality as especially important to women in relationships, and Carol Gilligan argued that for women the qualities of care and connection are fundamental to selfhood, organizers of identity, and moral development. According to Gilligan, men build towers and women build webs.

One of the enduring impacts of the work by feminist psychologists from the 1960s and 1970s has been a reaffirmation of gender differences—but now with a positive construction of the psychology of women. In her book *The Reproduction of Mothering*, Nancy Chodorow pointed out that because boys and girls are parented primarily by mothers, they grow up with different orientations to attachment and independence. Boys must separate themselves from their mothers to claim their masculinity, which is why boys of a certain age start shrinking from their mothers' hugs and why "sissy" and "mamma's boy" are still such powerful invectives. Girls, on the other hand, do not have to renounce their mothers' caring and connection to become women; they learn to become themselves *through* connection.

> Do you listen differently depending on the gender of the speaker? What assumptions might be at play?
>   How do you think your parents treated you differently because you were a boy or a girl?

In the wake of Nancy Chodorow and Carol Gilligan, the discourse on men and women appears to rely on an assumption that women have been socialized in such fundamentally different ways than men that they are probably better at listening. For people who accept this premise, life is simple: All the complexities of relationship can be dispensed with in favor of one all-purpose explanation. Men do this; women do that. End of discussion.

That wave of sexual typecasting was reflected in the popular reception of books that reduced every nuance, every polarity of conversation between men and women to one gender distinction: men seek power; women seek relationship. Sadly, even though the data suggest otherwise, a lot of people still take this for granted.

Back in 2005, the American Psychological Association published a meta-analysis looking at dozens of studies examining gender differences, The report begins: "Mars-Venus sex differences appear to be as mythical as the Man in the Moon." The lead author, Janet Shibley Hyde, concluded that, over a vast range of psychological variables, men and women are a lot alike.

So what are some of the differences worth noting? For one, researcher John Gottman suggests that because women live day to day with significantly more fear than men, it is much easier to frighten women. When a woman is startled, she responds anxiously; a man's natural response to being startled is anger and a desire to get even. During the course of an argument, though, men are more likely than women to get physically and emotionally overwhelmed—flooded—than women (though women can get flooded too). So Gottman recommends that couples try a "soft start-up" so no one gets stressed before the conversation even begins. Then, in conflict, the men might need to learn to behave in ways that attend to her feelings of stress and safety; the women might slow down or stop a conversation when he gets so flooded that he shuts down.

Importantly, also, men are significantly less likely than their wives to "accept influence" from the other, a capacity that is critical for healthy and enduring relationships. Wives accept the man's influence at high rates—in Gottman's research, it is the husband's rejection of influence, not the wife's, that predicts divorce. This issue of accepting influence has implications not just for the way it poses challenges for a particular marriage but also, more generally, for how we think about the role of power in relationships—who gets to speak and decide in a partnership can be political as well as personal. Listening, real listening, requires a capacity to allow the other person to have an impact on how you think and feel.

One of the most interesting ripples emanating from the #MeToo movement is the possibility of a new kind of conversation in which women also are seeking power—the right to be heard, to say "no," to talk about what has happened to them, and to give voice to upsetting and traumatic events that they have carried in fearful silence for years. In turn, this seizing of power over their bodies and voices has upset the social order and catalyzed men into asking more about the kinds of relationships they have had and are capable of having in the future.

After some backlash in which decent men have had to contend with feelings of being blamed for the behavior of others; angry sentiments shared by some women as well as men that #MeToo women didn't seem to make a sufficient distinction between a public hug and private molestation; newly troubled workplace politics; confusion about what might be acceptable—or not—in their own conduct; and disorientation due to a sudden and unexpected challenge to their extremely long run with power and privilege, there are encouraging signs that this movement is also generating conversation. We are beginning to listen more to each other across the gender divide. Many men appear more willing to believe the survivors in their lives and feel distraught. They are finding out how to ask for sexual consent and to understand that "No" is a complete sentence. They are more willing to "accept the influence" of their partners and view women as complex human beings— just like them.

If men and women are able to listen to one another and to embrace both power and relationship in their intimate lives, we will begin to connect more deeply. My point isn't that there aren't gendered differences in the ability to attend to intimacy or authority during conversations between men and women, but that perhaps it's time to stop exaggerating and glorifying them.

Why are so many women and men so willing to assume that we're separated by a vast gender gap, that we speak different languages, and that our destinies take us in different directions? Is it really true that it's a woman's nature to be caring and seek connection? Is it really just fundamentally a man's nature to be independent and seek power? Or do these polarities reflect the ways our culture has—thus far—shaped the universal yearning to be appreciated?

Sometimes social and political factors provide the underlying explanation for so-called gender distinctions. Might caring, for example, which has been represented as a gender difference, be more adequately understood as a way of negotiating from a position of lower power? Perhaps some women (and some men) are caring because of a need to please, which stems from a lack of a sense of personal power elsewhere. Thus the same woman who appeals to the need for caring in debates with her husband may emphasize rules in arguments with her children. The same social embeddedness that promotes caring may sometimes make it difficult for women to recognize their own self-interest when it is undermined by a relationship. Perhaps men, working to collaborate and be part of a team at work, come home after a day of feeling unimportant. They see the advantage of their power at home and use their status to disengage, to do less around the house and with the kids. Perhaps rather than making up explanations or apologizing for or celebrating gender differences, it would be more useful for us to talk *with* each other, instead of about each other, and to move toward partnership, not polarization.

Perhaps if we started listening to one another we could move toward greater balance, in ourselves and our relationships. There is encouraging evidence that more recent generations are, indeed, finding ways to value interdependence over the more polarized perspectives holding that women pursue and men distance, that women want to be connected and men want to stand on their own two feet. Women raised to believe that happiness is to be found in selfless service to others are learning more respect for their own strivings and capacity for independent achievement. Men who thought they might develop their masculine identity only in achievement are learning greater respect for the neglected dimensions of caring and concern. In the process of relaxing rigid definitions of what it means to be a man or a woman, fathers are circuiting the living room a hundred times trying to soothe a colicky infant and crying openly at their daughter's high-school graduation; mothers are juggling complex lives that include work, friends, engagement and activism in politics, and making sure there are cheese sticks in the fridge for a picky eater's lunch tomorrow.

As we let go of a misguided and unhealthy belief in gender differences as fixed and given, we can raise boys who can identify both with their fathers' power and their mothers' nurturance and care, who understand that girls are people too, and who will grow up to become more fully realized men and better fathers. In some ways, the path has been better lit for girls, who are more easily able to identify with their fathers as well as their mothers and increasingly feel entitled to be nurturing and independent persons with their own big dreams and stronger voices.

Comforting as it may be to blame a lack of understanding on other people's stubbornness or insensitivity—or on gender—the reasons we don't listen to each other turn out to be more complex. We have a path forward when we understand that, more often, it's complications of character and relationship that keep us from listening and being listened to.

A fuller appreciation of the dynamics of listening makes it a little easier for us to begin hearing each other. Is it necessary to dissect every misunderstanding and analyze it according to message, subtext, context, speaker, listener, and response? Of course not. The simple, heroic act of stepping back from our own injured feelings and considering the other person's point of view is quite enough of an accomplishment.

So why are we so sensitive to misunderstanding that we have trouble seeing the other person's side of things? To answer that question and continue to move toward hearing each other, let's look more closely in the next chapter at the emotional factors that complicate listening.

Quiz

To help you become more aware of your own listening habits, complete the following questionnaire. Answer the questions honestly and, because we listen differently to different people, think of a specific person you have a relationship with when you answer these questions. You might want to do this twice, once with a family member in mind and once with a coworker or friend in mind.

HOW GOOD A LISTENER ARE YOU?

When someone is talking to you, do you:

1—Almost never   2—Sometimes   3—Often   4—Almost always

1. Make people feel that you're interested in them and what they have to say?
2. Think about what you want to say while others are talking?
3. Acknowledge what the speaker says before offering your own point of view?
4. Jump in before the other person has finished speaking?
5. Allow people to complain without arguing with them?
6. Offer advice before you're asked?
7. Concentrate on figuring out what other people are trying to say, not just respond to the words they use?
8. Share similar experiences of your own, rather than inviting the speaker to elaborate on his or her experience?
9. Get other people to tell you a lot about themselves?
10. Assume you know what someone is going to say before he or she is finished?

11. Restate messages or instructions to make sure you understood correctly?

12. Make judgments about who is worth listening to and who isn't?

13. Make a concerted effort to focus on the speaker and understand what he or she is trying to say?

14. Tune out when someone starts to ramble on, rather than trying to get involved and make the conversation more interesting?

15. Accept criticism without getting defensive?

16. Think of listening as instinctive, rather than as a skill that requires making an effort?

17. Make an active effort to get other people to say what they think and feel about things?

18. Pretend to be listening when you're not?

19. Respect what other people have to say?

20. Feel that listening to other people complain is annoying?

21. Make effective use of questions to invite people to say what's on their minds?

22. Make distracting comments when other people are talking?

23. Think other people consider you to be a good listener?

24. Tell people you know how they feel?

25. Don't lose your cool when somebody gets angry at you?

Scoring

For the odd-numbered questions, give yourself four points for each question you answered "Almost always"; three points for "Often"; two points for "Sometimes"; and one point for "Almost never." For the even-numbered questions, the scoring is reversed: four points for "Almost never"; three for "Sometimes"; two for "Often"; and one for "Almost always." Total the number of points.

    85–96 Excellent
    73–84 Above average
    61–72 Average
    49–60 Below average
    25–48 Poor

• • •

1. If you got a high score on this questionnaire, congratulations. Read on to reinforce what you're already doing and perhaps get some additional ideas for improvement. If you scored less well, pick out one bad habit at a time and practice letting others finish talking, and then let them know what you think they're saying before you say what's on your mind. Just doing this will go a long way.

2. During the next few days, pick out a couple of relationships that are important to you and try to identify two or three things that get in the way of your listening. Common interferences include being preoccupied, trying to do two things at once, having negative thoughts about the speaker ("He's always complaining"), not being interested in the topic, wanting to say something about yourself, wanting to give advice, wanting to share something similar, being judgmental. Once you identify two or three of your own bad listening habits, practice eliminating one of those impediments for a week, but only in conversations that you decide are important to you.

PART TWO

The Real Reasons
People Don't Listen

4

"When Is It *My* Turn?"

THE HEART OF LISTENING:
THE STRUGGLE TO SUSPEND OUR OWN NEEDS

Forty-five years ago, I took my first course in how to be a good listener. I was in graduate school, and the course was called Elementary Clinical Methods. We learned about making eye contact and asking open-ended questions and how to parry personal inquiries with the therapist's famous evasion, "Why do you ask?" We practiced on each other, and I learned a lot of interesting things about my classmates. Then we went to the state hospital to practice on patients, and I learned that maybe I wasn't cut out for this work.

It was the first time I'd ever been in a psychiatric hospital, and I approached it with fascination and horror. Maybe I expected to see an axe murderer or perhaps a scene out of *The Snake Pit.* In those days before the widespread use of tranquilizers, some of the back wards *were* snake pits. But in the ward for new admissions, where they sent us, the patients were mostly just very unhappy people.

My first real patient was a young mother who'd become depressed after coming home from the hospital with her second baby. She looked disheveled and lonely, and I felt sorry for her. I asked her why she'd come to the hospital and why she felt so hopeless and where she grew up and things like that. She answered my questions, but the interview never really went anywhere. Every time I'd ask another question, she'd respond, but only briefly, and then wait for me to say something. Since I didn't have anything to say, it was an awkward wait.

It was my first interview, and I was very disappointed that it didn't go well. Eventually I learned not to ask so many questions and, if people didn't seem to have much to say, to comment on that, inviting them to explain their reticence rather than trying to fight it with questions. But the real problem in that first interview didn't have to do with technique. I wasn't really interested in that woman; I was more interested in being a therapist.

This troubling experience illustrates the most vital and difficult requirement for listening. Genuine listening demands taking an interest in the speaker and what he or she has to say.

Taking an interest can easily be sentimentalized by equating it with sincerity or caring. Sincerity and caring are certainly fine characteristics, but listening isn't a matter of character, nor is it something that nice people do automatically. To take an interest in someone else, we must suspend the interests of the self.

> Listening is the art by which we use empathy to reach across the space between us. Passive attention doesn't work.

Not only is listening an active process, but it often takes a deliberate effort to suspend our own needs and reactions—as Briana's mother so bravely demonstrated (in Chapter 1) by holding her own feelings in check long enough to listen to her daughter's fierce resentment. To listen well, you must hold back what you have to say and control the urge to interrupt or argue.

Kiana was enjoying going to the gym more now that she'd found a workout partner. Marilyn knew a lot about exercise and stretching and always seemed to have interesting things to say. Theirs was a nice, easy friendship, but so far it didn't extend beyond the gym.

One rainy morning, Marilyn came late and said that her basement had leaked and she had had to make an appointment with a handyman. Kiana was just about to say that she too had problems with leaks, but she held back her urge to talk about her own concerns to make sure Marilyn had finished.

Marilyn went from talking about her leaky basement to talking about problems she was having with her kids. Kiana appreciated Marilyn's opening up to her and felt that their friendship had moved to a more intimate level. After their workout, Marilyn asked if Kiana and her partner would like to get together for dinner. Kiana hadn't really needed to talk about the leaks in her ceiling, and now she was glad she hadn't.

The act of listening requires a submersion of the self and immersion in the other. This isn't always easy. We may be interested but too concerned with instructing or reforming the other person to be truly open to his point of view. Parents have trouble hearing their children as long as they can't suspend the urge to set them straight. Even therapists, presumably exemplars of understanding, are often too busy trying to change people to really listen to them. (Unfortunately, most people aren't eager to be changed by someone who doesn't understand them.) That failures of understanding occur in psychotherapy, just as everywhere else, is a fact often missed as long as therapists remain too wrapped up in their own theories to give themselves over to sustained immersion in the other person.

Although therapists may be less likely than the average person to interrupt, some are so anxious to be perceived as sympathetic that they offer sentimentality instead of compassion. "Oh yes," they say with their eyes, "I understand how you feel." Sympathetic or not, condescending kindness from a patronizing person isn't the same thing as listening. The superficially sensitive therapist doesn't have to listen because he already knows what he wants to say: "*Oh yes, I understand.*" Real listening is a strenuous but silent activity.

> There's a big difference between showing interest
> and really taking an interest.

Suspending the self does not of course mean *losing* the self—though that seems to be precisely what some people are afraid of. Otherwise, why do they insist on relentlessly repeating their own arguments, when a simple acknowledgment of what the other person says would be the first step toward mutual understanding? It's as though saying "I understand what you're trying to say" meant "You're right and I'm wrong." Or that to give someone who's angry at you a fair hearing and then say, "I see why you're upset with me" meant "I surrender." Ironically, when the fear of never getting your turn is so strong that you don't hear the other person out, it becomes a self-fulfilling prophecy.

Martina was trying to explain to Zach that when she gets upset about something she just needs to talk about it without him giving her the third degree. "I never get the feeling that you're willing to just listen to me when I get upset," she said.

"Yes, but," Zach said, "if I don't understand what's bothering you, how can I help?"

"I don't need you to analyze the situation," Martina said. "Sometimes I just need you to listen to me."

"I'm happy to listen to you," Zach said, "but if I don't understand why you're upset, I don't really know what the problem is."

Can you see that both Martina and Zach are doing a good job of expressing their feelings? And that neither is doing a very good job of listening?

I'll have some practical suggestions for breaking this pattern in Chapter 7, but first it's important to understand more about the difficulty involved in the simple art of listening.

Genuine listening involves a suspension of self. You don't always notice this because it's reflexive and taken for granted, and because in most conversations we take turns. But you might catch yourself rehearsing what you're going to say next when another person is talking. Simply holding your tongue while someone speaks isn't the same thing as listening. To really listen you have to suspend your own agenda, forget about what you want to say, and concentrate on being a receptive vehicle for the other person.

The listener's responsiveness is experienced subjectively by the speaker as—at least temporarily—vital to a sense of being understood, of being taken seriously. Listeners feel that pressure.

The Burden of Listening

Listening puts a burden on the listener. We feel the weight of the other person's need to be heard. Attention must be paid.

But, you might object, isn't empathy a natural response? Isn't listening something we automatically extend to each other as part of being human? Yes and no. Empathy is an active form of engagement. At times we're interested in what the other person is saying, and listening is easy. But there inevitably comes a moment when we cease to be engrossed. We lose interest or feel the urge to interrupt. It is at this moment that listening takes self-control.

. . . .

Genuine listening means suspending memory,
desire, and judgment—and, for a few moments at least,
existing for the other person.

. . . .

Suppressing the urge to talk can be harder than it sounds. After all, you have things on your mind too. To listen well, you may have to restrain yourself from disagreeing or giving advice or sharing your own experience. Temporarily, at least, listening is a one-sided relationship.

In everyday conversations, you may not notice that burden. But you can feel the pressure to be attentive whenever another person needs to talk for more than a few minutes. Even if you care about the person and are interested in what she has to say, you're caught. You need to be silent. You need to be selfless. You need to open your heart and be empathic.

Doreen asked her father out to lunch so the two of them would have a chance to talk a little more personally than they did when her mother was around. But when they sat down at the restaurant, he started in on his usual diatribe against the bureaucracy. His bosses were "morons," and none of his coworkers cared about anything but "putting in their time until retirement."

Doreen had heard it all before. She nodded and looked interested and thought about her upcoming sales conference. Once or twice she started to interrupt, but something about the way her father spoke with more feeling

than usual made her heart move. She stopped thinking about the sales conference and started listening to what he was saying. As she did, she began
to hear the hurt and disappointment underneath his carping. Suddenly she
was filled with sadness at her father's isolation. His unhappiness had less to
do with his frustrations at work than with the fact that his constant complaining had made other people in the family stop listening to him. Doreen's
annoyance gave way to a powerful feeling of sympathy and connection with
her father. For the first time, she understood how lonely he was. Later, when
she said so, her father's eyes filled with tears and he thanked her for listening.

Sometimes we're so touched by what people say that listening just happens. When your child bursts into the house and says, "Guess what happened!", you don't have to work at listening.

One day many years ago my son was sick and stayed home from school.
When I called at lunchtime to ask him how he was feeling, I didn't have to
make any effort to suspend my other preoccupations to tune in to his report.
Nor would anyone else have had to in my place. I was interested in his feelings, I intended to listen to him, and I did. We probably all listen without
much effort, dozens of times each day, at least for a few minutes.

Often, however, it's not that easy. Much of the time listening takes
work.

When I came home after work, my son was lying on the couch watching TV. Again I asked how he was feeling, but this time it wasn't quite as
easy for me to listen. As usual, he wasn't wearing a shirt or socks, and I had
to suppress the urge to nag him about that. He was watching two brainless
cartoon teenagers rating videos in which everything was either "cool" or "it
sucks," and I had to make an effort to ignore that. I had things on my mind
that I wanted to talk about, and I wanted to read the mail before it was
time to make dinner. None of these considerations was terribly pressing or
unusual. It took only a small effort to suppress them long enough to listen to
my son for a little while. Had he needed to talk for more than a few minutes,
however, I would have had to make a more active effort to suspend these
other agendas—or I would not have been able to listen.

Of course, suspending your needs in order to listen means more than just allowing the other person time to talk. It doesn't mean just letting a certain amount of time elapse while that person has his say, only to switch to your own agenda when he's finished.

We're not fooled by the feigned attentiveness of the restless narcissist, who may allow us a few minutes of airtime but is only waiting to take over the stage. On the other hand, when we open up to someone we expect to be interested and that person listens for a moment but then changes the subject to himself, we feel betrayed. It's like a slap in the face; we feel as though he didn't care about what we said.

Elena was worried about going back to get her master's degree after being out of school for six years. She'd been wanting to do this for a long time, and her friend David, who already had his degree, had encouraged her warmly. When she told him that she was concerned about doing the work, David was so enthusiastic about her finally having taken the big step that he jumped in to say how great it was that she was doing this for herself and that she'd gotten into such a good program. Elena got quiet and changed the subject. David's encouragement hadn't been very encouraging. Elena was trying to tell him that she was worried, and his saying how great it all was made her feel misunderstood. Ironically, David's expression of confidence in Elena felt invalidating and actually added more pressure, one more thing to live up to.

Like David, most people think they're better listeners than they really are. At best they allow the other person to state his case, and then they make their own interpretation of what the other person said. At worst they're preparing their own argument while the other person is still talking.

David thought he was listening, but wasn't able to suspend his need to have Elena not worry or for himself to be seen as supportive long enough to hear her out. A lot of us have difficulty listening when it means having to sit still and share someone's uneasiness or uncertainty. We want to say something to make the anxiety go away.

To listen well, you have to read the needs of the speaker and respond to the context.

For example, when parents ask, "What did you do in school today?", children often say, "Nothing." What follows is an exchange of questions and monosyllabic answers. The parent wants to hear what happened in school but doesn't listen to what the child is saying. The child might be saying something like "Nothing I want to talk about right now. I just want to be left alone."

A child at school is exposed all day. Other kids look at you and pass judgment on what you're wearing, who you're with, what you say, how your hair is fixed, and just about anything you might do. Teachers check to see if you did your homework and if you're paying attention and to make sure you're not making noise in the halls or generally having any fun. After being the subject of such scrutiny all day, some kids want nothing more than to be left alone. Their "nothing" isn't coy or withholding; it's self-protective.

The parents' side of this conversation isn't hard to understand either. They're curious about what goes on in their children's lives. They want to know if everything is okay. They want to know if their children are doing what they should be doing. They don't want to be shut out.

Sometimes kids say "nothing" but really do have something to say. Maybe you have to show them that you're really interested to convince them to open up. Asking them about their day, especially about specifics that show you're paying attention, and really being prepared to listen shows interest—and often leads to their sharing more important concerns.

Ask questions that demonstrate curiosity about their experience—"She said that?" "What happened next?" But don't expect to hear every last detail. Honoring their right to respond the way they want shows respect as well as interest—interest in them and respect for their feelings. Children who sense that their parents are interested in hearing what they have to say—as opposed to interrogating or prying or fretting—will open up when they're ready.

"What's Up?"

Questions that show an awareness of the other person's interests and concerns may help reticent people open up.

Ineffective Questions*	Effective Questions
How's everything?	How are you coming with that project you've been working on?
How was your day?	What's been happening with your headaches lately?

What's new?	How is your son doing in soccer?

*Note that most ineffective conversational gambits can be answered with "yes," "no," or "nothing."

If it's difficult to suspend the self with our children, imagine how much more difficult it is with another adult, whom we don't expect to have to indulge in any way—especially when we have our own problems.

Sometimes we fall into the habit of listening without effort because we put so much effort into other things. When we work until we're spent, we become preoccupied with our own worries and careless of concern for others. It's especially hard to listen when you feel that *you* haven't gotten the attention you need. Here's an example:

A woman who's having a bad day at the office wishes she could be at home with her five-year-old. She's envious of her college professor husband who, because it's summer, is at home all day with the boy. When she gets home, instead of complaining about her day, she asks how her husband's day went. He complains about the burden of having to amuse a five-year-old and the difficulty of figuring out what to do with all the unstructured time. She listens impatiently for a minute or two and then says, "Why are you complaining? You're lucky to have all this time off. Think of all the things you could do!" Her husband is hurt—first she asks him how his day went, then she criticizes him for telling her—and the woman herself is resentful. The woman in this example wasn't able to listen to her husband because she wasn't able to suspend her own feelings long enough to be receptive to his. After talking about this episode, the woman concluded that she needed to try harder to overcome or contain the stress of her work. (Perhaps it would be more reasonable for her to realize that when she comes home after a bad day she may need to talk about it before she's ready to listen.)

. . . .

A good listener may need to set aside his or her own needs
to tune in to the other person's, but completely selfless people
don't make good listeners. You have to get listened to yourself
to free you up to be receptive.

. . . .

"But I *Am* Listening!"

The selflessness of genuine listening is hard to sustain, and so in a number of ways we fool ourselves into thinking we're listening when in fact we aren't.

"That Reminds Me of the Time . . ." (Translation: "My experience is more interesting than your experience.")

When friends sit around having a casual conversation, they'll get on a particular subject and take turns telling their own stories. Carol will describe how her dachshund won't do his business outside in the winter because the minute he feels the icy snow on his paws he clickety-clicks back to the door and whines to be let in. Then Murray will tell about the time his Russian wolfhound lay at death's door for two days, until they found a small burr in his long silky fur, and when they removed it, Sasha suddenly made a miraculous recovery. Then I'll tell something fascinating (to me, at least) about my cat Ralphie's latest adventure.

In this kind of friendly exchange it's okay just to take turns. The person telling a casual anecdote doesn't need an elaborate response. However, there are times when someone has something important to say and doesn't want to hear your story until she's had a chance to finish hers—and get some acknowledgment. She needs a little time and attention. The woman who's just had her car towed away doesn't want to be interrupted to hear about the time that happened to you three years ago.

Interrupting someone to tell a similar story is a common example of how listeners don't restrain themselves. Sometimes this is annoyingly obvious, as when people draw attention to themselves by cutting in to say, "That reminds me of the time . . ." Most of us don't do that when it's obvious that someone really needs to talk. If someone needs to talk, we listen. At times, however, the speaker's need for attention isn't obvious, and instead of devoting ourselves to receptive listening, we respond from our own needs. A friend starts to tell us about an accident and, in an attempt to show empathy, we interrupt to tell her about ours—which, after all, was more upsetting to us, even though it happened six months ago. We might be trying to say, "You can share your experience with me because I am in a particularly good position to understand you"—but it might not come across that way.

> ### "Me Too."
>
> "I hardly slept at all last night."
> "Me too! I was up and down all night."
>
> When people tell stories, it's natural to be reminded of your own experience. Who do you know who frequently says "me too" when you're telling a story? When and how might such a response come across as empathy for you and make you feel understood? When does it feel like the spotlight has shifted away from you and onto the other person?

Why do people do that? Why do we interrupt to tell our own stories? Most conversation is interactive. We're engaged, and much of what people say to us triggers something in our own experience. If I tell you something annoying that my father does, you're likely to think of something annoying your father does. Or if I tell you about the time I fell in love for the first time, you're likely to remember your first love. Sharing these stories may feel like an effort to establish common ground. But listening to people means hearing them out—giving them sufficient time to say what's on their mind and taking sufficient interest to follow and acknowledge their experience.

"Oh, How Awful!" (Translation: "You poor, helpless thing. What *are* we going to do?")

Another example of listeners failing to restrain themselves is responding with excessive sympathy, a gift that usually means more to the giver than the receiver. Exaggerated concern may seem less selfish than turning the conversation around to yourself, but acting distressed isn't the same thing as listening. Listening means taking in, not taking over.

Real listening requires attunement—reading and acknowledging the speaker's experience—not the kind of effusive sentiment that may fool small children but comes across to adults as patronizing and false. Expressions of concern from a person who always makes a fuss over what you say become as meaningless as Muzak.

Once again, the problem is failing to suspend the self. Instead of holding himself back long enough to listen and to hear what you're saying, the excessive responder jumps in with an expression of sympathetic concern—as if to say, "Oh, *I* understand . . . (don't bother going on)."

When listening is genuine,
the emphasis is on the speaker, not the listener.

When something goes wrong, Christine no longer calls her mother for sympathy. She's learned that if she has the flu or one of the kids breaks a finger, not telling her mother is the only way to avoid an exaggerated show of concern. These things may not be very consequential, but she would like to share them. She doesn't, because when her mother says, "Oh, that's awful!" and makes too big a deal out of everything, she feels not understood, but that her mother is worried—as though *she's* the one with the problem. Then it seems that instead of thinking about her child, she's supposed to be taking care of her mother.

An empathic response is attentive, largely silent;
following, not leading, it encourages the speaker
to go deeper into his or her experience.

Part of the problem is confusing empathy with sympathy. Sympathy is more limited and limiting; it means to feel pity for someone's suffering without really trying to understand it. Nor does empathy mean, as many people seem to think, worrying about, praising, cheering up, gushing, consoling, or even encouraging. It means understanding.

"Well, If I Were You . . ." (Translation: "Stop bothering me with your complaining and *do* something about it.")

According to some experts, men show interest by giving unsolicited advice, while women show interest by sharing experiences. Unasked-for advice is annoying. It feels like being told what to do or being told that our feelings aren't valid because we wouldn't have to have them if we'd only do what the oh-so-helpful person we're talking to suggests.

Responding with a similar story can be equally unwelcome, especially if the person interrupts your story before you're finished or otherwise goes on without acknowledging what you've said. When I'm telling someone about an experience or a problem and he or she responds with unwelcome advice, I say, "Thanks, but I don't need any advice; I just need to be listened to." (At least that's what I'd *like* to say.) Do men give more unasked-for advice than women do? Maybe. Not in my experience. Perhaps in yours.

A few years ago I did something uncharacteristic for me and joined a men's group. It turned out to be a wonderful experience, largely because the other men in the group were all interesting and thoughtful people. One day we were talking about how we respond when a friend tells us about a problem, and I was surprised to hear most of the others say that they usually try to offer advice. I thought friends didn't do that, but just listened and tried to be understanding. I guess advice giving was trained out of me.

Of course, sometimes people *want* advice. Some individuals want advice all the time. They think other people should have an answer for their distress and should try to alleviate it. This emotional need stirs our expectations that advice is wanted. Even if it doesn't work (or get followed), giving advice may suggest that the listener takes the speaker's problems seriously.

The real issue in listening isn't whether we do or don't give advice, but whether or not our response is focused on reading and responding to the other person's feelings or is simply a way of dealing with our own. Telling the person with a problem to "do something constructive" reflects a listener's inability to tolerate his or her own anxiety. So too may be pushing others to "Express your feelings" or using imperatives such as "You should confront him about it." The difference between listening well and not listening well is the difference between being receptive and responsive on the one hand and being reactive or introducing one's own agenda on the other. Failure to suspend the self in favor of the other reflects a blurring of boundaries.

"Have You Heard the One about . . . ?" (Translation: "Never mind what you were saying; your concerns are boring.")

Another familiar failure to restrain the self is the jokester, who's always quipping, allaying his own anxiety and calling attention to himself instead of tuning in to the speaker. There are times when your fast-quipping friend is funny and you don't mind his joking. But there are other times when you're trying to talk and his wisecracking is annoying. What the jokester offers is the thin, unreliable rhetoric of distraction in place of authentic emotional engagement. This feeling of being distracted happens a lot when you're already having a conversation with someone and the jokester joins in. Only he doesn't join in. He doesn't tune in to you and what you're saying; he just uses something you say as a trigger to make a joke.

People who joke all the time are more or less annoying, depending on how funny they are. We can understand their constant joking by realizing that they have a lot of nervous energy and may have learned to make jokes as a defense against boredom. But, like other failures to restrain the self, someone who always interrupts our conversation with gags can be annoying.

"Don't Mention It." (Translation: "I'm embarrassed about wanting to be appreciated.")

Do you remember the last time someone did you a really big favor and you were so grateful that you wanted to express your thanks in a special way? Maybe you sent flowers or gave a nice bottle of wine to show your appreciation. Or maybe you put your gratitude into words. Did the person accept your thanks or say something like "It was nothing, don't mention it"? You can understand someone's feeling embarrassed about being thanked profusely, but it leaves you feeling slightly dismissed (as if being told that your thanks weren't necessary meant that your feelings of gratitude weren't warranted). Wouldn't it be nice to say, "Thank you," and have someone say, "You're welcome"?

"Don't Feel That Way." (Translation: "Don't upset me with your upset.")

You get a similar but perhaps stronger feeling of being dismissed when you tell someone about being angry or scared about something and she reassures you that there's no need to feel that way.

A lot of failed listening takes the form of telling people not to feel the way they do. It's frustrating when someone tells us we shouldn't worry or feel guilty or be so scared. The intention may be generous, but the effect is to cheat us out of having our feelings acknowledged. Most attempts to talk people out of their troubles are correctly understood as dismissive—namely, "Don't upset me with your upset."

Parents often wish their kids would act differently than they do, and who can blame them? A well-behaved child certainly makes life easier. But young children often need more than reassurance and redirection; like the rest of us, they also need to be heard and understood.

Alice was trying to talk with her mother about finding a nursing home for her father. Four-year-old Amy kept interrupting—perhaps she sensed her mother's anxiety—and Alice told her not to interrupt Mommy. Amy needed to go and do a puzzle in another room. But the interruptions continued until, finally losing her temper, Alice snapped at Amy and sent her to her room.

Alternatively: Alice was trying to talk with her mother about finding a nursing home for her father. Four-year-old Amy kept interrupting—perhaps she sensed her mother's anxiety—and Alice told her to go and do a puzzle in another room. When that didn't work, Alice bent down and picked Amy up and said, "What's the matter, honey?"

"How come I never get to talk to Grandma?" Amy asked.

"I know, honey, you love Grandma." Then she took Amy by the hand and walked with her over to her toys and said, "In ten minutes, you can take Grandma outside and show her your swing set."

Children don't whine just to be annoying. They have legitimate concerns. They whine because they're unable to express themselves in a more mature way. They're frustrated. They're tired. They're young. The parent who responds punitively—"Stop that noise!"—is inadvertently supplying the other half of the argument. The parent who ignores a whining child conveys—"I won't listen to you when you're upset." Or worse, "I won't listen to you until you get *really* upset."

When someone is worried or upset enough to talk about it, acknowledging those feelings is the best response—even if the worried person is only four years old. Reassuring the person that there's nothing to worry about or telling him to think about something else is not responsive to him; it's responsive to the listener's own uneasiness.

If someone tells you that she's worried about the future, and you can control it, then by all means do so. Otherwise, hear her out. Even if you *know* (or think you do) that things will turn out okay (in the future), saying so (predicting the future) doesn't erase the worry (in the present). Reassuring someone instead of hearing him out may ease his mind slightly, but the disconcerting effect of not being taken seriously is usually the stronger reaction. Telling someone not to worry doesn't make her stop worrying, but it may make her stop trying to talk about her feelings to you.

The best way to keep this section simple would be to say that telling people not to feel the way they do is not listening to them and leave it at that. However, there are times when it feels okay to be reassured. You're not too happy with your new haircut, and a friend says, "No, it looks good," or you're feeling bad about not having accomplished much, and someone reminds you of all that you have accomplished and you feel better. The line between wanting to be reassured and wanting to be heard may not always be easy to discern. The more a speaker expresses self-doubt or worry or concern in a questioning or tentative way, the more likely he is to want reassurance. The stronger the feelings, the more likely he is to appreciate being heard and acknowledged. When in doubt, listen.

"Haven't We Talked about This Before?" (Translation: "Why are you still hung up about this?")

It can be hard to hear the same complaints over and over again. My advice is to blame the person talking to you for your impatience. Try not to think about the possibility that the other person keeps talking about something because you haven't ever fully acknowledged his feelings. And certainly don't consider that the annoyance you feel is related to your sense that somehow talking to you hasn't made the person feel any better. When in doubt, always blame other people for your feelings.

Whether it's asked for or not, we expect that our advice will be followed. After all, it *was* great advice, wasn't it? We might even get a little frustrated when we discover that our pearls of wisdom were utterly ignored. In some circumstances—therapists face this so often that we should know better—even people who are asking for help seem intent on telling us why the advice won't work. It can be like skeet shooting—they ask, we throw out our wisdom, and they shoot it down. In fact, I tell my psychology trainees not to worry too much about giving good advice—because no one listens to it anyway. So when people in our lives continue to tell us the same sad story many times after we've done our best to fix things for them, we will probably feel a bit like throwing our hands in the air. We will struggle to keep listening.

But here's the thing: we can't change their story; we can only change how we hear it. Whether we like it or not, there are good reasons people need to tell us something again and again that have absolutely nothing to do with solutions. A man's wife leaves him after 10 years of marriage and he is devastated. He needs to talk about pain and bewilderment more than once or twice. A mother with a manic young adult son is frantic about his safety. She has no control over this—and neither do you—and she can think of nothing else. An independent woman gets a diagnosis that means she will need to have others take care of her for many months. In an instant, she has to change her whole life strategy, and she can't get over it. We may want to make it better, but what can we do? Listen compassionately; you can't make the woman's son take his meds, but you can bear witness to his mother's suffering, and that will give her comfort.

And people also tell us the same thing repeatedly because, to put it simply, we still don't get it, how hard it is for them. And by "get it" I mean empathize with their situation, understand their pain. Once they *feel understood,* they are much more apt to move on. They need to feel understood—not told "I understand."

· · · · · · · · · · · · · · ·

When we give advice before we really understand a problem,
we hurt more than help. After all, if it was that simple to fix,
she would have solved it already herself.

· · · · · · · · · · · · ·

"Guess What?" (Translation: "Never mind what's on your mind; whatever pops into my head is bound to be more interesting.")

Jack was talking to Gail about some problems at work when Woody came over and said "Guess what?" Then he proceeded to tell them about something unrelated to what they were talking about. Had they finished? Were they interested in what he had to say? Who knows? Certainly not Woody.

If Woody's interrupting two people's conversation to talk about what was on his mind seems like such an obviously insensitive thing to do, how different is it when someone is talking to us and we change the subject without making sure the person had finished saying what he or she wanted to say?

Going Through the Motions

A good listener is someone you look forward to being around. The good listener not only pays attention to what you say, but also encourages you to expand on your ideas and feelings.

. . . .

However it's phrased, a good listener's response
makes you feel understood and invites you to say more.

. . . .

Since we always want to be seen as good listeners, we sometimes just go through the motions. We nod and say uh-huh when we're not really interested, or we wait until the other person finishes even though we're not really listening to what she's saying. We all pretend to be listening occasionally, but some people make a habit of it.

Insincere listeners come in a variety of forms. Perhaps you'll recognize some of the following.

The Faker

These people feign attention. They fix their eyes intently on you when you're speaking. The intensity of their gaze reflects their concentrating on giving the impression that they're listening, rather than really listening. If you've never met one of these fake listeners (congratulations!), try meeting a politician or appearing on TV. Some Gen Z kids are brilliant at faking it: there's even a word, "phubbing," to describe their skill at typing on their smartphones while staring right at you, nodding while paying no attention to you whatever. Guess what: you are being snubbed in favor of a phone by someone—perhaps your very own teen—who is just pretending to listen.

The Self-Conscious Listener

Self-conscious listeners want to be seen as listening but are more concerned with the appearance than the listening. They're looking at you but thinking *Am I doing okay? Do I look all right? Does the speaker think I'm intelligent?* Preoccupation with themselves gets in the way of self-conscious listeners' concentration on what you're saying. (The ability to concentrate on listening was challenged further during the coronavirus pandemic in 2020, when video chatting became prevalent, and we had our own mirrored image in front of us throughout our conversations.)

The Amateur Therapist

Amateur therapists may be eager to play the role of listener, but they're more interested in the role than the listening. These people mistake the supporting role of listener for the leading part.

Young therapists often paraphrase everything they hear clients saying. While this sounds like a version of the acknowledgment I've said is part of good listening, it's often an attempt to pigeonhole the speaker's communication in some package of interest to the therapist—not feelings, but a summary of the facts, an analysis of some kind.

Carmen was telling her sister about the frustrations involved in arranging a conference at work. Instead of letting her explain the situation and how she felt, Mariana kept making little judgmental summaries. "Yes, these things should have been arranged well in advance." "So, your supervisor doesn't take charge of things." "I see, there shouldn't be so many people involved in the planning process." Mariana was probably trying to be helpful, but to Carmen her comments felt like a distraction. Mariana was saying how she thought things should be rather than responding to Carmen's feelings about the way they were.

The problem with the amateur therapist's comments isn't failing to acknowledge what the speaker says, but doing so in a way that focuses on the listener's helpfulness rather than on the speaker's feelings. "I know what's wrong." "Here's my expert analysis."

The Active Listener

Active listening is a useful technique whereby the listener paraphrases what the speaker says. The intention is to help listeners concentrate on hearing and acknowledging what other people are saying. Unfortunately, when "active listening" gets translated into simply summing up what someone says, the focus shifts from the speaker's expression to the listener's perceptiveness.

There's nothing wrong with active listening. Acknowledging what people say is part of the essence of good listening. The problem is that when listening is reduced to a laundry list of how-tos, some people make more of an effort to show that they're listening than to actually listen. Maintaining eye contact, nodding your head, saying mm-hmm, and paraphrasing everything you hear are mechanical listening skills. They may come naturally when you're really listening, but it's important to concentrate on listening, not demonstrating it.

There's an old joke in which a depressed patient is talking to a therapist who practices active listening. The patient says, "I'm depressed," and the therapist echoes "You're depressed."

The patient responds, "No, I mean it. I'm *really* depressed."

"You're *really* depressed," the therapist says.

Now exasperated, the patient says, "I'm so depressed that I feel like killing myself."

"You feel like killing yourself," says the therapist.

"I'll show you!" the patient says, and then gets up, walks over to the window, and jumps out.

The therapist goes over to the window, looks out, and, after a pause, says "Plop."

Obviously, this is a parody of how paraphrasing can be a mechanical operation—and how distressing it can be to hear robotic active listening like that. The important thing isn't to summarize what someone says but to understand what he or she is feeling. So, of course, the therapist should have said "Ouch!"

The Overly Sympathetic Listener

Some people make a show of listening sympathetically—"Oh, yes, I understand!" The person who interrupts with expressions of sympathy may not really be receptive to what you're trying to say; her frequent expressions of sympathy and elaborations may be an effort to assert herself—not in a competitive way, but as a particularly sensitive and sympathetic person. Many "supportive" people are like that. They don't say, "Look at me—I'm terrific"; they say, "Look at me—I'm supportive." Sometimes this kind of effusive interruption swamps the speaker; it can rob him of the chance to feel his own emotions and tell his own story, in his own way.

When people talk about feelings—what they're excited about, what's troubling them—they want to be listened to and acknowledged, not interrupted with advice or told that someone else had a similar experience. They want listeners who will take the time to hear and acknowledge what they're saying, not turn the focus to themselves.

Focusing on Yourself

This is what bad listening is all about. Listeners who remain focused on themselves may seem to be listening, but they're only waiting to tell their story or offer their opinion.

SPEAKER: "I hate my supervisor."

LISTENER: "Me too. My boss is so condescending . . ."

> **How to Overcome Focusing on Yourself**
>
> Sorry, but there are no magic answers here. The only thing to do is to concentrate on hearing the other person out. What you want to say may be perfectly legitimate, but saying it too soon skips hearing out and acknowledging what the other person was saying.

If someone says, "I hate my supervisor," and you want to say that you hate yours too, wait until it's your turn.

"I hate my supervisor."

"Gee, that's too bad. What does she do?"

Then, after that person has had a chance to elaborate, it's your turn.

But such efforts are doomed if the pressure to be heard is strong. Get the listening you need too.

EXERCISES

1. Ask someone you trust to help you check your listening skills. In the course of a practice conversation, summarize what the person said after the person has completed his or her thought. By summarizing, you will become aware of how well you heard what the person was trying to communicate. What's important isn't just repeating what the person said but articulating what you think the person was trying to express.

   If you're not able to do a good job of grasping what the other person was trying to get across, try to figure out what was getting in your way. Daydreaming, forming your own response, being critical of something? Were you bored? Thinking about something else? Did you get interested in some detail of what was said, and fail to concentrate on the main thing the speaker was trying to convey? These are the habits you need to overcome to become a better listener.

2. For each of the following statements from people expressing their feelings, check the response you are likely to make—not what you think you should say, but what you think you typically would say.

   a. "I've had a terrible headache all afternoon."
   - (1) Maybe you should take some aspirin.
   - (2) Maybe you shouldn't drink so much coffee.
   - (3) Gee, that's a shame.
   - (4) Gee, that's a shame. When did it start?
   - (5) I've had a headache too. Maybe it has something to do with a change in atmospheric pressure.

   b. "I can't decide what to wear."
   - (1) Why don't you wear—.
   - (2) Nobody is going to care what you wear.
   - (3) I know, it's tough to decide.
   - (4) I know the feeling. What were you thinking of wearing?
   - (5) I know what you mean. I can't decide what to wear either.

   c. "I hardly slept at all last night."
   - (1) Maybe you need to get more exercise.
   - (2) You fall asleep every night in front of the TV; no wonder you have trouble sleeping.
   - (3) That's too bad.

(4) That's too bad; any idea why?

(5) I didn't get much sleep myself last night.

d. "I hate staff meetings!"

(1) Do you just sit there and get bored, or do you try to participate?

(2) It's part of your job, isn't it?

(3) Yeah, I know what you mean.

(4) I hear that! What are yours like?

(5) At our meetings everybody has to put in his two cents' worth.

e. "I do twice as much work as everyone else, but I don't get any recognition for it."

(1) Maybe you should do a little less.

(2) It's your own fault. You're always doing things for other people.

(3) That's not fair.

(4) How long has that been going on?

(5) I know what you mean. I'm always the first person at work and the last to leave.

f. "I hardly made any progress on that project today. Every time I'd start to work on it, something would come up and I'd get sidetracked."

(1) Why don't you try shutting your office door and turning off the phone?

(2) You'll never get it done if you keep letting yourself get interrupted.

(3) That's too bad.

(4) You kept getting sidetracked?

(5) I'm getting like that myself lately. Whenever I have something important to do, I seem to find so many other things to do.

In each of these examples, choice (1) is advice, (2) is criticism, (3) is an empathic comment that closes off conversation, (4) is an empathic comment that opens up conversation, and (5) is talking about yourself. Is there a pattern to the responses you typically make?

Practice making empathic comments that invite people to elaborate or go deeper with what they are saying.

5

"You Hear Only
What You Want to Hear"

HOW HIDDEN ASSUMPTIONS PREJUDICE LISTENING

Listening, as we've seen, takes effort. But sometimes that effort is prejudiced: Our biases filter what we hear and how we respond. Those biases take the form of preconceived expectations and defensive reactions. I'll explain in this chapter how what we expect to hear filters what we do hear and then get to emotional reactivity in the next. To be clear, though, just as it isn't always easy to separate the speaker's and listener's contributions to misunderstanding, it isn't always possible to separate assumptions from emotions that interfere with listening.

How Our Attitude about the Speaker
Biases What We Hear

One way to learn something about the forces that influence listening is to hear the same story from two different sides.

Aisha was a special-education teacher who had a humiliating encounter with the principal of her school. When the principal needed to find space for a new reading instructor, she sent Aisha a memo saying that she would have to move to a small room in the basement, previously used for storage. Aisha prided herself on being flexible, but being banished to the basement made her feel humiliated and that the principal had little respect for the needs of her children.

When Aisha called to discuss this unsatisfactory arrangement, the principal made an appointment to see her that afternoon. But when Aisha showed up at four o'clock, the principal had gone to another meeting and left a note suggesting they get together later. Ten days went by before the principal finally made time to talk to her. By that point Aisha had to make an effort to control her anger to make the case, as calmly as possible, that moving to the basement just wasn't acceptable. Instead of listening, the principal, who'd obviously made up her mind, got defensive. At one point, when Aisha protested that the specially equipped classroom in which the children now met had always been her room, the principal said archly, "Oh, did you bring it from home?" Aisha left the meeting in tears.

As soon as she got home, Aisha called her sister, who since their mother's death was the only living member of her family. But when Aisha tried to explain what had happened, Katrine kept interrupting with questions. "What did you say that made that woman so defensive? You must have said something to set her off like that." Aisha couldn't believe it. Instead of being supportive, her sister was blaming *her* for the incident. It felt like a slap in the face. "Just listen, Katrine, will you!" she pleaded. That shut Katrine up for the moment, but Aisha could tell that her sister wasn't sympathetic and wasn't really listening, so she said good-bye and hung up.

When Aisha told me about this incident two days later, she said that her sister hadn't been there for her when she'd needed her. It certainly sounded that way. But by a strange twist of fate, I got to hear Katrine's version of the same event the following week.

According to Katrine, she's had lifelong problems talking with her sister. "Aisha has always dominated our conversations. She loves to talk about herself, but she hardly ever listens to anything I have to say. If I pause for a minute, she immediately jumps in with some comment or criticism." But what bothered Katrine most was that Aisha was always complaining. "She's always telling me about hassles with somebody—other teachers, neighbors, supermarket clerks, even the nice old man in the Chinese take-out place. And it's always the other person's fault. I used to try to listen—after all, she is my sister. But as I've gotten older, I just don't have time for her negativism."

According to Katrine, Aisha was hard to listen to because she'd used up her credit.

It's not uncommon for speakers not to be heard because their credibility is low. A father's credibility, for example, may be determined by whether his wife and children think he's tuned in to what's going on in the family or too preoccupied with his work or hobbies to know what's happening at home. If he's had an affair or drinks too much, they may not respect him enough to hear what he has to say even when he has good advice. A parent's status in the world also affects his or her credibility. A mother who is laid off and out of work may lose credibility. This may not be because her family is judgmental, but because people who have lost self-respect in their own eyes often express themselves with a bitter edge that makes them hard to listen to. Listening is always codetermined.

The minute you pick up the phone and hear some people's voices, you're on guard. They're asking you how things are going, but you're waiting for the pitch. They call only when they want something. Even if you want to be friends, the one-sided nature of these relationships wears thin after a while. When you answer the phone and they say hello, they can probably hear the enthusiasm drop out of your voice. Do they have any idea why?

Credibility is also influenced by whether you're viewed as being in an appropriate position within a particular setting. A colleague who's seen as not really caring about what goes on at work may not be listened to even when he has something worthwhile to say. A mother who talks to her adolescent children as though they were still six years old may be experienced as out of touch and therefore incapable of having legitimate concerns.

A lot of grandparents don't get heard when they give advice about childrearing. Their mistake isn't necessarily being intrusive but rather being out of touch with their children's insecurity about being parents. The grandparents aren't heard because their children perceive their advice as undermining their own authority. In this case, the grandparents' mistake may be treating their children as though they were *more* grown up, in charge and confident, than they feel.

Our credibility is also affected by whether or not our messages are clear and pertinent. If your father-in-law muddles his messages with malapropisms and tangential references, you may try to understand him as part of building a relationship with your spouse's family. But if you have to work too hard at it, after a while you may give up. If your father always changes the subject to talk about himself, you may get out of the habit of listening. People who abuse the privilege of our listening by going on and on or flitting from one subject to another may create the expectation that listening to them is too much work, so why bother?

When the speaker has lost credibility but the relationship has a good track record, you might pay attention even though you may not really hear. You might give the aunt who's always been nice to you the courtesy of your attention even though you don't respect her enough to really listen to what she's saying. But if there is relentless repetition of a message—any message— you're likely to withdraw even the courtesy of attention, replacing it with annoyance or distance.

If a friend can't stop blathering on about her fabulous ex-boyfriend, you may get tired of hearing it. And perhaps frustrated that she won't give it a rest. The same thing happens if a friend going through a divorce can't talk about anything but what a bitch his ex is. We have ideas about how long we should endure some kinds of conversations. Some people have saintly patience. Others may wonder resentfully as they labor to listen, "How many more times do I have to hear this?"

How Our Expectations Make Us Hypersensitive

Our relationships to each other depend on our capacity to transcend immediate experience by making a reproduction of it inside the mind, where we can then manipulate the possibilities. A simple example of this is a baby learning to tolerate his mother's absence by remembering her presence and relying on her return. This mental representation of experience can be the source of adaptive flexibility or of rigid inflexibility that sets some people at odds with the world around them.

From the start, our lives revolve around relations with others. The residue of these relationships leaves internal images of self, other, and self-in-relation-to-others. As adults we react not only to the actual other, but also to an internal other—the mental images we have of other people, built up from experience and expectation. That is, we relate to people in the present on the basis of expectations formed in the past. (A man who emerges from childhood with a clear picture of his father lording it over his mother may vow always to be kind and considerate to his own wife—at all times unstinting in his criticism and counsel.) A child who has been abused by caregivers is likely to be very cautious about trusting people later on. She may become quite skilled in figuring out whether someone is authentic or manipulative; her survival depended on knowing the difference.

Contemporary relationships and the earlier ones stored in our inner world interact in circular fashion. Life circumstances maintain internal expectations and are chosen because of them and interpreted in light of them. A bright girl who has been ostracized throughout her life changes schools for high school. She is greeted kindly by her new classmates. Expecting to be rejected as she has in the past, she responds coolly to them, and eventually they pull away. When that happens, she concludes that she was right not to trust their overtures of friendship. Her expectations for disappointment have been fulfilled.

Alison sometimes felt overwhelmed by all the people in her life who depended on her. She was the one responsible for taking care of her aging parents, even though her brother lived a lot closer to them than she did. Her thirty-year-old daughter called her three or four times a week to complain about something or ask for advice. Several people at work were always asking for her help on various things, even though she had her own projects to look after. What Alison sometimes forgot was that she liked doing things for people. It made her feel good. She had always sought out opportunities to be helpful. She grew up being rewarded for being the "good daughter" and was still playing that role, including with the two people who taught it to her in the first place. It was hard for her to imagine saying "no" even though she was exhausted by saying "yes." In some ways, Alison's ability to listen was too good; it depleted her and gave her little space in which to listen to herself.

Terry was an only child of older, quiet parents. He grew up accustomed to being on his own—doing his homework and practicing his clarinet. He was busy and successful, but he never had friends over or felt he was part of a group. He played in the student orchestra in high school, but he didn't go out after rehearsals with the other kids. College was no different. He did well academically but felt socially awkward and spent most of his time alone. He recalls that he might have felt lonely but justified his solitude by saying that he couldn't abide small talk that took him away from doing more important things. He came to therapy in his late twenties to figure out how to connect more with people and eventually make some friends. When he began to realize that he wanted his life to be different, he had to confront his expectations that he'd always be alone—and rethink the host of justifications that maintained his avoidance and isolation. Unlike Alison, Terry had grown up listening mostly to himself; he had to learn how to find space for other people too.

. . . .

The past is alive in memory—
and it runs our lives more than we know.

. . . .

Terry had lived cautiously up until this point. Like many of us, he'd kept doing what he knew how to do, possibly because he feared being seen as awkward or a loser. The devil you know is often preferable to the devil you don't know.

We are all sensitive to being wounded for some reason or another. Marina, growing up with a narcissistic and emotionally neglectful mother, had been cheated on and abandoned by a series of disappointing partners. Deep in her heart, she knew that love and pain were inextricably linked.

Roger's exposure to early childhood adversity left him with a desperate desire for love but the fear that he was unworthy of it. His adult relationships were unstable, swerving between extremes; some days they were "all good" and other days "all bad." Small miscommunications filled him with infantile rage. It is possible to imagine him as a frightened baby, crying to be picked up and somehow drawing this disappointing conclusion about the rest of his life when no one came to hold him. Even in middle age, he still swings back and forth across the two possibilities: What is wrong with me that you don't give me comfort? What is wrong with you?

Dylan's mother was in a constant state of worry and agitation about his cell phone use. They fought every single day about it, and about his disrespect, phone addiction, and rudeness. One day she told me some stories about her father, who had never had time for her. He hid his nose in the newspaper and got annoyed when she needed to interrupt and ask him something. It turned out that Dylan's preoccupation with his phone struck a very old and painful chord for Stacey. She noticed that he even sounded like her father when without looking up he said "Uh-huh" instead of actually listening to her.

To explain why some people caretake compulsively, some attack, and others withdraw, we might look to how their families responded to their narcissistic need for attention. Some people get attention for being good; in their families anger and assertiveness are beyond the pale. For others who get attention for achievement, vulnerability and weakness may be intolerable. When children have violent parents, some may become very careful and try to avoid attention as much as possible. Or, expecting the worst, they may act out in destructive ways so they have a modicum of control over what happens next, even if it's awful.

What's common to these scenarios is that we go into intimate relationships carrying the legacy of our pasts. We may look like well-put-together adults, but inside we do not feel equal. Indeed, it's useful to recognize that we are all fearful children intimidated not so much by the reality of other people as by imagined negative responses. Our expectations are there, unbidden, like wolves that only we hear howling.

How We Learn to Overreact

Some of the expectations we bring to conversations are acquired from the history of our relationships with specific individuals. But some of what we expect to hear is part of the deep structure of our personalities, the residue of our earliest relationships. To understand listening and the dynamics of relationship, it's necessary to consider not only what goes on between people, but also what goes on inside them.

. . . .

More than we like to realize, we continue to live
in the shadow of the families we grew up in.

. . . .

The sometimes vast difference between words spoken and message intended is nothing compared to the often vaster gulf between what is said and what is heard. Whenever someone seems to be responding unreasonably, it might be useful to ask: What would make that response reasonable? Once you start thinking this way—namely, that people act the way they do for a reason—you'll know something about the way they were treated by their parents.

> When was the last time you surprised yourself by saying something you hadn't meant to say or thought was uncharacteristic of you?
>   Where do you suppose that came from? Have you ever sounded exactly like a parent, perhaps in a way you vowed you'd never do? What did you say? What was that like for you?

One reason we carry sensitivities from childhood around with us rather than resolving them in a timely fashion is that growing up takes longer than most people think. The period of "emerging adulthood," lasting from about age eighteen through about age twenty-six, constitutes a kind of cultural developmental delay for a significant number of our young adults, most of whom will, I promise you, eventually, in their thirties, hit those traditional milestones for adulthood: completion of school, career, home, marriage, and kids of their own. The advent of the Internet and its increased ease of access across generations has further altered the landscape of grown up but not-really-away for subsequent generations. Add to the mix here economic uncertainty, an inhospitable housing market, longer stretches of time before a stable partnership fills in emotionally where parents leave off, and even a global pandemic sending emerging adults back to their childhood bedrooms in droves . . . and we have a whole new, glacially slow program for casting off the constraining childhood scripts that for too long have defined us.

Indeed, while once young people left home to forge an adult path in their early twenties, moving out is much less often the case today. Many millennials like the connection with their parents; they don't feel the pressure to grow away quite so fast.

People who decide to work on their relationship with their parents adult to adult often go at it with unfortunate expectations. They imagine themselves righting ancient wrongs like avenging angels, or waking sleeping intimacy, as though family ties, cherished, strained, or severed, could be refashioned overnight. The truth is, when you go home, even in your thirties or forties or fifties, you're more like one of nature's humbler creatures, and you have to keep your wits about you to avoid getting stuck on the family's emotional flypaper. Ram Dass says that if you think you are enlightened, you should go home and spend the weekend with your family.

Peggy and her parents agreed on many things—the value of hard work, the need to build something for the future, the importance of family. But agreement is something children and parents can always overcome, and Peggy and her parents managed to get into shouting matches on just about every visit. Most visits would start off well. Love and news would carry them through the first couple of days, but the inevitable blowup was like a ticking time bomb, set for three days and waiting to go off.

Peggy couldn't stop wishing her parents were different. She loved them, and they loved her; she just wished they would grow up. Her mother was loud and abrasive, eager for company but always complaining, never a kind word to say about anybody. Her father was quieter, self-possessed, cool, some would say aloof. He showed his love by offering advice, whether you wanted it or not, and by repairing things around the house, whether they needed it or not. Peggy found him impossible to talk to. When she tried to tell him what was going on in her life, he never really listened.

Unlike some people, who acknowledge the turmoil they feel on family visits but don't recognize their own contribution, Peggy was willing to look at her part in the conflict with her parents. First she figured out what it was that her parents did that made her reactive. Her mother assumed the right to criticize anything and anyone, but her meanest comments were reserved for family members who acted independently. When Peggy's sister-in-law went to work for an organization helping homeless people, her mother said, "Who does she think she is, putting herself in harm's way like that!" She was totally unsupportive when Peggy's cousin got remarried quickly after a divorce even though the first marriage had been a disaster. And when another cousin came to a family event with his boyfriend, her mother made insensitive comments he could probably overhear.

Next Peggy learned to see how her mother's small-minded negativism and intrusiveness triggered anxiety and rage in her. The fact that she'd learned to expect it made her hypersensitive. The minute her mother started in on someone, Peggy got upset, anxious, and angry at the same time. She felt she was being pressured to join her mother in mean-spiritedness, and if she resisted she felt as though she herself were under attack. She usually held her tongue, but the effort to repress her impulse to protest only put her anger under pressure, which eventually led to an eruption. The longer she held back, the more her rage would build. When she finally did blow up, her mother would get hurt and withdraw, leaving Peggy feeling helpless and despicable at the same time.

Peggy also began to see that although she rebelled against her mother's criticisms, she had incorporated her mother's habit of assuming responsibility for other people's feelings and reactions. Whereas her mother was critical and controlling, Peggy was benignly controlling—worrying excessively about her own children, always doing things for other people. The blurred boundaries between self and loved ones were the same for mother and daughter—only their way of showing it was different. The "nicer" and more "helpful" Peggy was, the more she expected there to be no walls between her and those she cared for. She felt guilty for not doing enough and suppressed her anger for not getting enough. Eventually, when her children, her friends, or her husband did something that made her feel shut out, she'd erupt in anger, just as she'd done with her mother. These scenes never changed anything. As you may have discovered, venting anger isn't the same as voicing feelings in a way that gets them heard. When she first consulted me about the relationship with her mother, Peggy said that she had tried everything. Her "everything" ran the gamut from A to C, appeasement to confrontation. The alternative, calmly stating her own point of view, never occurred to her, because by the time she finally responded to her mother's criticism she was too angry to be in control.

The word for unrestrained emotionalism is *childish*. The place where we learn (or don't learn) restraint is in our families. But it isn't in childhood that we overcome childishness; that isn't in the cards. As young children, we looked up to our parents. (But then we were short and looked up to everything.) Later, if they said something to incite or provoke us, most of us either absorbed it or cried. It was as teenagers that we began to see through our parents, stopped putting up with the exasperating things they said, and started fighting back.

Plenty of teenagers become so reactive to their parents that they flare up at the least hint of indignity, like kindling struck by lightning. (If you've ever had a teenager in captivity, you know what I mean.) If adolescence is a time for becoming your own person, emerging adulthood is a time for transforming relationships with parents from a childish basis to an adult one. Unfortunately, this transformation can take years.

It was a lot easier to sustain the illusion that we were grown up when we left home at eighteen, but the cost of that illusion was that our parents remained frozen in adolescent patterns. Now that emerging adults are staying home longer, returning home after college, or coming and going as they build their adult lives—and in touch by text more frequently the rest of the time—the shifting relationship can be confusing: one moment, a parent caring for a child, the next, a young adult helping out a parent; the next, two adults chatting in loving friendship; then wham, they're in a heated ancient battle that reignites teenage indignation and entitlement.

Only one thing robs Superman of his powers: kryptonite, a piece of his home planet. A surprising number of adult men and women are similarly rendered helpless by even a brief visit with their parents. Superman becomes mortal in contact with kryptonite; mortals become teenagers in contact with their parents. We revert to childish roles when we get anxious because we never fully learn to resist parental provocation.

· · · · · · · · · · · ·

Our parents may be the most important
unfinished business of our lives.

· · · · · · · · · · · ·

Our Divided Selves

We don't easily face our own shortcomings, and it's painful to confront our failures to listen. When we do, it's natural to get discouraged: "I'm a lousy listener," "I'm selfish," "I'm too controlling." Instead of thinking of ourselves in such global, negative terms, it's possible to realize that only a part of ourselves is having trouble listening. Using a little imagination to personify our parts as subpersonalities (residues of early relationships) may lead us to their source. Take, for example, a husband who finds himself shutting his ears when his wife tries to tell him that she needs more from him. With a little introspection, he might discover a part of him that feels like a little boy being reprimanded by his mother. The little boy doesn't want to hear it; his mother's criticism makes him feel scolded and controlled; he wants to be left alone. The husband can calm down his "little boy part" by realizing—really getting it—that his wife isn't his mother. She's not trying to control him. Even if she sounds critical, what she's trying to express is her loneliness and her need for him. It's not we who are afraid to listen; it's those fearful parts of us that, once triggered, reduce us to childish insecurity.

Some of our subpersonalities manifest themselves in warring inner voices that fuel those painful and tedious arguments we have with ourselves. The rival voices are normally apparent only when we're in conflict—facing a difficult decision or torn between two choices. This is when it's wise to remember that calm fosters unity; conflict fractures it. The next time you find yourself caught up in an internal debate, consider the possibility that the thoughts and feelings on either side of the argument aren't just situational. Maybe those competing voices have a lot to say. Maybe they've been saying similar things to you all your life, and maybe they've been fighting those same other voices that they're fighting now. We usually listen to one part, the one that represents the overdeveloped parts of our personalities. Here's an example:

Once or twice a year Richard takes time off from teaching at the university to spend a week by himself at a friend's house on Cape Cod. He likes to get away for some concentrated time writing and unwinding. But each time he goes he gets into a debate with himself about whether to spend most of his time working or relaxing. One voice says that he should concentrate on working because that's the most important thing. The other voice counters that he's always working and that this is his only chance to enjoy himself. Each time the debate is the same, and always quite frustrating. He really wants to do both, get a lot of work done and spend a few whole days swimming and fishing. But even though the debate is always hard fought, the voice that tells him to work always wins.

The people who know us can usually predict our choices, even if we still agonize over them. In Richard's case, the voice that says work always wins over the one that says play. His wife could tell you that. And she's learned, after much trial and error, that the only way for her and the children to get the attention of the part of Richard that likes to play is to reassure the part that worries about getting enough work done. She knows, for example, that he won't be able to relax on a family vacation unless he takes along some work to do in the morning. And if she tries to get him to visit her parents for the weekend, she always helps him find a little time to get some work done. She's not just thoughtful; she's smart.

> When you're torn between two (or more) choices, does one side usually win? What does that tell you about the dominant aspects of your personality? How is that helpful to you? How is it challenging?

> ### Asking for Advice
>
> The next time you find it necessary to ask someone's advice, take the opportunity to learn more about the opposing voices inside you. The need to ask is a sign that contending voices have a nearly equal claim on your attention. What is the nature of those voices? Does the part of you that asks and the part that is reluctant symbolize a debate between the dependent child and the self-sufficient one? And if you ask someone's advice, aren't you imagining what he or she will say? And do you sometimes seek out the right person to give you the answer that part of you really wants to hear?
>
> Do you have an advisor part who gives good counsel to friends and family? Have you ever asked that part to help you as you would a friend?

What does all this have to do with listening? Whenever someone asks your advice or shrinks from you or gets impatient with you, it's worthwhile to think about what parts of the person are coming toward you and what might be in conflict with each other. It may be useful to remember that you too have these conflicting voices when you're tempted to give obvious advice— telling people to stop drinking so much, start exercising, do their homework, or quit smoking—rather than listening for what they really want from you. Can you tell these people anything they don't already know? If not, how about trying to appreciate where they're at instead of pushing them to where you think they ought to go?

Giving predictable advice to adolescents—urging them to stop doing things that aren't good for them—is a classic mistake that most parents feel compelled to make. The voice of "no" is one that most teenagers are already well aware of. A more effective way to get through to them (or anyone else with self-destructive habits) is to adopt a more neutral attitude and simply ask them about the effects of whatever they're doing. Unfortunately, when this question comes from someone who is in fact anxious to make them change, it won't be heard as a curious and innocent exploration. Teenagers can smell manipulation a mile away.

Thinking in terms of subpersonalities can be especially helpful in heated discussions. Instead of thinking of being at odds with someone, it's more useful to think of parts of one of you trying to change parts of the other. In a typical scene provoked by a teenager's coming home late, his father gets mad and demands to know what happened. His accusatory tone makes the boy feel attacked, and he counters angrily, which drives up the father's rage to the point where his wife tells him to calm down and stop shouting. This infuriates the father, and he leaves the house. If you were the father, you would probably think of the boy as disrespectful and the mother as interfering. If you were the boy, you'd view the father as controlling and the mother as an ally. If you were the mother, you'd have trouble sleeping that night. Instead, think of the conflict as being waged among parts of them. A rebellious part of the boy activates a controlling part of the father, which in turn mobilizes a protective part of the mother to shield the boy from his father's temper. If you were any one of these people and you began to think this way, how difficult would it be to control your part? How might the problem be affected if any of you could stay calm and avoid letting your reactive parts take over?

Take another example. Does the question of whether or not to confront your partner with something that's bothering you represent the competing voices of a compliant child who believes that she shouldn't complain or people will get mad at her; a hurt part; and an angry part? Of the last two, which one is more afraid to speak up? Why? If you can identify those parts that have trouble speaking up, can you find a way to reassure them? Would it help to tell the person you have trouble speaking up to about the scared part of you? Would he (or she) be more understanding if you asked for his (or her) help to express this part of you? Sometimes it can help your anxiety about such a confrontation to name all the parts in the room and give them a share in the conversation. You might say, "Part of me is afraid that you'll be angry, and part of me feels really misunderstood. I think both parts might need to talk to you."

Let's take a look at a familiar interaction between intimate partners, using the notion of subpersonalities. A woman has trouble listening to her husband because he expresses himself in the form of tirades. Is this the sensitive and vulnerable man she married that she hears, or is it an echo of mounting anxiety and danger from long ago? And who is the "she" who's doing the hearing? The part of her who's strong and cares about her husband or a little girl part who trembled to hear her parents quarreling over her father's explosive temper and her mother's shame about it in front of others?

Getting to know more about our "parts" can help us better understand the obstacles and constraints that get in the way of listening. Once we know which part is struggling and why, we can increase our receptivity and release ourselves from these constraints. Having curiosity about our more immature and competitive parts, for example, is a very different way of thinking from accusing ourselves of being selfish or inadequate. It isn't that we're bad listeners; it's our hidden emotional agendas that crowd out understanding and concern. When we clear away automatic emotional reactions—criticism, fear, and hurt—we get to compassion, curiosity, and tenderness. Instead of condemning ourselves for being "bad listeners," we can learn to identify and relax those parts of ourselves that interfere. In so doing, we release ourselves for effective listening.

EXERCISES

1. Pick three people you see regularly. Write down what you generally expect them to say to you. Then write how you usually respond. How could you set aside those expectations to have a more in-depth conversation the next time you see one of those people? The most satisfying conversations with people we care about involve talking about our personal concerns and both getting a turn. If your conversations with someone are usually about things you care less about—the weather, the news, third parties— ask more direct questions about what you'd prefer to talk about. When

it's your turn, use an orienting comment—like "There's something going on with me" or "I'd like to tell you about . . ."

2. When you were growing up, what did you learn about the roles and rules for listening in your family? Who had the power to speak, and who was expected to listen? Were there differences based on age, gender, birth order, or temperament? How did people try to get attention and how successful were they? What did you learn about your right to be heard from this experience? Did you learn anything different from your siblings than from your parents? What did each of your parents do to make you feel they weren't really listening to you? How about your siblings? How do your family experiences with being listened to affect how you approach conversations now?

3. How could you approach either of your parents in some completely different way the next time you're in touch with them? What makes your child part afraid to try doing so now? Do you have a braver part who might be curious to change an old pattern?

4. Try to identify and personify the defensive parts (fearful, angry, hurt) that interfere with listening in the following examples.

   a. Ivan's boss is describing how they should handle a particular project, but Ivan doesn't hear any of the details because he thinks the boss's whole approach is wrong.

   b. Monica and Charlotte are eating lunch in a Chinese restaurant. Charlotte is talking, but Monica can't stop thinking about how annoying it is that the man in the next booth is talking so loudly on his cell phone.

   c. "Can I talk to you about something, honey?" Toni asks. "Not now, I'm busy," Rob says.

   d. Lorraine starts telling her father about a project she's working on when he interrupts to talk about something else. Lorraine doesn't say anything, but she doesn't hear a word he says.

   e. You want to tell someone how much he or she means to you, but you're afraid that kind of intimacy might make both of you feel awkward.

   f. Bev is explaining to Michael what kind of toaster she wants him to exchange for the one he brought home. Michael, who doesn't have the receipt, wishes she wouldn't make such a fuss about the toaster in the first place. When he gets to the store, he can't remember what kind of toaster he's supposed to buy.

g. Mindy's father is explaining where he keeps all his important papers and what Mindy will need to take care of after he dies. She knows these things are important, but her father is still in good health, so she doesn't really pay attention to what he's saying.

h. Sharon thinks that she and Carla should go to couples counseling, but she's afraid to bring it up for fear of how Carla will react.

Do you find it hard to identify the parts of these people that interfere with listening without knowing more about the people's backgrounds? The point of the exercise isn't to get the "right" answer, but to get you thinking about what kinds of feelings might be behind your and other people's problems in listening.

6

"Why Do You Always Overreact?!"

HOW EMOTIONALITY MAKES US DEFENSIVE

One of the reasons people don't listen is that they become emotionally reactive. Something in the speaker's message triggers hurt or anger, which provokes defensiveness and short-circuits understanding. Emotional reactivity is like throwing a switch and having the electricity come on, only instead of music you get static. The static is anxiety.

"What's *Really* Bothering You?"

The hardest messages for us to listen to without reacting emotionally are those that involve criticism. Most of us like to think that we can accept constructive criticism, and, on the other hand, most of us know people who can't. It takes practice to give feedback well and even more effort to hear it nondefensively.

Once a month the outpatient psychiatry staff at a hospital reviews patient charts to assess the treatment being provided at the clinic. This review may sound like a good idea, but it has become progressively more tedious as the need to monitor bureaucratic forms has crowded out time for considering the quality of patient care. At the last meeting the staff discovered that a few of the charts selected for review had already been examined at the previous month's meeting. When the director mentioned this fact to the administrator, she said, "Then get them yourself—I can't do everything!" and stormed out of the room.

If you believed that this kind of reaction was common from this woman, you'd have no trouble recognizing her as one of those hypersensitive people who can't take criticism. If, on the other hand, you knew her to be a very even-tempered person, you'd assume she was having a bad day. In this instance, you'd be right. Her assistant was out sick, and she'd had to stay three hours late the night before and come to work two hours early to get the charts ready. Of course she was on edge.

When people overreact uncharacteristically, we usually assume that something's bothering them. If our relationship with them has a history of goodwill, we give them the benefit of the doubt and try to find out what the problem is. But what about those people who regularly respond inappropriately? Are they having a bad life?

Corinne was a highly intelligent woman who couldn't allow herself to make mistakes. She had online subscriptions to *WaPo*, *WSJ*, and the *NYTimes*, but she also watched ESPN and wrote a baseball blog about her favorite team, the Atlanta Braves, that everyone at the office read. When the team's star pitcher injured his shoulder, Corinne wrote that this injury might turn out to be a blessing in disguise if it allowed a certain relief pitcher to prove that he would make a good starter as some insiders suspected. When Corinne read a draft of the piece over the phone to her cousin Drew, he said it was great, except for one thing: the pitcher was injured playing against Pittsburgh, not Philadelphia, as Corinne had written. Glad to get the facts straight, Corinne corrected the error. When the newsletter came out, a senior staff member told Corinne that he loved her piece, but it was Philadelphia, not Pittsburgh, where the fateful injury took place.

Corinne was so humiliated by this minor mistake that she was thrown into a tailspin. She cried and felt like a fool and couldn't bring herself to go to work the next day.

She was a shy person who preferred to express herself in writing rather than conversation; to her, being listened to meant having what she wrote appreciated. Being wrong made her feel humiliated. Instead of getting angry at her cousin for giving her the wrong information, she was ashamed of herself for not getting the story straight. Nobody likes to make mistakes, but clearly Corinne's reaction was excessive.

Another example of reacting inappropriately may be more familiar, in form if not intensity. Lenny was a hard worker, a devoted husband, and an engaged father. He did his share of household chores and coached his daughter's softball team. His wife Laila's one complaint was that he was too critical.

Apart from being struck by his belittling words toward Laila, I also noticed the degree to which she absorbed Lenny's criticism without answering with any complaints of her own. She seemed fearful of him, as if he was the lord and master and it was her job to cater to him. When Lenny said, "You should clean all the snow off the car before you start to drive," Laila protested feebly, "I was in a hurry to get to the cleaners." When Lenny countered, "You're always in too much of a hurry," Laila capitulated, "I guess you're right."

Experience has taught me to listen not only to what people say, but also for what they're not saying. I soon found out why Laila hesitated to protest. One time she said, "Don't you think you're being a little unfair?" and Lenny flew into a rage. He started shouting at her. "You *never* listen to anything I say! You have *no* respect for me. You say you love me, but it's a lie!"

It was awful. I don't really remember all of what he said because, frankly, I was too upset. What's more, the same thing happened every time Laila said anything Lenny took as critical.

Having read these two accounts, you can probably also guess something of what Corinne and Lenny felt. But clearly the intensity of their reactions was inappropriate to the situation. Let me also tell you that these are two instances when it's a lot easier to read about something than to witness it firsthand. Corinne's abject humiliation and Lenny's rage made listening to them almost impossible. What makes people respond in such extreme ways? Long memories.

From these brief descriptions, some people might say that Corinne was ashamed and Lenny was aggressive. Others might say that Corinne's turning her anger inward and Lenny's lashing out were typical of their genders.

In fact, these inferences are so general and judgmental as to constitute virtually meaningless clichés. For a more subtle appreciation of a person's overreaction you need to know its trigger.

A listener's emotional reaction seems inappropriate
only as long as you can't see his or her memory.

As a therapist, when I see someone responding "inappropriately," I ask myself what circumstances *would* make the response appropriate. (In my own relationships I just get upset like you do.) What would make it reasonable for a woman to feel worthless for having made a minor mistake? (Hint: Most of us manage to survive childhood, but not all of us outgrow it.)

Corinne was the last of four children in a talented and ambitious family. She had three older brothers "who were jealous and competitive" and "never liked me." Her father was cerebral and distant; her mother was a depressed underachiever who drank too much. Corinne was the baby, but rather than being doted on she was ignored. Early on, she decided that the only possibility of ever being loved was to be the perfect child, docile and mediocre—docile so as not to burden her parents, mediocre so as not to challenge her brothers. They tolerated her as long as she played the good little sister, but they couldn't acknowledge any sign of accomplishment from her. Deprived of acceptance themselves, they belittled their little sister's achievements and mocked her mistakes. They called her "lardass," "Miss Piggy," "stupid," and "retard." Even the smallest slipup could trigger their scornful laughter. Years later Corinne was still so hypersensitive to humiliation that she sank into despair whenever she made the slightest error. The man who pointed out her mistake did not say "retard," but that's what she heard.

When you're a little child, it's hard to fight back.
When you're an adult made to feel little,
it's also hard—but not impossible.

What made Lenny so critical of others and yet unable to tolerate criticism in return? Not the kind of cruel treatment you might expect. Lenny's parents were decent, loving people. But their lack of involvement outside the family led them to expect a lot from each other and from their children. When they didn't get what they wanted, they criticized and complained. This alone might not have made Lenny so unable to tolerate criticism. But his parents, for all their basic goodness, never gave him the empathy that would have solidified his sense of worth. Without a store of loving memories, without a sense of being taken seriously and appreciated just for himself, and without expectations of more understanding to come, Lenny harbored deep and ugly fears of worthlessness. Hard work and family devotion kept these feelings at bay, until, that is, someone said anything remotely resembling what Lenny himself feared in his heart of hearts—that he was no good.

I once had a gray-and-white cat named Tina who was perfectly friendly, except that once in a while she'd lash out violently with her claws. These attacks were totally unprovoked. One minute Tina would be purring to have her head stroked; the next minute you'd have a bloody scratch on the back of your hand. Eventually we took her to the vet and learned that she had an injured hip—possibly from a car accident when she was a kitten—so that what seemed to us like a harmless touch could actually be quite painful.

Shame and insecurity are the wounds that make people react violently to criticism. Some people retreat from hurt feelings, others attack. The most shame-sensitive individuals flare up at the slightest sign of criticism. Such people are hard to live with. But reacting to criticism with hurt and anger is something we all do. What varies is only the threshold of response.

The universal vulnerability to criticism is related to the universal yearning for love and approval. What we really want to hear is that we're terrific (sometimes "okay" will do).

Our sensitivity to criticism varies with the situation and the way it is delivered. We're hurt most by criticism of something that feels like an important part of ourselves—our motives, for example, or the products of our creativity, or, during adolescence (and sometimes slightly beyond), our appearance. We're especially sensitive to criticism from someone whose opinion we care about. The right person saying the wrong thing can puncture your ego like a pin bursting a balloon.

Getting criticized by email or text is also distressing; however, the hurt is sometimes accompanied by bewilderment about whether we have screwed up in the first place. When I send six colleagues an email describing how I've handled a challenging departmental task, I might get three responses. Do the nonresponders think I did a terrible job? That's possible, though who knows if they even read the email in the first place? If my department chair replies merely saying, "Okay," does that mean she's satisfied, or is that the kind of faint praise that implies that what I did wasn't all that important? Then one colleague merely writes, "Good job," without an exclamation point. Did she mean that as a lukewarm response, or did she just not bother with punctuation? I'm not offering this example to demonstrate how thin-skinned professors can be but just to describe the multitude of ways the digital age has complicated communication—especially when we are hoping for positive feedback.

We read a lot into emails and texts because we have so few cues about the writer's intent when he dashes off something tepid or cryptic. In the absence of contextual information, our anxiety fills in the gaps.

How to Listen to Criticisms

Do you often find yourself interrupting someone who's criticizing you before the person has a chance to finish? This understandable but counterproductive impulse robs the other person of a sense of having been heard. You don't have to agree to hear what someone has to say.

To avoid getting defensive, concentrate on listening to the entire criticism. Then ask, without sarcasm, "Is there anything else?" Finally, offer your understanding of what the person was trying to say—*not a paraphrase* but what you think the other person was trying to get at.

Why Do People Complain to Us?

Behind every complaint is a request. Listen for the request and then ask if that's what the person would like.

Respond to the request by accepting it or making a counteroffer—in the spirit of trying to give the other person what he or she is asking for.

How to Complain Nicely

Consider these two ways of complaining:

1. You never do the dishes.
2. I'm feeling exhausted after cooking dinner; can you help me with the dishes?

Or these:

1. I can't believe you burnt the popcorn again.
2. Do you think the popcorn would come out better if we used a different kind of oil?

In both versions, the criticism is there and so is the underlying request. Which version do you think would be easier for you to hear?

What Makes Us Intolerant?

When you're trying to figure out why you or anyone else overreacts, keep in mind one of the great ironies of understanding: We're likely to be as accepting of others as we are of ourselves. That's why those lucky enough to be raised with self-respect make better listeners. Still, you needn't be stuck where you find yourself. If you learn to respect other people's feelings, you will learn to treat your own feelings more kindly in the process. It might work the other way too: if you become more compassionate toward yourself, you may find your generosity overflowing.

> What we can't tolerate in others
> is what we can't tolerate in ourselves.

We can't listen well to other people as long as we project the mistaken idea that parts of us aren't good enough to be loved, respected, and treated fairly. A wider respect for human dignity flows from and enhances respect for ourselves. Tolerance and appreciation of our own and other people's feelings helps us hear and understand the hurt that inevitably lies behind anger and resentment. When our feelings aren't heard, our spirits are bruised.

What Turns Conversations into Arguments?

Reacting emotionally to what other people say is the number one reason conversations turn into arguments.

If you're not sure what emotional reactivity is, take inventory of your feelings, the next time you rush out of the bathroom to catch the phone on the last ring—and it turns out to be somebody selling something. That agitation, that anxious upset that makes you want to scream at the caller, is emotional reactivity. Is it wrong or unjustified? No, of course not. But it's that feeling, in relationships that do count, that makes it hard to listen, hard to think straight, and hard to say what you want to say.

Reactivity is like a child interrupting an adult conversation—it isn't bad; it's inopportune. Our intrusive emotions may need to be hushed, but they may also need to be listened to later. Why are we reactive? What are the reactive parts of ourselves, and what are they reacting to? Disruptive feelings are messages from our inner spirit about something we need to change or pay attention to in our lives. Our reactivity can lead us to parts of ourselves that we haven't yet befriended—angry and resentful parts, frightened and lonely parts.

If Corinne were to tell a friend how stupid she felt for screwing up the newsletter, the friend might try to reassure her by telling her not to worry. Everyone makes mistakes. Yes, but when Corinne made a mistake, she could hear her savage brothers sneering "Lardass! Retard!" And she'd feel again what she'd spent her whole adult life running away from: that she was ugly and stupid, nobody loved her, and nobody would ever love her.

Lenny's dishing out but not being able to take criticism might seem less unreasonable if you realized that deep down he too felt worthless and inconsequential. Inside him were dark and ugly voices he anxiously shut his ears to lest he get in touch with the part of him that still felt like a little boy who was never good enough.

What turns conversations into arguments for some people (not infrequently mothers on the front lines) isn't so much something inside of them as the fact that they are being asked, perhaps many times a day, to deal with certain distressing things about people close to them.

One of my patients doesn't want to hear what's going on in her daughter's life. It's too upsetting. Madison was arrested for prostitution at age fifteen. Despite her mother's heroic efforts, Madison continued to get into trouble, using drugs, hanging around with a motorcycle gang, coming home drunk night after night. Finally, when Madison was eighteen, her parents insisted that she get her own apartment. They supported her for a while, then gradually stopped paying her expenses. Madison now works as a cocktail waitress, when she works, but her parents are reasonably sure that she's using drugs and that she probably still prostitutes herself from time to time. They know she occasionally gets arrested for drunk and disorderly behavior, because they've had to go to the jail in the middle of the night to bail her out. Her mother still loves her but finds it necessary to cushion their relationship by visiting infrequently and avoiding the details of her daughter's activities, which she finds too upsetting to listen to.

This mother's avoidance is based on a correct assessment of her own vulnerability. It isn't just worry that she's avoiding; she can't listen to her daughter's troubles without feeling her heart breaking and the need to rescue her. The temptation to tell her daughter to stop taking drugs and hanging around dangerous characters (as though these were novel ideas) interferes with listening; yielding to that temptation triggers shouting matches. She has to avoid her daughter because the alternatives—fixing the problem or listening impassively to her daughter's distress—are just not possible for her.

The worst thing about reactivity is that it's contagious. When anxiety jumps the gap from speaker to listener, it escalates in a series of actions and reactions, which may eventually lead to an emotional cutoff. The cutoff may be as simple—and simply frustrating—as walking out of the room or as sad as someone walking out of another's life.

The next time you have the misfortune to witness two people arguing without hearing each other, notice what each of them does to keep the argument going. (If you're one of the parties to the argument, just notice what the other person does; the alternative is too demanding.) Notice how the argument could end if either one of them would let go. In the runaway logic of arguing, both parties feel compelled to get in the last word.

. . . .

The world is divided into people who think they are right.

. . . .

The ability to listen rests on how successfully we resist the impulse to react emotionally to the position of the other. The more actions we feel compelled to take to reduce or avoid our anxiety, the less flexible we are in relationships. When you are preoccupied with not blowing your top, you aren't in the best place to listen to anything else. If your pulse is racing with fear or rage, or you're just feeling overwhelmed, it's almost guaranteed that only regrettable things will come out of your mouth.

Let me give you an example from the wide perspective of a public situation—before focusing on the more anxiety-arousing settings of personal exchange. The next time you attend a lecture or observe a news conference, notice the hostile questions. You'll note that many "questions" aren't really questions at all, but rhetorical attempts to prove that the speaker is wrong and the listener is right. Observe how the speaker handles these questions. Some speakers try to remain calm by finding something to agree with; others get defensive and counterattack.

A speaker is likely to get defensive if she feels that the questioner is trying to make her wrong and himself right. "Excuse me, but haven't you overlooked . . . [you dummy]?" Few such "listeners" really want answers to their questions; they just want to be right. The speaker who gets defensive and tries to counter (put down, really) the questioner often hopes to "win" the exchange by saying "No, actually . . . [I am right; *you're* wrong]." In rare instances a clever speaker can succeed in putting down a hostile questioner with superior intellect or knowledge of the subject. More often the questioner, who maybe wanted to make a point, feels dismissed, cheated out of the opportunity to have his voice heard.

. . . .

When neither party to an exchange is willing to break
the spiral of reactivity, both are likely to end up
feeling angry and misunderstood.

. . . .

How to Alleviate Arguments

I don't know about you, but I hate arguments. Why do some people always have to say the opposite of whatever we say? In the interests of understanding, I've made a list of some reasons people argue with us.

- **They have bad memories.** "My partner and I argue all the time about whether one of us said something or not. I wish I could record our conversations. I should know what I said, shouldn't I?"
- **They're selfish.** "My boyfriend insists that we spend Christmas with his parents. Why can't we spend Christmas with my family?"
- **They're ignorant.** "We interviewed three job candidates last week, and I thought one of them was clearly the best. So it was a shock when two-thirds of the group voted for one of the other candidates."
- **They're old-fashioned.** "My father doesn't have a cell phone. So I often have to call several times to catch him at home just to give him a simple message. When I suggest that he get a cell phone, he says, 'What do I need one of those for?' "
- **They're stubborn.** "My wife says we should keep the car for another year before buying a new one. When I remind her that a new car will cost less now than next year, she insists that it will be cheaper in the long run to keep our present car for another twenty-five thousand miles."
- **They're naïve.** "My daughter wants to study creative writing in college. She has no idea how hard it is to make a living as a writer."
- **They're emotional.** "When I tell my boyfriend that it's too expensive to visit each other every single weekend, he gets all hurt and angry."
- **They're bossy.** "My husband insists on going out to dinner almost every night. Why can't we eat at home once in a while?"
- **They don't really listen to what we're saying.** "Whenever I bring up some chore that my roommate doesn't like doing and say that we don't have to do it right away, he never hears the don't, and he's always getting needlessly upset."

It's easy to see what these explanations have in common: They underscore the basic fact that when other people argue with us, it's *their* fault. Naturally, it's our responsibility to straighten them out.

Why, some of you sticklers for fairness might be thinking, is it never we who are selfish, stubborn, or naïve? Because what we say makes sense!

There are, of course, two sides to every argument. But when we argue, we insist on repeating our side without listening to the other person's position.

Listening with a Clenched Mind

Listeners anxious to avoid conflict may not listen because they're too busy protecting themselves to be open to what someone else is trying to say. Listeners intent on talking speakers out of unhappy feelings or independent inclinations won't hear what others think because it might be threatening. Even speakers who have something worthwhile to say may not get heard if they make the other person feel criticized or misunderstood; the listener is likely to become defensive or angry and counterattack or withdraw, making listening the last thing on his or her mind. Misunderstanding is perpetuated when each one broods over the awful things the other one does and one or both of them eventually finds someone else to complain to.

Silent Arguing

Misunderstanding and disagreement can persist and even escalate even when only one person seems to be engaging in the conflict. In some families, the old adage "You have not converted a man because you have silenced him" constitutes a reliable strategy of defense for the passive resister.

People living under the same roof often have disparate ideas about how important someone else's agenda should be for them. Teenagers in particular can be gifted "silent arguers," but they probably learned that skill watching their parents maneuver around certain pressures and expectations.

Todd walked into the living room where his son Daniel was sprawled on the couch watching TV. "Danny," he said, "tomorrow is garbage day. Will you please take out the garbage before you go to bed?"

"Uh-huh," Daniel replied.

The following evening when Todd came home from work, he was annoyed to see the garbage bag still sitting in the kitchen where he'd left it the night before. He was irritated not only because the garbage hadn't been taken out, but also because Daniel had broken yet another agreement with him.

As should be obvious, Todd didn't really have an agreement with his son. He asked Daniel to do something while he was watching TV, and Daniel mumbled whatever it would take to get his father to leave him alone. Daniel probably didn't intend *not* to take out the garbage, but he never really made a conscious commitment to do so. If Todd thought about it, he'd probably admit that he'd done his share of silent arguing in his marriage over the years. You can't fight about everything, and silent arguing offers a path of least resistance.

Not all negotiations in families are explicit. Like Todd, we may ask one another to do things for us and make assumptions that the answer is going to be "yes" when we've gotten no such commitment. The people we need to do those things may grunt, shrug, sort of agree, or do whatever they must to avoid being hassled. Their "okay" doesn't mean "Okay, I'll do it" as much as "Okay, I hear you, now leave me alone." When confronted, the silent arguer will say, "I forgot" or "Okay, I'll do it later."

When someone repeatedly fails to do what you expect, it's a safe bet that he or she doesn't want to. That much may be obvious. But what may be less obvious is that silent arguers often "forget" because they don't think something really needs to be done, or they don't think it's fair that they have to be the one to do it. One way to find out is to ask.

> The reason for silent arguing is not believing
> that the other person is open to your point of view.

"It seems like I always have to remind you to cut the grass. Do you resent having to do it?"

"I need you to be ready to be out the door by eight. Is that okay?"

"I have a late meeting on Thursday; I wonder if there's a reason you haven't told me you can pick up the kids at the sitter's?"

"You didn't get around to putting on the water for pasta. What happened after you read my note asking you to start dinner?"

Subjects Too Hot to Handle

Couples famously have trouble talking about money, sex, and children. The problem with these subjects isn't differences of opinion but the emotional reactions those differences trigger. Even though both partners may be equally reactive, they might show it in different ways. One may press for more dispassionate analysis, while the other may feel shushed and press for more emotional honesty. Each is sensitive to slights, hurts, and criticism. Some people's radar is so good that they pick up these signals even before they're sent.

And it's not really the content of the fight that sends couples off the rails anyway. John Gottman's research concludes that the number one thing that couples fight about is *nothing*. Partners don't usually sit down and say, "We need to hash out our budget." More often, some conflict flares, out of nowhere, maybe in the middle of some other conversation. One person says something that's hurtful or upsetting; the other has to figure out how to handle his upset. And so the actual problem isn't even the fight itself. Indeed, the hot topic and the disagreement about it are probably both less important than how the angry feelings get handled afterward.

After DeShawn and Shannon have a blowup, he becomes distant. After a while, he calms down and tries to make amends. He says he's sorry for what he said. But she never apologizes. She either accepts his apology or, if she's really mad, takes it as permission to say more about what he did that upset her. DeShawn's least favorite version of this is "You *always* do that, and I hate it!"

Finally, DeShawn told Shannon that he truly was sorry when they argued and often could see his part in it, but it really bothered him that she never apologized. "It's like everything is my fault, like you don't have any role in our problems. It's not fair."

Shannon blew up. "What am I supposed to say, 'It's *my* fault you're so grouchy'? 'I'm sorry *you* don't like my driving'? 'I'm sorry the baby was sick'?" At this DeShawn threw up his hands and walked out of the room.

What Makes It So Hard for Some People to Apologize?

Here are some possibilities:

- Shame
- Guilt
- Difficulty distinguishing making a mistake from being bad

- A narcissistic need to never admit to doing anything hurtful or wrong
- Worry that an apology will be used against them
- Self-righteousness
- Fear of losing the person they have hurt
- Fear of losing the battle and letting the other person be the winner
- Thinking it won't make a difference anyway
- It shouldn't be necessary when someone knows you love him or her
- Belief that it would let the other person off the hook
- Being afraid of the vulnerability they'd feel
- Low self-esteem and not feeling worthy of forgiveness
- Confusing humility with humiliation

Truth be told, Shannon probably had trouble apologizing for many of the reasons on this list. But not because she felt blameless. In her heart of hearts, Shannon blamed herself for everything that went wrong in their relationship. She blamed herself for DeShawn's moods (if she was *really* a good wife, he'd be happy); she blamed herself for not enjoying sex with him more (she must be inhibited); she even blamed herself when the baby got sick (if she were a better mother, nothing bad would ever happen to her child). She came from a family that specialized in blame. The result was extreme sensitivity to anything anyone might say that triggered her own inner self-blame. That's the nature of reactivity.

> We're most reactive to the things
> we secretly accuse ourselves of.

"How Come You Listen to Everybody But Me?"

Partners often complain that their mates never listen to their ideas, but come home and announce that they just heard something very interesting—and that something is precisely what their spouse has already told them.

Recently, for example, when Marilyn told her wife that she'd decided to see a friend's chiropractor about her back, Cara hit the ceiling: "I've been telling you to see a chiropractor for years! Now all of a sudden when your precious friend Mary Elizabeth tells you, you listen. How come you never listen to me?"

Marilyn was taken aback by Cara's outburst. But even if she'd known what to say, Cara didn't stick around to hear it. She stormed out and slammed the door. Later, Marilyn did answer Cara at length, in her head, where most of us make our best comebacks.

True, Cara *had* told her to see a chiropractor. But she hadn't asked Cara's advice. When she complained to her about her back, she wanted sympathy, not advice. Cara was always telling her what to do. Why couldn't she just listen?

When Marilyn told me about this episode, I thought her assertion that she wanted sympathy, not advice, from her wife was true as far as it went, but that it was missing something. It turned out that when Cara gave advice, it was usually in an intense, pressured way—Cara's amped-up response to the anxiety Marilyn's complaints generated in her. Marilyn usually ignored Cara's advice, not just because she wasn't in the market for advice, but because it was delivered with an emotional pressure that made her defensive.

This is typical of how messages get deflected. It isn't always the content that makes people deaf; it's the pressure it comes packaged in. A speaker's eagerness or anxiety is often felt by listeners as pressure to make them wrong or to change their way of thinking. As if it weren't hard enough to tone down one's own reactivity, doing so is often made even more difficult by the condition of the relationship.

How Some Speakers Make Us Hard of Hearing

We've all had experience with listeners whose emotional reactivity makes them defensive or argumentative instead of hearing what we're trying to say. An equally important barrier to understanding is the speaker's emotionality. A speaker who talks in a highly emotional way makes listeners anxious and therefore hard of hearing.

* * * * * * * * * *

Some people have no idea how pressured and provoking
their tone of voice is; they come at you like a bad dentist.

* * * * * * * * * *

The hardest people to listen to are those who treat us with dictatorial disregard of our feelings. The pressured speaker may not know how he comes across, but his urgent, anxious tone of voice, emphatic hand gestures, or conclusion of every other statement with "Right?" (implicitly demanding agreement) makes us feel backed into a corner.

A Charged Atmosphere

The emotional climate between speaker and listener has a lot to do with the quality of understanding that can pass between them. If the atmosphere is calm, especially if it has a history of being calm, the listener can usually hear what the speaker is trying to get across. But if there's anxiety in the air—or even just intense feeling—the listener may be too tense to take in what's said. The listener may be anxious about being blamed, or pressured to change, or proven wrong. Speakers who trigger such feelings, venting emotion in a way that makes listeners feel backed against the wall, may not get heard, even though they have something important to say. It's the way hard things get said that determines whether or not they get heard.

The emotional state of a relationship depends not only on the way individuals express themselves, but also on the extent to which they remain differentiated as individuals.

A differentiated individual is a mature and autonomous person who knows where his or her skin ends and other people's begin. In emotionally less-differentiated relationships, anxiety becomes infectious and the partners increasingly reactive to each other, especially on hot subjects. Among some couples, money is such a charged issue that sparks fly at the first mention of it. A mother who is poorly differentiated from her child may be so threatened by the childish retort "I don't love you!" that she either reacts punitively or gets sucked into a pointless discussion that begins with "But I love you." A more well-differentiated parent doesn't feel so threatened by her son's or daughter's protests. Such a parent has enough distance to realize that "I don't love you!" means "I'm angry that you won't let me have my way." Differentiation is achieved by learning to separate what you think from what you feel—and by learning to be yourself while respecting other people's right to be themselves.

When boundaries are blurred, individuals become emotionally fused and almost any agitation from the speaker will make a listener reactive. As differentiation decreases, individuality is less well defined, and emotional reactivity becomes more intense. Poorly differentiated and highly reactive people tend to come across as either emotionally demanding or avoidant.

An "independent" husband may be aware of his "dependent" wife's emotional reactivity but blind to his own. He sees her dependence because she shows it directly. When she objects to his wanting to go off by himself, he says, "You're so dependent! Why don't you develop some interests of your own and quit hanging on me?" She cries and accuses him of being selfish. As far as he's concerned, she's emotionally immature. She's so dependent that he can't even complain without her getting all worked up. What he doesn't see is how dependent *he* is on her feeling positively toward him, so much so that he's unable to hear her complaints as an expression of her feelings. He hears what she says only as a threat to himself and a constraint on what he wants to do. And so he goes off and broods in self-righteous resentment about his wife's inability to respond to him without reacting emotionally.

Hallie had to talk to Leon about needing help around the house. She knew it was a sore subject because they'd both grown up with the expectation that housework was something wives did. But, damn it, with both of them working and the kids to look after, their family couldn't afford the luxury of one parent officially designated as housekeeper. For three months since beginning her new job, Hallie had put off asking Leon for help because she didn't want to start a fight. But she was finding it impossible to get dinner on the table before the kids started getting cranky, and so she just had to talk to him.

So that night after dinner Hallie told Leon how unfair it was for her to have to do all the cooking and cleaning now that she was working. As she spoke, the anger and frustration she'd been sitting on for three months came pouring out.

Leon, who knew he wasn't doing his share, listened as Hallie talked about how hurt she was that he hadn't offered to help. But as she went on about all she had to do and how little he did, Hallie started talking faster and more urgently, waving her arms as though her words couldn't keep pace with her feelings. Leon listened with growing upset.

What started out as a legitimate request turned into a tirade. Instead of listening and feeling like cooperating, Leon felt attacked and got defensive. "Why do you have to go on and on about everything? And why do you have to exaggerate so: You do *everything*, and I do *nothing*. Who earns the real money in this family? Who keeps the cars running and takes out the trash?"

That did it. Hallie burst into tears, and Leon, who couldn't take it anymore, stormed out of the room and slammed the door. Hallie was left alone crying in the living room, feeling how unfair it was that Leon was too selfish to care about her and no closer to getting the support she desperately needed.

A lot of complaints turn into confrontations
because people wait too long to speak up.

Fear is contagious. Sometimes a speaker's powerful emotion generates corresponding anxiety in the listener, making it particularly difficult for the listener to be the receptive vehicle that the speaker requires. When it comes to telling your side, particularly in a relationship with a history of tension, the best way to be heard is to tone down your emotionality. Even if you don't make the mistake of blaming the other person, he or she may feel attacked if you express yourself in an anxious or pressured manner. The trouble is, sometimes it's hard not to.

We don't recognize the impact of our tone of voice,
because we hear what we feel like, not what we sound like.

Elise gets annoyed because Jay takes the other side of almost every issue she brings up. This is a common complaint. Most subjects are complex enough to have two sides; when someone points to one side, we have a natural tendency to think of the other. The trouble is, it doesn't feel good to say the cup is half empty only to be told "No, it's half full." Jay's tendency to take the opposite position made Elise feel not just disagreed with but negated.

Once she commented that the neighbor's porch railing looked to be in bad shape and might break; someone might get hurt. Jay looked at the railing—which was in halfway good shape—and said, "I don't think so; it looks okay to me." When Elise said, "I hate it when you disagree with every-thing I say," Jay felt attacked. "Must I agree with everything you say?" he wanted to know. Like many reasonable couples, they discussed the issue without raising their voices or hearing each other.

Elise could understand Jay feeling that it wasn't fair to have to agree with everything she said, but that wasn't what she wanted. She just wanted her feelings to be acknowledged. Jay heard that, sort of, but didn't know what he was supposed to do. "If you say the railing looks like it's going to break, and I don't think it is, how am I supposed to know that you're just expressing your feelings and that I'm only supposed to acknowledge them? How do I know what you want if you don't tell me?"

One reason Jay had trouble hearing Elise was that she expressed herself with anxious emotion. Even clear, meaningful messages were so charged with feeling that Jay reacted to her anxiety rather than to her statement. Instead of getting through to Jay, she became something to brace against.

Elise gets excitable and raises her voice because she's been holding things in and is eager to get them out. But when she gets anxious, Jay gets tense, and he's more aware of the knot in his stomach than of what Elise is trying to tell him. When she told him how much it bothered her that he always disagreed with her, it was the upset she conveyed that made him defensive, not the message.

No matter how they tried, Elise and Jay were never able to hear each other in heated discussions. Only when I interrupted and talked to them one at a time were they able to listen without a defensive response. It turned out that Elise had grown up with a father who demanded adherence to his rules and dismissed his children's opinions. Both Jay and Elise recalled her brother and his habit of responding to even the most insignificant disagree-ment as though it were a declaration of war: "Either you're with me, or you're against me!"

Jay and Elise aren't very different from many couples who sometimes despair of ever really being listened to by each other. If you want to be heard, consider how much emotionality and anxiety you have—or how much gets churned up when you talk about certain things. Listeners react to that emotion. If you can reduce your emotional pressure, you may get heard, even when the subject is difficult. Remember: it isn't so much what you say as how you say it that determines whether or not you get heard. That's one reason people are often more open to what they read than to what someone says to them. (At least I hope so.)

Let's take another look at the interaction between Jay and Elise. Jay had trouble hearing his wife because she expressed herself with anxious emotion, her sentences flapping at him like flags in a high wind. When her voice rankled and Jay shrank into himself, he didn't hear the sweet, eager girl he fell in love with but an echo of harshness from long ago. The "he" who was doing the hearing wasn't the part of him who was strong and loved his wife but a little boy part, the one who could never stand to hear that harsh and powerful voice telling him that he couldn't go out to play, that he had to stay in the house all afternoon buried alive in chores.

Is it Medusa that turns men into stone, or is it the little boys inside them?

Hurt Feelings and Broken Connections

As a family therapist, I'm often consulted about impasses in relationships. Even though much has changed in family structure and functioning in the past few decades, there are some things that seem to cross time and culture: Wives still complain that their husbands don't care how they feel; husbands continue to grumble that their wives make too many demands; parents forever worry that their children are not happy; siblings insist that they're singled out unfairly; and adult children lament that they are feeling increasingly responsible for their aging parents. Many of these individuals come to therapy by themselves because the people they're concerned about refuse even to talk about the problem.

Michael's sister Susan moved to the West Coast after a bitter divorce. When she called from Los Angeles to talk to him, her ex-husband, who just happened to have stopped by, answered Michael's phone. Susan was furious. She felt betrayed and stopped speaking to her brother. When Susan didn't return Michael's phone calls, he got so upset that he took a plane to California the next day to straighten things out. But when he got there, Susan had already left town for the weekend because she wasn't ready to talk to him. Michael was livid. He could understand that she was upset, but he hadn't done anything wrong. And to refuse to see him after he had gone all the way to California—that he could not forgive.

The first step to healing a ruptured relationship is to understand the other person's point of view. Try to figure out what that person might be feeling and then say it in a way that invites him to elaborate. Until you acknowledge the other person's position, he is unlikely to be open to yours. He may listen, but he won't hear.

> When you demonstrate a willingness to listen
> with a minimum of defensiveness, criticism, or impatience,
> you are giving the gift of understanding—
> and earning the right to have it reciprocated.

Michael tried to apologize to his sister, but his heart wasn't in it. After all, he hadn't done anything wrong. So although he said he was sorry that she was upset, he just had to add that he hadn't done anything wrong. Unfortunately, when someone feels aggrieved, any attempt to justify your own behavior, no matter how innocent or well-meaning, may cancel your acknowledgment of her feelings. Michael was infuriated when his sister refused to see him, but she rightly intuited that his attempt to make up carried the pressure for her to forgive him. If Susan had been less upset, Michael's attempts to heal the breach might have worked. But when someone is really hurt, the only thing he or she wants to hear is an apology, not an apology coupled with self-justification. The greatest lesson in humility may be learning to say, "I'm sorry I hurt you" without having to protest your innocence.

I saw Michael a total of three times over several months. In our first meeting I made exactly the same mistake I am preaching against here. Instead of acknowledging his resentment, I advised him to reach out to his sister. Since he felt that he'd already done so and been spurned, he rejected my advice.

Our second meeting occurred five months later. He'd been getting on with his life and had calmed down about the falling-out with his sister. Time and distance had softened his bitterness, and he was ready for suggestions about how to patch up the break. I advised him to write a snail-mail, handwritten letter acknowledging the hurt and betrayal Susan felt and say that he was sorry. I cautioned him that the letter must be absolutely devoid of two elements that would render it ineffective: any hint of self-justification, expressed or implied, and any suggestion, expressed or implied, that his sister needed to do something about his apology. It had to be an unconditional apology—"I'm sorry I hurt you"—nothing more and nothing less. I also warned him that his sister's first response might be an angry one— something that can be hard to take when you apologize. He understood that and said he could accept it.

Four days after Michael wrote to his sister, he received an email from her saying how betrayed she felt when her ex-husband answered the phone at her own brother's house. How could Michael have been so insensitive? After that, Susan's note lightened. She wrote about her job in California and a new friendship and asked Michael what he was up to. Not every rupture can be fixed, of course, but a heartfelt apology is usually an excellent first step when it matters enough to try.

"He Never Talks to Me"

How can you be a good listener when certain people seem to withhold themselves from you and resist all your efforts at intimacy?

People are reticent in relationships because they don't want to get hurt. The reticent person moves through life in a protective bubble of psychological distance, not because his need for attention has ceased but because he's ceased to allow himself to feel it. Inside the prison of his avoidant defenses he preoccupies himself with other things. He keeps busy, he reads, he thinks, and he has long conversations in his head, where no one else can mess them up. Like many prisoners, he can be comfortable in his limited and protected routines, but the idea of parole into the wide world of other people and emotions terrifies him.

Although the emotional reticence of someone you care about can be powerfully frustrating, the reticent don't feel powerful. They feel vulnerable.

In fact, their stress levels are every bit as elevated as their more emotionally expressive counterparts; they just don't show it. People who withhold themselves from us are trying to insulate themselves from their own sensitivity to criticism or rejection. It isn't all them, either. In the process of trying to get closer to someone who doesn't say much, we often set up a pursuer–distancer dynamic.

Pursuers and Distancers

One of the most easily observed conversational patterns between intimate partners is the pursuer–distancer dynamic.

As you may have noticed, pursuing distancers only makes them feel pressured and inclined to pull farther away. It's a dance between one person who moves forward and another who moves back. The pursuer–distancer dynamic is propelled by emotional reactivity—in both participants. The people who pull away from us aren't just "shy" or "withholding"; they're responding to the pressure with which we approach them. I can almost hear the protests: "I don't put any pressure on so-and-so; he [or she] just won't open up."

We rarely feel the emotional demands we put on others. What we feel is their response to it. The people who resist conversation with us may indeed be more reticent than most. Still, their backing off is both habit and response.

Unfortunately, some of the people we find hardest to listen to are an important part of our lives: They are our partners, our parents, our children, our bosses, or our colleagues, and they arouse our reactivity because our need endows them with the power to please and distress us. When the frustrations of trying to listen and be heard get to be too much, we may be tempted to give up.

Facing encounters that raise your anxiety tests your maturity, strengthens you if you have the courage to stand fast and let matters unfold, or weakens you if you fall back into reactivity and defensiveness. Making contact, letting others be themselves while you continue to be yourself, and learning to resist automatic reactions strengthens you and transforms your relationships. Staying open and staying calm—that's the hardest part. You do the best you can.

If all of this seems obvious—to listen well, you have to resist the urge to overreact—it's only obvious from an objective distance. Up close, when you're caught up in the pressure to get the words out or the aggravation of listening to someone saying something you don't want to hear, objectivity is in short supply. Emotionality takes over.

EXERCISES

1. To test your flexibility in a pursuer–distancer relationship, try the following for a week. If you are a pursuer, try backing off and see what happens. Don't pout or get passive–aggressive; just spend more time on your own. If you are a distancer, try initiating some mutually enjoyable activity before the pursuer has a chance to approach you.
   Note: These experiments are not designed to cause any kind of permanent change in the pattern; they are merely experiments to help you explore the possibility of becoming more flexible.

2. To practice dealing with criticism, find an occasion to invite it. Plan in advance to respond without getting defensive. Listen without arguing. Invite the critic to say more. Then acknowledge what you think you heard and invite him or her to elaborate or correct your understanding.

3. Go back through your old text messages where you might have had a disagreement with someone. Can you see where the conversation started to heat up? Knowing what you know now about yourself and the person with whom you were struggling, try to:
   - Imagine what you might have said differently if you had cooled down first.
   - Jot down three possible reasons the person responded to you that way.
   - Think about apologizing for your contribution to the text fight if you haven't already. If not, go back and look at the list of why people don't apologize and figure out how come you didn't do it. Consider giving it a try.

PART THREE

Getting Through
to Each Other

7

"Take Your Time—I'm Listening"

HOW TO LET GO OF YOUR OWN NEEDS AND LISTEN

Real listening requires *attention, appreciation,* and *affirmation.* You begin the process by tuning in to the other person, paying attention to what he or she has to say. Put no barriers between you. Turn off the TV, put down your cell phone, ask the kids to play in the other room, shut the door to your office. Look directly at the speaker and concentrate on what he or she is trying to communicate.

Practice listening whenever your partner, family member, friend, or colleague speaks to you, with the sole intention of understanding what he or she is trying to express. People need to talk—and be heard—to feel understood by and connected to you.

Paying Attention

You take the first step to better listening by making a conscientious effort to set aside whatever is on your mind long enough to concentrate on hearing what the other person has to say.

Listening to each other never seemed to be much of a problem for Tony and Joan before the baby was born. They had lots to talk about and, maybe

151

more important, plenty of time for it. Then the baby came, and the pressures of parenthood squeezed the intimacy out of their relationship. They got out of the habit of going out together, and neither of them had much energy for conversation in their brief and hectic evenings at home.

Tony made an effort to ask Joan about her day, but when she responded only perfunctorily, he didn't pursue it. Anyway, he was so tired when he came home that he didn't really mind getting off by himself with his laptop. They weren't angry or upset with each other, but they were drifting apart.

When Tony sought my advice about the lack of intimacy in the marriage, he described his failed attempts to talk to Joan at the end of the day. I could see two mistakes he was making. The first was timing. Trying to have a serious conversation when he first came in the door, while Joan was cooking supper and the baby was winding down like a little clock, just didn't work. The second thing was that Joan didn't respond well to global questions like "How was your day?" Such questions may work when someone is relaxed and ready to talk, but they aren't effective when someone is worn out or distracted. Joan needed him to ask more specific questions, like "How did it go at the pediatrician's?" or "What did the baby do today?"—questions specific enough to show that he was aware of what was going on in her life.

I did not, however, say any of this to Tony. Instead I turned to Joan and asked if she felt lonely. She said yes. Then I asked if she thought Tony was really interested in hearing what was going on with her. "Maybe . . . ," she said softly, "but I don't feel it."

All I said to Tony was "I guess you better try harder."

. . . .

Better listening doesn't start with a set of techniques.
It starts with making a sincere effort to pay attention to what's
going on in the other person's private world of experience.

. . . .

My challenge to Tony—"I guess you better try harder"—turned out to be a one-session cure. He did try harder. It didn't occur to him to ask more specific questions; he just didn't give up so easily. Instead of offering Joan a brief moment's attention, he started showing real interest in her feelings. In response, she began to feel once again loved and cared for—and much more like being intimate with Tony in return.

When you're trying to have a conversation with people who aren't revealing much of their thoughts and feelings, it may help to make empathic guesses about what's going on inside them. Comments like "Tough day?" or "Are you worried about something?" or "Is something bothering you?" may show enough awareness to make the other person feel that you're really interested. But it isn't any particular comment or technique that gets people to open up. It's taking a sincere interest in what they have to say. Listeners who pretend interest don't fool you for long—even though they sometimes fool themselves. The automatic smile, the hit-and-run question, the restless look in their eyes when you start to talk—all these are giveaways to the fact that they're more interested in being taken for good listeners than in really hearing what you have to say. Real listening means setting all that aside. Good listeners don't make a show of being compassionate. They don't charm, flatter, provoke, or interrupt. None of that *look at me, listen to me, admire me, appreciate me.* None of that. They suspend the self and listen.

> Research shows that just having a phone visible nearby, even if it is off, will be distracting. If it's within reach, the quality of your social interactions will be reduced—along with empathy, closeness, and trust. Some studies suggest that if the phone is just in the same room—even if it's in a bag and out of sight—it reduces your capacity to give your full attention and focus on the task at hand. If you really want to listen well, don't have the phone easily accessible.

Appreciating the Other Person's Point of View

Understanding one another is a give-and-take process. The best way to get the listening you need is to make the other person feel listened to first.

· · · · · · · · · ·

Most people aren't really interested in your point of view
until they become convinced that you've heard
and appreciated theirs.

· · · · · · · · · · ·

Even when you're the one initiating a discussion, the best way to ensure that you'll be heard is to invite the other person to explain his viewpoint before you present yours. Suspending your agenda so as to hear the other person out enables you to understand what he thinks, helps make him feel understood, and clears the way for him to be more willing to listen to you.

Let the other person know you're interested in what he has to say by inviting him to say what's on his mind, what his opinion is, or how he feels about the issue under consideration—and then giving him your full attention.

"Can we talk about . . . ? What do you think we should do?"

"I'm not sure I really understand how you feel about . . . What is your point of view?"

"I'm sorry we had this misunderstanding. I'd really like to hear what happened as far as you're concerned."

"You seem upset with me. Am I right about that?"

Elicit the other person's thoughts and feelings about the subject at hand by asking specific questions that show your grasp of what she's said and encouraging her to elaborate.

"So what you're saying is . . . Is that right?"

"I think I understand, but I want to make sure. You think we should . . . ?"

"I'm not sure I know exactly what you mean. You said . . . , but I wish you'd say a little more about it so I'm sure I get it straight."

"I think I understand where we disagree, but I'm not sure. Did you mean that . . . ?"

If you feel yourself getting impatient or defensive while the other person is talking, restrain your urge to respond until you've heard her out. Just keeping your mouth shut and pretending to listen may be better than interrupting, but it isn't the same as really listening. To really listen, try hard to appreciate what the other person is feeling. Imagine how you would feel if you were in her shoes.

> When you're listening to someone but thinking about your
> own reactions, you're really talking to yourself, not listening.

Suspending your needs long enough to hear the other person out is part of being a good listener. But suspending your needs isn't the same thing as becoming a nonself.

Sometimes you need to recognize that you can't suspend your needs effectively unless you also find a way to fulfill them. So while it might seem selfish, telling your partner that you want to hear about his day but you have to get your own problem off your chest first may not be. By the same token, there are times when the most considerate and honest thing you can say to someone who wants to talk when you aren't up to listening is "I can't concentrate on what you're saying right now. Can we talk after supper?" Trying to listen when you're not up to it saps your capacity to empathize. But do try to remember to ask later when you feel up to it.

Some listeners are so fearful of asserting their own needs that they do become nonselves, tucked into others, embedded in a framework of obligations and duties. These people find it easier to accommodate than to deal with conflict, threats of rejection, arguments, or signs of distress in others. Their anxious, demanding partners are frequently unaware of how much their selfless mates accommodate to preserve harmony. They take it for granted and want more. Such compliant people may seem like good listeners, but you aren't really listening if you're nothing but a passive receptacle, a reluctant sponge.

> Listening well is often silent but never passive.

Instead of listening passively, and maybe feeling a little trapped, get involved by asking questions that help the other person express his feelings or elaborate on what he's thinking.

"What does he do that bothers you the most?"

"What do you think she should do?"

"That sounds great! What was the best part?"

"What did you feel like saying to her?"

"What would you *have liked* to hear him say?"

Real listening means imagining yourself into the other's experience: concentrating, asking questions. Understanding is furthered not by knowing ("I understand") but by investigating—asking for elaboration, inquiring into the particulars of the speaker's experience. The good listener isn't a passive receptor but an active, open one, attuned and inquiring.

When you ask the same old questions time after time—"What's new?" "How are you?"—you'll get the same old perfunctory answers. Here are some more specific sorts of questions that suggest you're really interested in what's going on with someone.

"What's going on at work? At school? What are you working on?"

"What are you looking forward to this week? This month?"

"What are you worried about?"

"What's happening with your family?"

"What's the thing that you're most enthusiastic about these days?"

"What are you facing at home and at work?"

"What's been the highlight of your week so far?"

"How is the transition to middle school going for Jake?"

"What's new with your mom?"

"What are you reading?"

Listening and Texting

When Miranda and her teenage son have a disagreement in the morning, they often continue to sort it out over the course of the day via texting. She's usually the one to try to resolve the situation: "Sorry for the rough start this morning. Good luck on the math test." Sometimes Trevor will send her a note in the afternoon, as if to clear the air before he gets back home: "Hey,

Ma, I'm stopping at Jake's on the way back from soccer. Home by five." They have a reasonably good strategy for smoothing out the inevitable minor irritations this way.

But they don't do as well resolving big fights by text—Trevor's rudeness to his stepfather, for example, or Miranda's worrying about his study habits. These more emotionally loaded conversations are better handled in person.

Rosie tore her ACL playing softball and is facing surgery and rehab. Her team captain, Nellie, calls the night before the procedure to hear how Rosie is doing, and Rosie starts to tell her how worried she is about anesthesia, frustrated to be missing the rest of the season, and annoyed at the prospect of navigating on crutches during the hot summer weeks ahead. Nellie, who hadn't really expected this outpouring of distress, offers some perfunctory reassurances and promises of help with rehab exercises before rushing off the phone. Rosie can't believe it; how could her friend be so callous? Nellie has a chance to think over the conversation too. She shoots Rosie a text in the morning: "Thinking about you, honey. I know you have a lot to deal with. Hope it goes well up there. Let me know when you're home." It would have been better if Nellie had been able to listen more receptively at the time, but maybe it was still nice to know she understood some of Rosie's anxiety and took the time to write a note like that.

Texting can be a legitimate supplement to listening, repairing small ruptures, or sustaining a connection that feels a little fragile. Still, it usually falls short when it becomes a primary mode of dialogue. A text message instead of real conversation, no matter how well intended, still runs the risk of misinterpretation: Is it an easy substitute for real engagement? Does it open up the door to a richer consideration of someone else's perspective—or shut it down? Is Trevor's text saying when he'd be home evidence of caring or just the appearance of caring, perhaps more a sweeping gesture to get a problem like Miranda to go away? Does Nellie's text seem as much a way to alleviate her guilt for not listening in the first place as it is a kindness? Much has been made of the problems of misunderstanding *content* in texting. But the *process* also creates some new challenges to clear communication. Good listeners don't just use their ears to understand words; they engage with their hearts—and that's best done in person.

Affirming Your Understanding

Sometimes we pretend we're listening when we're not. In spite of this, we're taken aback when someone accuses us of not listening. One reason people wonder if we're listening is that we fail to let them know we heard them. Silence is ambiguous.

Without some sign of understanding, the speaker begins to wonder if what she's saying makes sense, if it's worth talking about. Doubts surface. *Maybe I'm boring him. Maybe I shouldn't be complaining like this.* Without some evidence of empathy, people don't trust us enough to tell us the simple truth about their feelings, much less reveal potentially difficult truths. Everyone is vulnerable in this sense, and everyone holds back in some ways.

Ordinarily we take turns talking. The roles of speaker and listener alternate so naturally that it may seem artificial to call what one person says "the listener's response." Responding turns listeners into speakers. But listening well is a two-step process: First we take in what the speaker says, then we let him or her know it. Failure to respond is like being ghosted when texting; you never know if you got through.

Repeating the other person's position in your own words is the best way to show that you understand. But effective listening is achieved not by summing up what the other person said as though that should be the end of it, but as a means of inviting him to elaborate so that you can *really* understand.

> Effective communication isn't achieved
> just by taking turns talking; it requires
> a concerted effort at mutual understanding.

The best way to promote understanding is to restate the other person's position in your own words, then ask her to correct or affirm your understanding of her thoughts and feelings. Remember: it isn't your paraphrase that's important; it's inviting the other person to expand on what he or she is saying. If you work on this process of feedback and confirmation until the other person has no doubt that you grasp her position, she will feel understood—and will then be more open to hearing from you.

"So you're saying you don't think Kevin should join Little League, because it will put extra pressure on him and because you'll be the one who gets stuck driving him to all the games?"

"Let me make sure I understand what you're saying. You feel like you're always the one who calls to get together, and that makes you wonder if I really want to spend time with you. Is that right?"

"Okay, I want to make sure I understand. You're saying that we should hire Gloria, but we should make it clear what we expect, we should be serious about the probationary period, and if she doesn't do the job we should let her go at the end of six months. Have I got that right?"

"So all this time you've been thinking that I'm mad at you, and that's why you thought I didn't want to be affectionate. No wonder you're upset. You must have been feeling hurt for a long time."

"You Just Don't Get It, Do You?"

When one person says, "The world is round," and the other replies, "No, it's flat," it's clear that the second person got the first person's point and disagreed. But when the subject is more personal, disagreement—without some acknowledgment of the other person's point of view—can come across as invalidating the speaker's feelings. If people spoke in therapeutic jargon, they might say, "I see what you're saying, but I don't agree." But since most of us not only don't speak like self-help manuals, but often react in heat and haste, many conversations take on the form of two-part disharmony.

. . . .

The simple failure to acknowledge what the other person says explains much of the friction in our lives.

. . . .

The more heated the exchange, the more important it is to acknowledge what the other person says. When two people are talking about something important to them, each feels an urgent need to get his or her point of view across. Without some acknowledgment, each may continue to restate his or her position, thinking *If only he [or she] would listen to what I'm saying, we wouldn't have to keep arguing like this.*

Two friends who are having an argument text back and forth about some misunderstanding, and it escalates quickly, each digging in deeper and not even really waiting to read what the other is writing. If you saw a split screen of this, you'd see two young women with their heads down, frantically typing, with barely a moment's pause. After several rounds of accusation and counteraccusation, the communication actually devolves still further. Now it is all in capital letters (virtual shouting). Then, when one pointedly *copy-pastes* her last comment (the point when, in person, someone might be yelling the same insult over and over again), the other replies "NVM" (Never mind—she's virtually walking away in a huff). It will be a few weeks before they speak again, when, as often happens with trivial spats, they can't remember what got them so burned up in the first place. That disagreement might have gotten resolved face-to-face, the friends seeing the impact of their words on each other. By text, it never had a chance.

One Friday night, after a long and tedious week, Jason said, "We never go out." "That's not true!" said Rob, feeling attacked. "We went out last week." This just upset Jason more, and he renewed his attempt to get Rob to understand what he was feeling. "You mean when we went with Jada and Darnell for pizza? I don't call that going out. You never want to do anything but sit around in front of that stupid TV." Now Rob was pissed. "I work hard all week, and if I want to relax on the couch, what's so wrong with that?" By this point Jason felt completely invalidated. "You just don't get it, do you?" Then he went upstairs and slammed the bedroom door.

Maybe you can identify with Jason. Or Rob. Or both of them. The choice between going out and vegging out is one that most of us have feelings about. But what was unfortunate in this quarrel that left both Jason and Rob feeling so misunderstood was that neither took the time to acknowledge the other's point of view.

- - - - - - - - - - -

You don't have to be responsible for someone's feelings
to acknowledge them.

- - - - - - - - - - -

When Jason said, "We never go out," he was expressing a feeling—he's bored and lonely—and making a request: he wishes that he and Rob could have a little more fun, do something together, maybe be a little closer. But something about the way Jason said it (or Rob heard it) made Rob defensive. Instead of showing that he understood what Jason was feeling, he just felt criticized. Rob heard him saying that Rob was lazy, selfish, uninvolved—just the things he worries he might be—and so he didn't listen to Jason's feelings, much less respond calmly to his request.

Dueling Points of View

When two people keep restating their own positions without acknowledging what the other one is trying to say, the result is dueling points of view. One is tempted—especially if one is a therapist—to think of two people involved in dueling declarations as simply lacking a communication skill, that of paraphrasing what your conversation partner says before responding. The trouble with this communication-as-skill perspective is that it leaves out conflict and anxiety, precisely the things that make understanding so difficult. The partners who don't acknowledge what each other says are afraid to. They're afraid that acknowledging the other's position means surrendering—"You're right, and I'm wrong."

When the subject isn't too emotional, the result is a mildly unsatisfying sense of at least having said what you mean even if the other person didn't acknowledge it. But when feeling runs high, dueling declarations escalate into painful misunderstandings.

Professional advice givers often talk as though couples could get along fine if only they'd learn "to communicate"—making "I-statements" and all the rest. That's nice, but it overlooks the existence of real conflict.

Although they hadn't really discussed it, Charlotte assumed that when Alberto finished his PhD they would move back to New York. But Alberto liked where they were living, and when he announced that he might take a teaching job at the university, Charlotte felt betrayed.

Because the question of where to live was so important to both of them, they found it difficult to discuss without disparaging each other's point of view. When Alberto presented his arguments for staying, Charlotte would try to discredit them or say that he had a responsibility to make up to her the sacrifice she had made in leaving the city for the sake of his career. He'd respond by talking about the sacrifices he'd made for her. Later, after months of estrangement, Charlotte said that if at any point in the process Alberto had acknowledged that she had given up a lot for his schooling or had said that she would get her turn later, she could have agreed to stay. But instead of listening and acknowledging her right to feel the way she did, Alberto responded by saying that his career was more important than hers.

For another couple who faced the same issue, both wanted to move; the problem was where. Raymond was an accountant, and Joyce was the dean of women at a small college. Both agreed that since he would be able to find work more easily, her search for another deanship should be given priority. Raymond, however, felt strongly about *where* he wanted to live. It wasn't so much a regional preference as wanting to live either in a big city or well out in the country—anything but suburbia, where Lawn Doctor reigned. And so half the time when Joyce told him that she'd read about a job opening, he'd respond by saying, "I'd never live *there*." She'd feel defeated and angry and think he was being totally unreasonable.

Why did Alberto find it necessary to put Charlotte down by saying that his career was more important than hers? And why did Raymond have to reject so many of Joyce's possibilities so quickly? What made it so hard for these two husbands to acknowledge what their wives were feeling?

Alberto was apparently afraid that acknowledging Charlotte's feelings would automatically lead to giving in and acting on their dictates. Likewise, Raymond didn't seem to have the confidence that he could still say no to a potential new place after he and Joyce had visited it. Otherwise, why wouldn't he agree to at least take a look? Why weren't these two men able to listen better to their wives? Is it simply "selfishness" or "masculine insensitivity" or "immaturity" that prevents people from hearing each other? Maybe Alberto and Raymond had trouble listening to their partners because they felt anxious and insecure about their own ability to assert themselves. Maybe we—men and women—always have reasons for not listening, not understanding one another.

Listening is hard because it involves a loss of control—
and if you're afraid of what you might hear,
it feels unsafe to relinquish control.

He Says, She Says

He says, "You should have said something," she says, "You should have asked," and neither feels heard. She talks about the things she'd like to do, and he talks about being tired. He never hears what doing these things means to her, and she never hears that he hates his job. Arguments escalate, feelings go unrecognized, and minds don't meet as long as we fail to acknowledge what the other person says—or is trying to say—before we respond with what we have to say.

A behavioral strategy widely employed by couples therapists involves teaching how to paraphrase what partners say before going on to give their side. This "active listening" practice serves to interrupt the cross-complaining that keeps family members in conflict from ever feeling understood, much less actually doing anything about each other's complaints. If a wife tells her husband that she wishes he would cook something different for supper, and he complains that she's impossible to please—and she gets defensive and withdraws to brood over how unfair he is—neither one of them will feel understood. This misunderstanding—and many others like it—has less to do with being unable to resolve conflict than with being unable to tolerate it. If instead of getting defensive and attacking, either person would simply acknowledge what the other said, it might not prove so difficult to come together.

Even when conflict is serious, we all feel better if we can at least say how we feel—what bothers us, what we wish—and have the other person say those magic words: "I understand." You don't have to agree with people to be able to acknowledge their feelings.

Why do people need a therapist to have these conversations? They don't—*if* they can each say how they feel about the situation, and the other can hear *and acknowledge* these feelings before going on to say how he or she feels.

The Importance of Relinquishing Control

As I've said, I don't like to be interrupted in the middle of a story by someone giving advice I didn't ask for or "sharing" a similar experience. Interruption is interruption. What's missing in both cases is some expression of understanding, something like "Gee, that's lousy." What's going on with interrupting is that the listener won't relinquish control of the exchange. Many of us are convinced that we're good listeners because we say all the right things. But are we? Often the speaker ends up feeling unheard, because what we're really doing is going through the motions.

"Why Don't You Just . . . ?"

A wise supervisor once told me that my treatment of a shy, overweight young man was bogged down because I was trying to change him before he felt understood by me. To me it seemed so simple: if the young man would only make a little effort to initiate conversations with people, at the same time we explored the roots of his insecurity, he could work toward change on two fronts. He, however, felt that my suggesting that he simply start doing what he found so difficult proved that I didn't understand how painfully self-conscious he was. The supervisor's technical recommendation (which had to do with transference and countertransference) was: "Shut up and listen."

A Gaping Silence

If everyone followed my supervisor's advice, the world would be a better place. But if listening were only a negative accomplishment, you could concentrate (as many therapists, and people playing therapist, do) on simply not interrupting. Speakers may be gratified at being allowed to say what's on their minds but frustrated by the absence of curiosity and appreciation. This means that, taken too literally, "shut up and listen" isn't enough to convey understanding. If you're telling someone at a party about what kind of work you do and she's listening without interrupting, but her eyes are wandering around the room, you hardly feel listened to.

Whether or not someone is really listening only that person knows. But, on the other hand, if you don't feel listened to, you don't feel listened to. We judge whether or not others are listening to us by the signals we see. Are they showing that they're paying attention by setting aside distractions and turning toward us? If they are "listening" via email or text, are their responses sufficiently detailed and prompt that we can be confident they actually read what we sent them?

Before they comment on what we're saying, people show interest and attention by maintaining eye contact, smiling with pleasure or frowning with concern, and making little interjections like "uh-huh" and "really?" Head nods also show attention; larger and repeated ones show agreement. You don't have to take Elementary Clinical Methods to learn these responses; they follow from taking an interest.

The Leading Question

Questions convey interest, but sometimes the interest they convey is tangential to what the person is trying to say. Sometimes the distraction is obvious. If you're telling a friend all the inconsiderate things your boyfriend did on your vacation and she interrupts with a lot of questions about where you stayed, you won't feel listened to. At other times people seem to be following but can't help trying to steer. These listeners impose their own narrative structures on our experience. Their questions assume that our stories should fit their scripts: "Problems should be denied or made to go away." "Everyone should be together." "Men are insensitive." "Bullies must be confronted." "Women are enablers." By finishing our sentences, pumping us with questions, and otherwise pushing us to say what they want to hear, controlling listeners violate our right to tell our own stories in our own way.

Responsive Listening

Responsive listening is a technique designed to reduce arguments by hearing the other person's side of the story before giving your own. Responsive listening allows you to shift from an adversarial stance, reflexively countering what someone else is saying, to a receptive stance, allowing the other person to express his feelings, while you put your feelings on hold. Responsive listening was developed to resolve arguments. However, as you'll see in subsequent chapters, responsive listening will enable you to improve your listening in almost any situation.

Here's how responsive listening works.

RESPONSIVE LISTENING

1. At the first sign of an argument, check the impulse to argue back and concentrate on listening to the other person's side of the story.

2. Invite the other person's thoughts, feelings, and wishes—without defending or disagreeing.

3. Repeat the other person's position in your own words to show what you think he or she is thinking and feeling.

4. Ask the other person to correct your impression or elaborate on his or her point of view.

5. Reserve your own response until later. On important or contentious issues, wait a day or so before giving your side of the issue. On minor matters, pause and ask if the other person would be willing to hear what you think.

When someone starts to argue with what you've said, your first impulse might be to explain or restate your ideas. But when two people insist on talking, neither one is likely to listen.

To break that pattern before the argument escalates, remind yourself that you're going to draw out the other person's *feelings* before responding with your own. Don't even start to argue; stay in control by listening.

Arguments are like Ping-Pong games:
It takes two to keep them going.

To really hear another person's concerns, you have to suspend your own agenda, at least temporarily. It isn't possible to listen effectively when you're just waiting to respond. It may take some effort, but the active decision to postpone responding to explore the other person's thinking is the first step in breaking the chain of argumentation.

"I don't remember saying that, but you may be right. What do you want to do about this situation?"

When is an argument not an argument?
When you don't argue back.

Because most people expect arguments to focus on the outcome, it may take a little time for people to learn that you really are interested in understanding their feelings. On the first few occasions you try responsive listening, the other person may be the one who is impatient to get to a resolution. The ability to resist being drawn too quickly into making a decision begins with a conscious effort to focus first on the other person's feelings.

"Do we have to go out to dinner every night?"

Repeating the other person's position in your own words is the best way to let him know that you understand. Don't sum up what you've heard as though that should be the end of it, however, but rather as a means of inviting the other person to elaborate so that you can *really* understand.

"Let me see if I understand. You'd like to eat healthier. You don't like going out to dinner every night because the places we go to have rich food and overcooked vegetables so you don't feel like we're eating healthy enough?"

Notice how this paraphrase is expressed with a question. The point isn't to convey that you understand but to convey that you're trying to.

The fourth step of responsive listening is tied directly to the third. I list it separately to emphasize the importance of getting the other person to elaborate on his or her position. The point of responsive listening isn't to reach some conclusion—or to cut off the discussion—but to allow the person you're talking to tell her side of the story—and to feel that you're listening to it. The longer the other person talks, the longer the cycle of arguing is avoided. The goal is communication.

"I think I understand what you're saying, but I want to be sure. Do you mean . . . ?"

"I'm not completely sure I understand what you mean. You're saying _____, but I wish you'd say more about [your position] so I can get it straight."

"Is there more? Are there other reasons you'd like to eat out less often?"

Responsive listening is as important a skill for supporting children as it is in conversation with adults, but it can take more time to read between the lines and hear what deeper concerns a child is conveying.

Sadie, age nine, comes home beaming. She runs up to her mother and says, "Mommy, Mommy, guess what! I got an A in spelling!" "That's nice, dear," her mother responds, sounding pleased, but not very, as she finishes emptying the dishwasher. Sadie tries again. "There's *twenty-nine* kids, and I got the second-highest score." "That's good, honey." The conversation continues for another couple of minutes. Sadie is so proud and excited that she's trying to drive up her mother's enthusiasm. Her mother is, of course, glad that her daughter did well, but she's also worried that Sadie is getting too focused on grades. She doesn't want Sadie to get hooked on achievement (like her father). Still undaunted and full of pride, Sadie persists. Finally, her mother admonishes her, saying, "Don't brag. It isn't nice."

One minute Sadie is bursting with excitement. Getting an A was a wonderful accomplishment. She couldn't wait to tell her mother, to share her delight. You could say she met with misunderstanding, but it was worse. Because a child seeking appreciation is reaching out, exposed, a failed response is an emotional head-on collision. Responsive listening allows us to take time to see what's important to someone else. Sadie's mother's empathic failure was painful and shaming; it's likely Sadie will think twice about sharing her great news next time.

Emotional Validation

Responsive listening entails not just taking the time necessary to understand another person's reasons for being upset or frustrated, but also to work to be sure you actually can empathize with how he might feel that way. This means that your inquiry might also include clarifying questions and comments that focus on his emotional state—or what you sense it might be. Remember: you don't have to agree with how someone is feeling to connect emotionally with what it's like for him. Indeed, you might even suspend your own agenda long enough to imagine that if you were that fellow, you too would feel exactly as he does.

"You seem discouraged."

"I can see you're upset about this."

"What do you wish would happen?"

"That sounds really lonely."

"How else did you feel?"

"I imagine that must have been hard for you."

"So you really felt _____?"

"Are you feeling disappointed?"

Sometimes, after showing that you understand the other person's reasons for not agreeing with you *and* how the person feels about the situation, you may simply want to reaffirm your position. The conversation now switches from understanding to reaching a decision. At this point, any attempt to justify your position as anything other than your personal opinion or preference only invites further debate. Just say, "Well, this is how I feel," and then if a decision is required, the two of you can negotiate an agreement that hopefully takes both of your preferences into account. I'll have more to say about negotiating later.

As often as possible, it's a good idea to separate the conversation in which you try to be understanding from the one in which you have to reach a decision. Doing so makes the other person feel that you are considering his or her position, and it gives you time to review your options with less pressure. Responsive listening isn't magic. It doesn't automatically eliminate differences of opinion. It's a way to reduce the argumentativeness of disagreements. But you'll find that it is very useful—if you remember that the goal is to draw the other person out and really listen until he or she feels felt and understood.

There are a variety of other approaches that encourage listeners to acknowledge the speaker's feelings, but most of them are designed to bring the conversation to a quick conclusion.

"I understand how you feel, but now I want to tell you what I think."

"I guess we'll have to agree to disagree."

This "yes, but" approach doesn't work very well. Responsive listening is designed not to summarize conversations but to open them up. Even if your primary goal is to get the other person to accept your position, getting him to talk at length about his point of view is the best way to put him in a receptive frame of mind. A perfunctory acknowledgment of feelings usually doesn't work.

When you're trying to empathize with someone's feelings, saying, "I understand" isn't very understanding. It implies that you know what the other person is trying to say. Since you already know what she's thinking and feeling, there's no need for her to talk about it.

Imagine how you'd feel if you were worried about an upcoming presentation at work, and you said to your mate something like "Honey, you know I'm a little worried about how I'm going to handle that project I've been working on," and he responded with a perfunctory expression of sympathy, "Yeah, I know what you mean," and then turned back to what he was doing. How would you feel?

Actually, a more useful thing to say when trying to appreciate what someone is feeling is:

"I *don't* understand."

"I'm not sure I really understand how you feel. Can you explain it to me?"

"I think I understand how you feel, but I'm not certain. Can you tell me?"

- - - - - - - - - - - - -

The difference between saying "I'm not sure how you feel"
and "I know how you feel" is the difference between
showing an interest in listening and not showing an interest.

- - - - - - - - - - - - -

The point of responsive listening isn't to get to the point where you can paraphrase what the other person has said. The point is to get that person to talk. It's the talking—the communicative act of expressing feelings to someone who cares enough to listen, not the accuracy of the listener's perception—that makes people feel understood. When it's genuine, responsive listening is a way around arguments, and a way inside other people's feelings.

Responsive Listening in the Digital Age

Responsive listening by text and email is harder to do, even if you double-check that your missives are as clear as possible. For one thing, these devices are really most efficient when they convey small bits of information that can be digested quickly. On the small screen, time and effort required to read a lengthy text or email can be daunting, and, sadly, the reader is apt to scan it superficially—even if the sender obsessed over every word.

And then there's the sheer volume of correspondence to keep up with. Let's pause a moment to consider this level of distraction in the face of our enormous need to connect and desire that others pay attention to us and really listen when we speak. Somewhere in the midst of keeping up with our social networking sites, emails, texts, instant messaging, and hours of compelling screen time, we also might have a partner who had a staff meeting from hell and really needs our undivided attention for seven minutes. Do we have it to give?

One way to use these dastardly devices to ensure better listening is via video chatting apps like Skype, Zoom, and FaceTime. Even if you can't be there for someone in a physical sense, you can still see her, and she can still feel your attentive gaze—a feature that became that much more appealing during the 2020 coronavirus pandemic. By seeing her, you can get more nonverbal information about how she is feeling than via text or phone. If you are looking right at her and nodding, she can tell she has your attention; she'll know you're not on your computer playing video games or folding laundry while she tells you about the crazy stuff that happened at the office.

GUIDELINES FOR GOOD LISTENING

1. Concentrate on the person speaking.
   - Set aside distractions.
   - Suspend your agenda.
   - Interrupt as little as possible. If you do interrupt, it should be to encourage the speaker to say more.

2. Try to grasp what the speaker is trying to express.
   - Don't react to just the words—listen for the underlying ideas and feelings.
   - Try to put yourself in the other person's shoes.
   - Try to understand what the other person is getting at.

3. Let the speaker know that you understand.
   - Use silence, reassuring comments, paraphrasing.
   - Offer empathic comments that convey you both understand what the person is saying (or trying to say) and the feelings that make this important for you to hear.
   - Make opening-up statements (tell me more, what else) versus closing-off statements (I get it; the same thing happened to me).

How to Get the Listening You Deserve

(The devil just whispered in my ear that maybe I should make that " . . . the Listening You Want." Maybe we already get the listening we deserve. But I'm not going to listen to that old devil.)

How to Ask for Support
Without Getting Unwanted Advice

One way to get the listening you need is to tell people what you want.

> "I'm upset and I need to talk to you. Just listen, okay?"

> "I have a problem I need to discuss, but I'm not ready to decide what to do, so it would be helpful if you could just listen to me."

If you don't want a reactive or intrusive response, anticipate your listener's expectations.

> "I'm not asking you to agree with me, but can you understand where I'm coming from?"

> "I want to tell you something, and I don't want you to get mad at me. Just listen and think about what I'm saying, will you?"

> "I want your opinion about something, but I'll have to figure out what I want to do about it. I'd like to hear what you think, even if I don't end up following your suggestion."

If someone gives advice when you just want to be listened to, by all means say so. But put the emphasis on what you want, not on how intrusive she is: "Thanks for the advice, but right now I just want to tell you about what happened" works better than "I didn't ask for any advice" or "Can't you just listen for once, without always having to tell me what to do!"

How to Handle Interruptions

If you're driving down the road and someone cuts in front of you, there's not much you can do about it. Oh, you can hit your horn and call that person something you sit on. But you pretty much have to yield unless you want to get into an accident. The same isn't true when somebody cuts in when you're talking. You can't be interrupted unless you allow it. When you're talking, you have the right of way.

If someone starts to interrupt, you can:

- Hold up your index finger.
- Say "Wait a minute, I'm not finished."
- Just keep talking: "What I was trying to say is . . ."

If someone does cut you off:

- Instead of getting upset (or instead of *just* getting upset), practice saying, "I wasn't finished; please hear me out." Then go back to what you were saying and finish saying it.
- Comment on feeling cut off, but without lecturing or attacking:

  "I wish you'd let me finish what I was saying."

  "I'm sorry, but I can't pay attention to your story because I wasn't finished telling mine."

  "I was trying to tell you something that's important to me. When you start talking about something else, I feel like you're not interested in me or what I have to say."

  "When you keep looking at your phone instead of me while I'm speaking, it feels like you're not listening to me."

  "I do want to hear what you have to say, but I really want to finish what I'm telling you first."

  "I was listening to that story on the news. I wish you'd wait a minute before breaking in."

Resisting the Temptation to Turn Away

Some people are so self-involved, boring and repetitive, politically wrong, or otherwise insufferable that we might actually try not to listen when they speak. There are many situations when it would be easier to act as though a person wasn't even there. At times when we want to control others' access to us, we may even avoid looking at them. A teen ignores her fretful mother's repeated texts. A man watching television may avoid looking at his wife when she tries to speak to him. Or a waitress may evade a customer's glance to prevent his initiating a request she's too busy to fulfill at the moment.

A paradoxical example of this responsive unavailability occurs in psychoanalysis, where the analyst sits behind the recumbent patient. The result is disconcerting. Unable to see how the therapist is responding, the patient is unsure of being understood and sympathized with. The therapist may feel equally uncomfortable in not being able to offer visible evidence of interest. Eventually, this constrained arrangement turns out to be liberating. The patient, who gets to trust that he won't be interrupted, learns to follow his own thoughts more fully and to express them more freely. The therapist discovers that looking away with no pressure to demonstrate interest enables her to listen more freely and to think about what's being said.

What is to be learned from the analyst being liberated to listen by not having to appear attentive? We've noted that listening well means suspending our needs, including the need to *do* something—to solve problems, to say the right thing, even to act attentive. Better to *be* attentive. Be interested. Listen hard. Overcome the need to get credit for listening.

It may not be possible in everyday life to offer that focused and silent listening in which analytic patients are encouraged to reveal and reconstruct themselves. If people have learned not to expect careful listening from you, you may have to reassure them of your interest. But if you listen carefully, people will learn to trust you. Just listening, without interrupting or turning away, goes a long way toward establishing that trust.

EXERCISES

1. The next time someone you care about has something to say, give him or her your full attention for three minutes. How long did those three minutes seem? How hard was it to stay tuned? How hard did you have to work to suppress what you wanted to say? What were the consequences of devoting that time to listening?

2. Note the next time someone responds to you with advice instead of

listening. Write down later how you felt and why you think he or she couldn't hear you out.

3. Is there someone you can listen to without jumping in with advice or correction? If so, why? Does it have anything to do with respect?

4. Think about someone from your childhood who really listened to you. Try to remember what that was like for you and how that person let you know you had his or her attention. Can you remember a specific conversation that still sticks with you today?

5. Practice responsive listening twice in the coming week. First with someone who's easy to talk with. You probably won't be defusing an argument; you'll just be using responsive listening to draw the other person out a little more than usual. Second, pick someone you're likely to have a disagreement with. Plan in advance to use responsive listening and avoid giving your side of the argument until at least a day later.

8

"I Never Knew You Felt That Way"

EMPATHY BEGINS WITH OPENNESS

Among the unhelpful expectations we bring to listening are preconceived notions about what the speaker is going to say and how communication should take place. Assuming you know what someone is going to say means you don't have to bother to listen.

Our assumptions about how people should talk to each other aren't usually conscious; they're part of the way we were brought up. Assuming that your way of communicating is the right one means you'll have trouble relating to people with different conversational styles and sensitivities. Such assumptions come in pairs of opposites, such as:

"Polite people make requests indirectly" versus "Honest people say what they want."

"Explanations should be short and sweet (rambling on is boring)" versus "Explanations should be thorough and complete (make sure the other person understands what you mean)."

"It's best to be logical and calm at all times" versus "If you have a strong feeling about something, the emotion adds to understanding."

The listener who settles for confirming his expectations is like the museum goer who looks at paintings only long enough to verify the name of the artist; he'll never get closer to another person's experience. There is no bridge of understanding, no touching. The listener who remains open, on the other hand, sometimes experiences surprise and insight as his assumptions topple and he discovers the speaker—child, lover, friend—in a deeper, fuller way.

. . . .

The essence of good listening is empathy,
achieved by being receptive to what other people
are trying to say and how they express themselves.
Empathy takes a mind open to other sensibilities.

. . . .

Although most people would improve their listening by setting aside preconceived notions and remaining receptive to what others are trying to say, a complete absence of assumptions is neither possible nor desirable. Anticipation is both useful and inevitable. Anticipating how someone might react can help you express yourself more effectively; anticipating a speaker's needs and style of communicating can help you hear all levels of messages being sent. So, what am I saying? Are expectations a help or a hindrance to listening?

Expectations hinder communication when they take the form of fixed assumptions and egocentric perspectives. Such expectations are unexamined and close us to other points of view. Expectations promote communication when they take the form of sensitivity to other people's styles of communicating. Such sensitivities make us aware, thoughtful, and receptive, not biased.

Creating a Climate of Understanding

One of the most common expectations we bring to conversational encounters, especially at home, is that we will be able to communicate by doing what comes naturally. Unfortunately, the listening we do on automatic pilot is often perfunctory, precisely the kind of halfhearted listening that makes our relationships less fulfilling than they could be. If you want to make any relationship more rewarding, practice *responsive listening*.

Responsive listening involves stopping what you are doing long enough to hear the other person out, then letting him know what you understand him to be saying. If you're right, the speaker will feel a grateful sense of being understood. If you didn't quite get what he intended to say, your curious feedback allows him another chance to explain. (See Chapter 7 for details.)

Responsive listening can be practiced like any other skill if you're willing to put in the effort. If.

Listening Takes Practice

Why is it that we can admit we don't dance well or can't draw, but we won't admit (even to ourselves) that we aren't good at listening? Because being a good listener doesn't seem like a skill; it seems like a character trait, related to being a nice person, someone interested in others. If you're not a good tennis player, it's because you haven't practiced. If you're not a good listener, you're a bad person. In reality, people who are good listeners work at it every day.

Think of how many situations where familiarity, tension, or distraction has made you fail to be attentive, considerate—concerned. The next time your partner comes home at the end of the day, or your child runs to tell you something, or someone at work wants to talk, try making an extra effort to be attentive. Paying attention goes a long way. Your effort to listen a little longer and more carefully to others will initiate a positive spiral in all of your relationships.

Put down your device, pause the video, silence the TV, shut your laptop. The odds are close to 100% that you will be distracted by your screens; they were designed to be more alluring and diverting than anyone in your family is.

"I Know What You're Going to Say"

"Like hell, you do!" Have you ever felt like saying that when someone finishes your sentence?

The person who starts a sentence
should be the one to finish it.

Unfortunately, jumping to conclusions is something we all do at times. You may not actually make the remark I've used as a heading for this section, but one of the bad listening habits we all need to break is making assumptions about what people are going to say.

Rachel got home at six-thirty instead of six as she'd promised and said, "I'm sorry I was late, I—"

"That's okay," Patrick broke in to say. "The kids and I made spaghetti. It's all ready."

Rachel was grateful not to have to cook supper but still felt cut off. She was about to say that she was late because her boss dumped a last-minute assignment on her, but Patrick's assumption that she was about to apologize for inconveniencing him made her feel that he didn't care. All he was interested in, it seemed to her, was his supper.

She could have told him anyway, right? Maybe. But if he's in the habit of cutting her off, she may get tired of trying to force him to listen to her.

Cutting someone off to take over conversational control can certainly be annoying, but so can jumping in before a speaker is finished with words of encouragement or agreement or to tell a similar story.

At first Hank appreciated Sharon's habit of interjecting little expressions of support when he talked to her. Her *wows*, *gees*, and *what a shames* made him think she was tuned in to his feelings. But after a while these expressions seemed trite and predictable. They began to make him feel that she was more interested in coming across as supportive than in really listening to him.

Being supportive means neither anticipating nor exceeding a speaker's own expression of feeling. I knew a woman who was so supportive that waves of compassion radiated from her like hot air from an oven. She may have been trying to be sensitive, but after a while it was all too much.

"Oh, I know what you mean!" Celia said. "My principal treats me the same way." Though she intended to establish empathy, Todd was annoyed. He doubted that her principal really gave her as many last-minute assignments as his boss gave him. Besides, that wasn't his point. He never got to make his point because Celia cut him off to demonstrate that she understood.

The best way to avoid cutting people off is to concentrate on what they're trying to say. Give them a chance to make their point, acknowledge it, and *then* say your piece. Don't pounce at the first pause. Curb the impulse to switch the focus to you and what's on your mind. Don't tell every story that crops into your head. (I wince as I write this.) Stop and consider whether your comment would encourage the speaker to say more or would take over the conversation.

"When Is It My Turn?"

Sometimes we don't listen because we've developed habits that interfere with openness. We make assumptions, we react emotionally, and we focus on what we have to say. We seem to be listening, but we can't resist giving our feelings, our experience, our advice, our opinion.

How do you overcome focusing on what you have to say? Make an effort. Often what you have to say is fine, but it skips hearing and acknowledging what the other person was saying.

Not: "I hate my job."
   "Yeah, me too."

But: "I hate my job."
   "Gee, that's too bad. What's going on?"

Always listen first. Then acknowledge what the other person said. Whether and when you take a turn depends on whether the relationship is one of equals. If your child complains, usually just listen. If it's a friend, listen first, then tell your story. But "equals" aren't equal when one person is upset. That person gets preference. It's like when someone you live with gets sick. He or she needs the attention. Put your needs on hold.

It's not like pie: listening to someone else doesn't mean there will be none left for you.

> Not: "I felt all alone when you left me at your office party for a half hour to talk to your boss."
> "What could I do? He pays my salary. He wanted to talk. I had no choice."
>
> But: "I felt all alone when you left me at your office party for a half hour to talk to your boss."
> "I'm sorry."

If you make a habit of talking out of turn, people will consider you intrusive. If you get excited and jump in before the other person has finished, try to catch yourself and back off politely. Say, "Go ahead" or "I'm sorry, I didn't let you finish." If you prefer quick repartee and find yourself restlessly waiting out the musings of a slow or deliberate talker, you may be particularly tempted to jump in to move things along once you get the gist of what the speaker is saying. Try then to take a deep breath and hear the person out.

Even if you *do* know what somebody is going to say, he or she still needs to say it—and have you acknowledge it—before feeling understood. If conversation were an aerial dogfight, it would be wise to anticipate the other person's moves so you could shoot them down as fast as possible. But conversation shouldn't be like that. The person who has something to say wants to express both an idea and a feeling. Listening with an open mind gives you a chance to discover what's on her mind and gives her a chance to clarify her own thinking and feeling. The gift of your attention allows you to understand—and the other person to *feel* understood. Taking seriously a bid for your attention actually gives the speaker a double satisfaction: you were there when he needed you *and* you cared enough to stick around to hear him out.

Developing the Empathy
to Become a Better Listener

Most of us are born with some capacity for empathy, but we've gotten by, more or less, without really developing it. We tend to assume that empathy comes naturally, and so we may not realize that it takes effort. The sympathetic response we feel when people talk about their problems isn't the same thing as empathy. Empathy requires a deliberate effort to understand what that other person is feeling. It's not automatic, and it's not always easy. Besides, we have our own feelings to deal with.

> There's a difference between reacting and responding. When we get hooked by someone's emotions, we are apt to *react* automatically, adding our own feelings to what we've just taken in. If we take a deep breath and think about what got us to react, we can then distinguish our own feelings from the other person's and have a better chance of *responding* both empathically and intentionally.

Becca's son, Otis, was having a tough adjustment to his new high school. When the family moved a couple months ago, she worried this might happen; he had always been a kid who struggled with transitions. But Otis was actually dealing well with the new situation, joining a club where he'd met a couple like-minded classmates and kicking around his soccer ball after school to burn off the day's tension. Unfortunately, Becca was so wrapped up in her concern that she couldn't hear him describing how he was working through this transition. She kept texting Otis a couple times a day to let him know he wasn't alone, until her son snapped at her one day that she was "blowing up his phone with her anxiety." Becca started dealing with her own and became much better able to listen to Otis's distress empathically without becoming flooded by it—and could start to notice what he was doing to find his own way.

The Parent's Gift of Empathy

A parent's empathy—understanding what a child is feeling and showing it— builds a bridge of understanding, linking the child to someone who listens and cares, thus confirming that the child's feelings are legitimate. The sharing of emotional experience is the most powerful feature of true relatedness.

Foremost among the obstacles to listening are those that stem from our need to *do something* about what someone tells us: defend ourselves, disagree, or solve the other person's problems. Parents are prone to offer advice; it comes with the job description. But if a father's first response to his son's painful sunburn is that he should have used sunblock, the boy will feel blamed rather than commiserated with. Likewise, if a little girl complains that she doesn't have any friends, and her mother tells her that if she acted friendlier, other children would be more friendly in return, the girl might conclude that even her mother doesn't like her.

Psychologists use the term *empathic immersion* to describe the intense and focused listening that therapists use to understand their patients' experience. It's an evocative metaphor, but it is of course hyperbole. Perhaps a better metaphor for empathy would be taking someone's hand. Two clasped hands are still two hands—but they are also two hands touching, the warmth and pulse of one in contact with the other.

To be better listeners parents should lead less and follow more. If a child shows signs of distress, a simple statement like "You feel bad, don't you?" is more likely to make him feel understood than pressuring him to explain what he feels. If an exasperated child indicates that she wants to be alone, let her. She may need time to pull herself together. If someone is having a hard time putting something into words, it's more empathic to say, "It's hard to explain, isn't it?" than to guess what the person is trying to say. A parent who finishes a child's thoughts for him may feel empathic but comes across as impatient.

. . . .

Listening well is more midwifery than dentistry.
In the presence of an empathic listener, children are able
to discover their own minds rather than having to resist
or succumb to what someone else expects them to feel.

. . . .

The empathic failure that saps self-regard isn't the kind of child abuse we usually hear about; it is a silent, invidious lack of responsiveness. Empathic failure doesn't batter, bruise, or injure children physically; it deflates and silences them.

Empathy is energizing. Being listened to releases us from brooding self-absorption and mobilizes us to engage the world around us. With insufficient empathy children grow up uncertain about the legitimacy of their needs; in turn, they will be less likely to know how to extend such concern to others. Some of these children become compulsively self-reliant. Their experience has taught them that people don't care what they think and feel, and they try to stop needing that kind of attention. Others may amp up the effort to get people to listen; they become preoccupied with their own distress and symptoms, seemingly determined to do whatever it takes to arouse empathic concern. These empathy-hungry kids tend to be well known by school nurses, who will ask them all about how they feel and may let them lie on a cot nearby for the rest of the period. A child's bid for attention is also a bid for relationship. The unlistened-to child remains locked in thwarted conversation within himself and will be unable to engage robustly and confidently with others.

Listening empathically to babies and toddlers often evokes magnification of feeling. An infant who giggles a little gets back a delighted chuckle from his mother; he learns about his feelings by seeing them reflected in her face and hearing the echo of his expression in her laughter. A toddler who comes inside with a scraped knee may be comforted knowing that her woes are fully understood; the offer to "kiss the booboo" really does make it better. When we listen empathically to older children and teens, we convey our emotional engagement through a similar (if less cute) immersion into the experiences they are sharing with us. We meet them where they begin their stories and listen to the feelings beneath what they are saying. "No one moved over to make a place for you to sit? That's awful! What did you do?" "You said that? Oh my god, that's hilarious! Did everyone laugh?" Like everyone else, our kids live in the details of their lives. Our willingness to really engage with those small shared moments gives children the kind of listening that they need to feel understood.

Listening Empathically to Your Partner's SOS (Same Old Story)

At the other end of the life span, within long-term family relationships, partnerships, and friendships, we face a completely different empathic listening challenge: the SOS. Some people who consider themselves fine listeners the first couple times they hear about a girlfriend's case of poison ivy or a mother's reminiscence about the gross jelly omelets she ate long ago lose all patience the third, fourth, or fifth time the tale is told.

Our capacity to be good listeners over time depends, in part, on figuring out how to handle the SOS in our most important relationships. Why is this so hard for us to do? Most stories just take a few minutes to tell. A perfectly nice dinner conversation turns south when one person begins, "Did I ever tell you about the time that . . . ?" In a relationship that has lasted many decades, the odds are good that, indeed, she has. The people we love the longest can be so exasperating, not only due to the way they handle conflict or misunderstand us, but also through sheer repetition of conversation. Perhaps hearing the SOS leads you to feel oppressed, invalidated, fatigued, bored, or just plain exasperated. You've listened to this one *so* many times, you could relate it verbatim. Must you endure it again? Yes, probably. But you can learn how to be less aggravated by it.

First, understand the motivation behind the repetition. Is the person lonely and just needing to talk? Is she so self-involved she doesn't care, as long as she gets to say whatever she likes? Is it possible he's actually forgotten he's shared this with you before? Is she a gregarious yarn spinner who delights in storytelling? Is he anxious about something more current that's harder to talk about? Is she filling an uncomfortable silence? Does he love the response he gets even if it's a collective groan from everyone at the table? Is she beginning to have memory problems? Does he feel you haven't sufficiently heard or appreciated how important this story is to him? What else might be the cause? Your explanation will guide your response. If you believe she is launching into an SOS just to vex you, you will be vexed.

Second, consider what you'd like your response to accomplish. Do you want him to change, understand your frustration, accept your limit setting, listen to your feedback, or just know how long you've suffered? Do you want to vent or problem-solve? Do you think it's going to be hopeless to have any impact after all these years or imagine there might be a better way for you to listen and respond?

Third, think about how you usually react and consider how well it's working for you and your relationship. Perhaps you have an approach that is both effective and kind: "I remember that one—you made the jelly omelet with strawberry jam, right? So gross!" Or you and the person embarking on the SOS have agreed that you can say, "Honey, I've heard this story" and agree to move on, no hard feelings.

If, by contrast, you feel like nothing you've tried has worked, it's no wonder you're looking for a new approach. It is toxic to your relationship if you feel reduced to the point of disrespectful commentary and eye rolling, heavy pained sighing, sarcasm, criticism, bored silence, or a hasty departure. It might be useful to take a few minutes and think about what's going on.

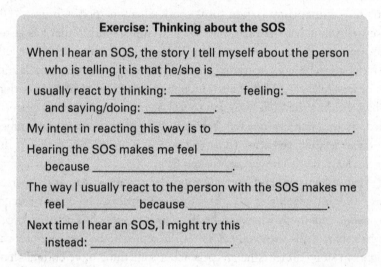

Exercise: Thinking about the SOS

When I hear an SOS, the story I tell myself about the person who is telling it is that he/she is _____.

I usually react by thinking: _____ feeling: _____ and saying/doing: _____.

My intent in reacting this way is to _____.

Hearing the SOS makes me feel _____ because _____.

The way I usually react to the person with the SOS makes me feel _____ because _____.

Next time I hear an SOS, I might try this instead: _____.

My friend Lisa has an admirable strategy. She has been married to Jim for many years. Instead of getting all worked up when Jim starts in with an SOS she's heard dozens of times, Lisa smiles, sits back in her chair, and says cheerfully: "I love it when you tell this story." Jim is going to tell it, and telling it gives him pleasure. It's true that Lisa is a gifted listener, but if you are in a long-term relationship, it's pretty much guaranteed you'll also have plenty of opportunity to practice this skill. With effort, you can get better at listening to your dear one's SOS with something approaching tolerant appreciation. If you haven't started repeating yourself yet, one of these days, you probably will. Trust me on this. And it's a great practice: listening empathically to someone's SOS is the very definition of loving kindness.

Empathy and Technology

Up until now, I've been talking about the challenges to empathic listening in intimate relationships when two people might be in the same place, adjusting responses automatically through verbal and nonverbal cues without any conscious exertion, and registering, in real time, the impact of their words and tone on the other person. This is already challenging for most of us. How, then, do you transfer these skills to email and social media? How do you learn to be an effective listener communicating through all of the obstacles of time, distance, speed, autocorrect, email overload, and the tendency of humans to read anxiously between the lines in the absence of evidence to the contrary?

It's not as hard to listen well online as you might think, though you might want to add on a few steps to be extra careful. For most adults, our "virtual empathy" turns out to be a lot like our thoughtfulness in our face-to-face encounters. We may need to supplement emotional cues that aren't evident by attending to punctuation (the exclamation point is widely used to convey enthusiasm), emoticons (thumbs up), and shorthand cues to ensure the reader knows we're just kidding (JK), enjoying the humor of the exchange (LOL), speculating (IMHO), or not wanting the words to be as heavy as they might seem (the emoticon with sunglasses, among thousands of others, works well here).

Indeed, research seems to suggest that we digital communicators are, overall, managing our relationships online about as well as we do anywhere. The available research suggests that those of us who balance our social online and real lives tend to be as kind in cyberspace as we are in person. Your abrupt boss is unlikely to send out sensitive emails; your fabulous big brother is going to text you the perfect words of encouragement before you take your baby to college.

You're probably listening online as well as you can, and many of the skills you are learning in this book will help you develop your virtual empathy too. Here are a few commonsense suggestions for minimizing online miscommunication:

- Don't send any written messages that would be hard for you to receive.
- Think about the person to whom you are writing. Be sensitive to his or her particular feelings of vulnerability.
- Take at least ten minutes before you respond to social media of any kind that makes your blood boil and would otherwise lead you to answer thoughtlessly. Remember that it's more dangerous to react in writing than to speak impulsively. Once a missive is out there, you can't take it back. You also won't be able to amend it as quickly or see its impact on other people. Be careful.

- If you try to clarify a confusing email or text through responsive listening, and after two rounds you sense that you're still not grasping what someone is saying, pick up the phone. Or better yet, arrange for a face-to-face exchange. The medium has limitations; some enduring misunderstandings need workarounds—like actual voice contact.
- Never end a friendship or a romantic relationship by text. It's cowardly, rude, and mean. Just don't.
- Don't rush to the worst conclusion even if you have an emotional response to what you are reading. You might be wrong. Or less right anyway.
- Never send anything without proofreading first.
- Don't assume you have the same expectations for the conversation as the other person. Don't assume she will respond as quickly, carefully, fully, or kindly as you do. As in the rest of our lives, our assumptions about relationships online can really interfere with connections.

Here's an example of the problems we can create when we ignore these guidelines. Just a few days ago, I failed to follow my own advice. A colleague wrote me an email reminding me of a piece of work I hadn't sent her yet. I dashed off this note: "So sorry; you're at the top of my crazy list." I didn't hear back from her, which was surprising since she usually replies quickly. I went back and reread my email. Could she have thought the word "crazy" referred to her rather than, as intended, the length of my to-do list? I immediately wrote again to clarify. Then she got right back to me, grateful for my apology and explanation; she laughed it off. But taking five more seconds to proofread would have been better.

How to Move Beyond Assumptions to Openness and Empathy

To listen well you must set aside memory, desire, and judgment. This is a formula for openness, calling as it does for listeners to suspend preconceptions, assumptions, and their own needs. Real listening is an act of self-transcendence.

However much the people in our lives care about us, they're still largely preoccupied with their own agendas: worries, problems, projects, grudges, hopes, dreams. Even (or especially) if unspoken, such personal agendas are compelling and absorbing. As long as they remain private, these preoccupations have a tendency to separate us from each other. Shared thoughts and feelings are a step toward each other. Empathy is the bridge.

An empathic listener inquires and acknowledges what we're thinking and feeling and thus confirms our experience. In this way the receptive listener vitalizes us by emotional participation and reflection—feeding back to us what we sometimes experience as inchoate.

People live in their own personal and subjective worlds. To meet, truly meet, means that they must open up parts of themselves and share them. And they must be received. Much of the time we hide away our real feelings, sometimes even from ourselves. As a result, our conversational encounters, like our relationships themselves, often consist of shadows dancing with each other.

Empathy bridges the gap between us, but it requires an effort at openness. Too many assumptions are inimical to understanding. You can hardly take in anything like the full richness of someone else's experience if you're just waiting for your turn. Empathy takes restraint; it takes work.

The empathic listener offers a bond of understanding in a deep sense. It's more than the dutiful sympathy you might get from your hairdresser. It's a deeper resonance of understanding. Perhaps you remember a time when you were hurt or scared and a friend put a hand on your shoulder. Empathy is like that.

Empathic listening means working a little harder at understanding the other person before asking him to do the same for you. It means demonstrating your understanding with comments that draw out the other person's thoughts and feelings: "Uh-huh," "I see," "Yes." Simple empathic comments express understanding and help bring out something unexpressed in the other person's experience. This helps break down the withholding of feeling that keeps us apart. Withholding is unnecessary with someone who cares and understands.

- - - - - - - - - - - - - -

The empathic listener celebrates the naturalness
of what is felt—"No wonder you were mad!"—and helps
to overcome the other person's tendency to hold back.

- - - - - - - - - - - - -

Empathy is achieved by suspending your assumptions and placing your-self attentively at the service of the other person, being alert to what he or she is saying and to the emotional subtext. It means listening without being in a hurry to take over.

Empathy requires two kinds of activity. The first is receptive openness, like a moviegoer who allows himself to be absorbed in a film and moved by the actors. The second is a balance between thinking and feeling. This requires a deliberate shift from feeling *with* a speaker to thinking *about* her. What is she saying? Meaning? Feeling?

Suppose your mate comes home and says he's had a bad day. You know what that feels like. You're sympathetic. So you ask what happened. He says he has to go out of town next week. His boss wants him to represent the agency at a meeting in Buffalo, and he's not looking forward to it.

You know how he feels. All that travel. And Buffalo of all places!

Maybe that's how *you'd* feel. You don't look forward to business trips because you don't like to be away from home.

Our own feelings make us sympathetic. But empathy, real empathy, requires a second step: thinking *about* the other person. How does his "not looking forward" feel?

Maybe he's excited about being chosen to speak for the agency. It's a chance to show the boss he can handle more responsibility. But maybe that makes him nervous. Speaking in public is a lot harder when your agenda is trying to prove yourself.

Whether or not your partner gets to talk about these issues, to clarify and share his feelings, depends on how empathically you listen. If you want to know how someone feels, ask.

· · · · · · · · · · · ·

Do you rely on sympathy and presume you understand,
or do you use empathy and work at it?

· · · · · · · · · · ·

Remaining open to what other people have to say is easier in the absence of conflict. Being at odds with someone means that you have your own agenda, and the conflict makes you anxious to press your point of view. But since two force fields can't occupy the same space at the same time, even if your only objective is to get your ideas across, the most effective way to do so is to hear the other person out first—make him feel understood and taken into account. Here are a couple of examples:

A few years ago a colleague who was editing a book on psychoanalytic therapy changed jobs and asked me to take over for him. I was delighted—until I saw that most of the chapters weren't very good. It was hard for me, a young and relatively unknown psychologist, to convince the authors, who were big shots, to do the necessary work. One of the authors, however, was very solicitous. He called every week to ask how the book was coming and even offered to be my coeditor. Then I read his chapter. It wasn't the worst, but it was close. Trying to be diplomatic, I returned the manuscript, praising its strong points and asking for a few minor changes. Three months went by. Then I received a letter thanking me for my "suggestions" but saying that a couple of his friends had read over his chapter and agreed with him that it was just fine the way it was. Arghh!

After counting to ten (about twenty times), I wrote saying that he seemed upset about something and I was interested in hearing about it. He called the day he received my letter and told me with a lot of feeling how hard he'd worked on his chapter and how much rewriting the previous editor had already put him through. I didn't really have to say anything. He was so appreciative of my listening to him that as soon as he finished complaining he thanked me for being understanding and said he'd be glad to make the changes I'd asked for.

With someone you do care about, empathic openness is more than a useful strategy. It's the essential means of discovering what things look like from inside that person's world.

Linda was certain that Andrew didn't like to spend time with her. He was married to his career. That's why she'd developed so many outside interests over the years. Now that the children had gone off into the wide world, Linda began to sense the marriage was over. Maybe it was time to turn off the life supports. She dreamed of freedom from the disappointment. What had she expected when she married? Attention, shared interests, affection, conversation. What she had was what she did on her own.

And Andrew? After years of professional success, his loneliness made him feel like a failure anyway. He longed to be closer to Linda, to share something more than domestic arrangements. He dreamed of love.

Unfortunately, they'd gotten out of the habit of talking. He went about his business wearing the armor of indifference.

When Linda came to see me—maybe a therapist would tell her what she wanted to hear—I tried to point out one reason she felt stuck: she wasn't open to the possibility of trying to talk to her husband, trying to rekindle some basis for staying together other than sharing children.

Linda had assumed that Andrew didn't want things to change and so it would be a waste of time talking to him. When Linda tried to open up and talk to Andrew, she found out that he had assumed she no longer wanted to be involved with him, so he didn't say anything.

Such assumptions are protective. They keep us from getting our hopes up and our feelings hurt. But they also keep us from getting through to each other.

> Most of our assumptions about why
> communication breaks down are about the other guy.
> We take our own input for granted.

After their talk Linda and Andrew did get a little closer. Not a lot, but enough to make a difference. Shared understanding was the first step.

Openness may be the key to listening, but not total openness, as in a blank screen. Real receptivity must be informed by sensitivity to other people.

Sensitivity: Expectations at Their Best

One of the things we learn after a while—sometimes a long while—is that different people have different emotional needs. If, for example, you need time alone when you're upset, it might be hard to remember that in the same circumstances the first thing your partner wants is to talk. People also have different ways of communicating. To be a good listener you have to be sensitive to other people's conversational styles. The automatic rhythms and nuances of a person's conversational style include such things as whether descriptions are detailed or abbreviated, whether the pace of speaking is fast or slow, and whether who-said-what-to-whom or what-I'm-working-on-now is the preferred topic. Cultural norms as well as personal styles guide how people approach listening; it helps to understand there is no single way to communicate that would or should work for all of us.

To Naomi, loud, overlapping talk was an indication of enthusiasm and mutual involvement. To Wardell, it was a sign of rudeness and not listening.

Yuki wants details; Makiko feels interrogated.

Rick wants Sherry to get to the point. To her, it feels like he isn't interested in what she has to say.

Veronica likes to talk things over. She complains that Steph is always leaving the room. Steph replies that Veronica says something and she responds, then when she goes to finish what she was about to do, Veronica gets mad.

Listening between intimates often erodes over time because the only way they know to solve problems is to talk things out or to bury them under the recycled newspaper. But when communication styles clash, talking this way doesn't help, and neither does the silent treatment. Trying harder, if it means doing more of the same, only makes matters worse.

People who communicate indirectly feel that people close to them should understand how they feel. Direct communicators think, "We should be able to tell each other what we want."

Being sensitive to other people's conversational ways doesn't mean you have to have them all figured out. It means you should be receptive. If you're used to a New York City pace and you're listening to a languid southern speaker whose conversation is like an old hound dog that stops at every tree, relax. Be patient. You might even get to enjoy the differences.

Unfortunately, when conversational styles differ, misunderstandings multiply. It's difficult to straighten out such differences if you're convinced of the rightness of your position and the wrongness of the other's.

Belinda was with her husband at a New Year's Eve party at his parents' house. Halfway through the evening, Belinda's mother-in-law came over and whispered, "Loosen up, have some fun. Don't be so formal!"

Belinda was annoyed. She had been having fun. She'd had several enjoyable conversations with her husband's cousins. She wasn't being formal; she was being herself.

Then Belinda was pissed. *Who does that woman think she is? Did I say anything to her about laughing hysterically whenever anybody said something?* In fact, Belinda found the mother-in-law's loud show of emotion and high-pitched chatter jarring. It wasn't her style.

Both of these people were behaving in self-evidently appropriate ways, the ways they were brought up to behave.

Some people consider their restrained style of speaking "polite." They find people with a more expressive style "crude," "loud," "histrionic," "vulgar." More emotive speakers think of themselves as "open and honest," "warm," "friendly," while they think of more restrained speakers as "aloof," "standoffish," "distant."

(Notice, incidentally, how Belinda and her mother-in-law each addressed their differences in character. The mother-in-law was "honest" or "rude," depending on your point of view. Belinda was "polite" or "aloof," as you see it.)

Sensitivity means being responsive to other people's feelings. It doesn't mean assuming you know what they're going to say; it means being interested enough to find out. On the other hand, sensitivity does mean using your knowledge of other people to understand their perspective and respect their individuality.

Some of the ways you can show sensitivity are:

- Paying attention to what the other person is saying
- Asking how the other person would like you to listen: "Do you want to vent or problem-solve?"
- Acknowledging the other person's feelings
- Listening before giving an opinion
- Listening without offering advice
- Suspending judgment and blame even if you've known each other forever
- Listening without immediately agreeing or disagreeing
- Asking "Is there more?" to be sure you've heard everything the person has to say

- Noticing how the other person appears to be feeling—and then asking
- Asking about his or her day, both before and after
- Respecting a person's need for quiet times
- Tolerating the other person's silence during a conversation as he gathers thoughts and gets on top of strong feelings
- Respecting a person's need to address problems
- Listening to but not pushing too hard for feelings
- Checking in some more at a later time

Maybe you won't get through to some people as long as you keep approaching them the same way you always do.

We're Most Insensitive to Those We Love

What makes someone insensitive to what others are saying? To figure out why a listener becomes reactive instead of listening, consider where the person's anxiety might be coming from. Sometimes anxiety comes from stress—real or imagined. People resist both actual and threatened change. We think of powerful people as dominating relationships and perhaps therefore not willing to listen, but in fact the powerless also have trouble listening. A man who feels that his opinions about the children aren't respected may resist his wife's efforts to talk about them. An elderly parent living in a three-generational home may not feel entitled to say what she wants (and doesn't want) so may be reluctant to participate in family decisions. Most people begin to listen better once they realize what power they do have in a relationship.

On the other hand, sometimes a person who clearly seems to have power in a relationship—a parent, say, or a dominating spouse—still doesn't listen. When a dominant person doesn't listen, it's usually because some hidden emotional issue is present, making him or her anxious.

One afternoon Tommy came home from school with so much restless energy that he decided to mow the lawn. The machine plowed into the deep grass, releasing its familiar sweet smell. But Tommy hadn't gone ten feet when the mower stalled, its blade clogged with wet grass. After several frustrating starts and stops, he shoved the insubordinate machine back into the garage, stomped into the house cursing and banging, went upstairs, and slammed his door.

By this time Tommy's stepfather, Jerome, came home. When Jerome asked what was the matter, Tommy told him about his lousy day at school, then coming home and the lawn mower not working. He was frustrated and angry.

Instead of empathizing, Jerome gave him a lecture. "When you have a problem, it doesn't do any good to lose control and start yelling. You have to stop and be calm. Nothing is accomplished when you get upset." As Jerome went on, Tommy's head sank slowly to his chest.

"You can't cut grass when it's a foot high and be in a hurry. You've got to go through it very, very slowly. You can't bull your way through anything— including life."

Tommy tried to explain. "Yeah, but when you've had a bad day at school and you come home and everything goes wrong, your anger keeps building. You've got to let it out somehow."

"Remember what we talked about last night? About problems? What did I say?"

"You said you've got to swallow your tongue." Tommy had stopped looking for sympathy and was now just trying to hang on to some of his pride.

But Jerome wasn't finished. "I also told you that problems when they're compounded make bigger problems. But if you take that problem and break it down, and make individual problems out of it, you can usually solve them very easily. Remember we talked about that?"

Tommy gave up trying to explain himself, and the conversation was finished.

This is a story of a stepparent's failure to listen—and worse. Jerome asks Tommy why he's upset and then, when the boy tries to tell him, instead of listening, gives him a speech on the futility of anger, a lecture for a course the boy didn't sign up for. Tommy attempted to explain his feelings because he was looking for understanding. Instead he became a captive audience forced to listen to an account of his own inadequacies and endure his stepfather's tedious pedantry.

What's so hurtful in this encounter (and others like it) isn't that Jerome has a different perspective from Tommy; it's that, because of the feelings Tommy's behavior arouses in him, he tries to allay his own anxieties by pushing his perspective on the boy. In this scenario, he's trying to play the part of father knows best; Tommy's perspective carries no weight. It's never even acknowledged. The real impact of these insensitive lessons for living may be that Tommy grows up to be one of those people, like Jerome, with didactic views on everything—and unable to listen.

But *why* was Jerome so unable to listen to him explain why he was upset? What was so threatening? Anger (and perhaps a shadow of anger: shame).

Emotional intolerance is a huge impediment to listening. Some people, like Jerome, are so uncomfortable with anger that they can't tolerate even normal amounts of this basic human emotion. They may get so involved in managing their own emotional reactivity that they feel the need to disconnect not only from the distressing feelings but also from the person who caused them. The superlogical stepdad who offers information instead of comfort is probably doing the best he can under the circumstances; however, he's only passing along his own feelings of shame and disconnection. And sadly, the boy will learn to keep his feelings to himself next time.

It's sad that we're so reactive to the people closest to us. The closer the relationship, the more engaged our own needs, and the more we need, the harder it is to be receptive.

Sensitivity to Other People's Inner Voices

One example of failing to be sensitive to other people's need to be heard is giving unwanted advice. When you're tempted to give advice, remember those conflicting inner voices. Doing so may not only stop you from wasting your breath (and credibility), but also might give you a fresh perspective on the person's feelings and how to approach him or her about a sensitive issue.

What if the issue has already touched off a tirade? The ideal response to the person who goes into a rage about something is to acknowledge what he's feeling. Something's bothering him, and he's trying to tell you that. But there are times when most of us find it impossible to listen to someone who's shrieking at us. As John Gottman has pointed out, we won't be able to hear what someone is saying no matter what we do if our heart rate is soaring. In that case, better to take a twenty-minute break. The question then might become not how to defuse the blowup but how to repair things afterward.

That's when thinking about the other person's rage and your reaction in terms of subpersonalities can help you gain a little empathy and insight. Seeing a person's tirade as a childish tantrum may help you figure out that he feels weak and helpless, not powerful. Powerful people don't scream. But if screaming scares you (welcome to the club), when you calm down, if you consider what kind of person the screaming reduced you to (a scared kid yourself, say), that in itself may help you recover your objective adult self when it comes to addressing the incident later.

"Have You Got a Minute?"

One way to use sensitivity to *get* better listening is by checking to see if the person you want to talk to is busy. People signal their openness to conversation by their posture. The person who looks up expectantly when you enter the room or shuts his laptop with a smile, or who walks up to you and says hello is probably open to talking. The person with her head down in her phone, looking away when you approach, checking email, or reading, or tending to a demanding toddler, or otherwise preoccupied may not feel like chatting. If you really want to talk to someone who might be busy, ask if he's available. "Have you got a minute?" It's like knocking to enter.

Recently Glenn started getting home from work an hour earlier. On the first day of the new schedule he looked forward to having a chance to talk with his sixteen-year-old son before dinner. He came in the door and called "Hi!" but there was no answer. Too bad, Charlie must have stayed after school. But then a few minutes later, he heard Charlie's speakers blaring upstairs.

Glenn climbed halfway up the stairs and called out, "Hey, Charlie, it's me, Dad. Come on downstairs. I want to talk with you."

A few moments later Charlie came into the living room and said, "What did I do?"

Glenn felt bad. Is that what their relationship had come to?

No, not really. Charlie just felt off guard and misconstrued what his father meant. So now on days when he expects to be home early, Glenn shoots him a text before leaving work. "I'll be home around five-thirty. Maybe we can hang out while I fix supper."

. . . .

Expectations about how and when
communication should take place work
not when they're right or wrong but when they're shared.

. . . .

Self-Reflective Observation

Consideration for others helps make you sensitive enough to be a better listener. But even more important is developing self-reflective awareness. When you have trouble hearing someone or getting someone to hear you, step back and examine the process of communication between the two of you as just that—a *process*. You'll need to get beyond brooding about personalities to thinking about actions and reactions. And you'll need to get beyond the linearity of thinking that the other person *makes* you respond the way you do to seeing the process as circular.

Say that your teenage daughter never talks to you. Oh, she'll let you know when she needs new jeans or a ride somewhere, but you miss the talks you used to have when she was younger. Now she's so sullen. You can write off this uncommunicativeness to adolescence if you like, or you can think of it as part of a circular process.

To reflect on your part in the process, ask yourself what might cause your daughter's reticence or what might reinforce it. Do you pry into things that she isn't going to divulge, like which of her friends gets high or vapes? Are most of your "conversations" about undone chores, incomplete homework, the disarray of her room, or being nicer to her little brother? Do you bombard her with questions when she wants to retreat to the sanctuary of her room? Do you start conversations when she's tired or trying to do her homework? And when she does open up, do you show respect for her opinions or argue with everything she says?

How Well Do You Listen to Yourself?

The respect for other people's feelings that makes you listen to them can be turned around to yourself. How well do you respect your right to think and feel what you do? How well do you listen to yourself?

Kate suffered from chronic headaches but had given up going to doctors because it never did any good. None of them ever figured out what was wrong, and few of them bothered to listen carefully to her complaints. Finally, at her sister's urging, she went to the headache clinic at a leading hospital in Boston.

One of the tests they did was a CAT scan of her brain. Afterward, Kate waited anxiously for the radiologist who would explain the results. When he finally arrived, it was clear that he was rushed. He introduced himself, but Kate didn't catch his name. Then he showed her the pictures from the CAT scan, and she saw a small white spot on the film. "That's just a normal calcification of your pineal gland," he said, "nothing to worry about."

As the doctor headed for the door, Kate felt unsatisfied and wished the conversation could have gone on a little longer. But she wasn't sure how to frame her questions and was embarrassed that she didn't remember the doctor's name.

Halfway out the door, the doctor turned and said, "Any other questions?"

Kate answered in a subdued voice, "No."

Kate heard the doctor's anxiousness to leave. But she was far less well tuned in to her own needs. Her fear and uncertainty, combined with the doctor's rushed manner, had created a cloud of fog surrounding her own needs.

> If you don't listen to yourself,
> it's unlikely that anyone else will.

Listening to yourself means not only respecting your own feelings, but also getting to know something about your style of communicating. This isn't always easy, and it isn't always pleasant.

I, for example, have a penchant for making jokes and wisecracks in social situations. Maybe some of my jokes are funny, but they're often distracting. Joking around may be a defense against social anxiety, or maybe it's just an outlet for restless energy. Whatever the reasons for it, there are times when I have to make an effort to suppress the smart remarks that pop into my head.

You may find it easier to recognize other people's conversational habits you wish they would change. But the effort to understand your own ways will enable you to relate more effectively to other people, regardless of what they do.

In Chapter 2, I mentioned that one of the reasons people seek solitude is that they haven't learned to handle their anxiety around other people. But solitude has its uses, especially if it isn't frittered away checking email, playing video games, or posting images on social media. Being alone without distractions gives you time to listen to yourself. To hear your own thoughts. To think them through. Among the things you may find yourself thinking about are feelings you haven't been aware of and conversations that didn't go as well as you would have liked.

Most of us run around doing things all day. All too often, our actions are driven rather than undertaken with awareness. When you get caught up in a river of obligations, it winds up submerging your life as it carries you along. If you are waiting for a cup of coffee, sitting on the bus, taking a walk, or engaging in any other solitary mundane activity, the temptation to check your phone may be overwhelming. But then, when you grab for it, you aren't alone any longer. It's no wonder we struggle to listen to other people when we have so much trouble tolerating our own company—the voices in our own head deserve attention too.

"I Don't Have a Minute to Catch My Breath."

Well, here's your chance. Find a couple of times during the next few days to sit down with yourself without distractions. Tune in to your breathing. Concentrate on one full inhalation as it comes in and one exhalation as it goes out. One more in, and one more out. Relax and breathe. After you quiet down, listen to what's going on inside of you.

. . . .

Do you have the patience
to wait till your mud settles and the water is clear?
—LAO-TZU

. . . .

I always regretted that I didn't go to a psychoanalytic institute after graduate school. So, after practicing for a number of years, I decided to go back and do it. At the institute I took classes and received supervision on my cases. In supervision you find out what you should have said, so that, hopefully, you'll do better next time. Supervision made me a better therapist, and it also made me feel a little stupid every week. *Why did I say that? Why didn't I see this?*

After finishing my course of study, I returned to my practice and became my own supervisor. I was by then much more aware after a session of things I missed or wished I had said. But instead of feeling stupid (or just feeling stupid), I started writing letters to patients between sessions. I might sum up what we talked about if I thought I hadn't made something clear, and sometimes I'd put things in the letter that I just hadn't thought of in the session.

Maybe you too are your own supervisor. Maybe you come away from certain conversations wishing you'd said something differently or wishing you'd been a better listener. You can try to do better next time, or you can seek out the person you have unfinished business with and try again to hear what he or she was saying and then clarify what you meant to say. Asking for clarification and feedback—even days later—will convey the caring you feel, open the opportunity to repair a conversation that could have gone better, and help to make you a better listener in the long run.

EXERCISES

1. Once or twice in the coming week, think about what you will be doing and whom you will be talking with. Predict what might happen if you made a concerted effort to listen to those people. Pick someone you care about. Consider what might distract you from listening. At the end of the day, take five minutes to reflect on what happened in those

conversations. How well did you listen? What made it difficult? What was the result of your efforts?

2. Practice not interrupting people who are talking to you. Try to come up with two or three lines that invite people to finish what they're saying. You could say, "mm-hmm," or "tell me more," or find something that seems to work for you. You may or may not find this device helpful. The point is not to interrupt. Cultivate patience.

3. Try asking "Do you have a minute?" before telling people what's on your mind. What effect does this seem to have on the quality of the listening you get?

4. We develop empathy for others when we know what it feels like ourselves. Indeed, it is much harder to experience compassion for someone else's joy or pain when we don't feel we are deserving of it. Sit and breathe deeply with each of these sentences for a moment. What does it feel like to say them to yourself or to imagine someone speaking these words to you? Where in your body do you feel the impact? See if your curious attention leads to feelings like sadness or wistfulness or even anger. Stay with whatever the feelings are and see what happens next. If you are having skeptical thoughts, take time to study those too.

- I want to support you.
- You are a good person.
- You have done enough.
- I understand your pain.
- I will protect you.
- You are important.
- You are interesting.

9

"I Can See
This Is Really Upsetting You"

HOW TO DEFUSE EMOTIONAL REACTIVITY

We come now to the number one reason people don't listen: reactive emotionalism. As we saw in Chapter 6, when someone says something that triggers anxiety, understanding goes out the window. If failing to acknowledge what the other person says turns discussions into conversational Ping-Pong, overreacting can turn them into the Battle of the Bulge. If the war metaphor seems melodramatic, take inventory of your feelings the next time a series of attacks and counterattacks leaves you wounded.

Some people are so provocative that it's almost impossible to listen to them without getting upset. But regardless of what other people say, your problem is how you react.

And what about those thin-skinned individuals who fly off the handle at the slightest sign of criticism? Sure, they're overreactive, but unless your relationship to them is expendable, your challenge is finding a way to get through to them.

Empathy Turns Defensiveness Around

We're all insecure to some extent. Therefore, when we feel threatened, we tend to react defensively rather than being open to the other person's point of view.

One reason people pay thousands of dollars to psychotherapists is simply to be listened to. (Good therapists may do more than just listen, but they certainly do no less.) When people complain about other people in their lives, a therapist doesn't feel blamed and therefore doesn't get defensive. But when you talk to the people you're close to about your upsets, they feel implicated. That's why their response is often reactive: "No, don't feel that way!" An accepting, nonreactive response feels like "Yes, is that how you feel? Tell me more."

People Are Defensive for a Reason

When someone says, "You pay more attention to your parents than you do to me," a reactive response might be "I hardly ever see them!"

What imagined threat might the reactive partner be defending against?

What would be an empathic response to "You pay more attention to your parents than you do to me"?

How might an empathic response put you in a more vulnerable position? A more empowered position?

Empathy is permission giving. Receptive, nondefensive listeners allow us to get our feelings out. They welcome unpopular parts of us to speak (which allows us to do the same for ourselves). They recognize that even on those occasions when what we're saying about them may not be true, our feelings are.

> Feelings are facts
> to the person experiencing them.

The simple—and often enormously difficult—act of not becoming reactive has a tremendous impact on relationships. It enables you to handle difficult conversations—and it empowers you to remain in control under pressure.

How to Avoid Reacting Emotionally
When Provoked

Every so often Nadine lets out her frustration in the form of an emotional outburst about Tim's many failings:

"You're selfish and inconsiderate."

"You *never* think of anyone but yourself."

"You don't care about me; all you want is sex!"

Tim can't stand these tirades. *If she's unhappy, why can't she just say so without calling me every name in the book?* Tim tries to listen to Nadine's complaints, but by the time she's through dumping, Tim just wants to go away and hide.

When Gordon complains about Paul's handling of a customer, Paul gets furious. First Gordon leaves everything to him, then he criticizes Paul for doing what he thinks is right. *Gordon's always right, and he's always wrong.* So Paul lets Gordon know just how he feels.

All four of these people have a right to their feelings. The trouble is, no one is listening. To listen without flying off the handle, you have to learn to tolerate a certain amount of anxiety—and to resist the "fight or flight" urge.

"Don't Get Defensive!"

The trouble with this famous advice is that it's harder to *stop* doing something than it is to *start* doing something else. If you're trying to cut down on coffee, it's easier to pour yourself a cup of tea than to sit there not drinking coffee. If you want to stop eating junk food, it's easier to grab a carrot than to try to avoid the urge to tear open the potato chips. If you want to reduce your emotional reactivity, concentrate harder on listening. (If "listening harder" seems abstract, just try listening longer.)

You probably know how it feels to be berated or found fault with by someone who's better at criticizing than helping. But getting reactive only makes things worse. Tim thinks his problem is Nadine's emotional exaggeration. But a fuller description of the problem would be that when Nadine feels ignored she tries not to say anything until she can't stand it anymore and then her feelings come pouring out—*and* Tim isn't able to pick up her signals of unhappiness before she explodes or, when she does, to listen without getting angry and pulling away. Likewise, Paul's problem isn't just that Gordon leaves the difficult customers to him and then complains about his handling of them. Paul's reaction—getting mad and counterattacking—is part of what keeps Gordon from getting more involved.

A full description of any listening problem
must include both parties.

What defeats us isn't the provocative speaker but our own defensive response.

The best way to master emotional reactivity is by having the courage to engage emotionally intense situations and tolerate the anxiety associated with that engagement. Avoiding such encounters affords only the illusion of self-control.

Ginny didn't call her mother after being in a car accident because she didn't want to have to deal with her mother's frantic questions and exaggerated concern. So she burdened herself with another secret and reinforced her own inability to deal with emotional pressure.

Learn to resist the impulse to act out your usual defensive response—avoiding, arguing, stonewalling, blaming, rebelling, dominating, or accommodating to achieve peace at any price. These reactions are driven by anxiety and designed to mask it by avoiding issues and defying, avoiding, or appeasing others. Facing up to people and situations you'd prefer to avoid, and learning to contain your own reactive reflexes, leads over time to a reduction of your anxiety.

In Chapter 6, I talked about hostile questions. Something a speaker says (or maybe it's just sitting there being lectured to) makes someone in the audience restive, and he or she attacks the speaker in the sublimated form of a question.

"Excuse me," said the eminent French deconstructionist Claude Nasal-Passages, who just happened to be in the audience, "but isn't everything you've just said total blather and you're full of nothing but helium?" In big words, of course.

Unfortunately, having just stood up in front of an audience for an hour or so pouring out their ideas, some speakers get a little touchy at such moments. And I've noticed (in other people, you understand) a certain unfortunate tendency to respond in kind.

"Well, yes, Professor Nasal-Passages, that's an intriguing point. But you're a pompous ass, and so is the horse you rode in on." Big words, again.

A better way to respond to hostile questions is to apply Formula Number One for resisting reactivity: hear the person out. Instead of agreeing or disagreeing, invite the questioner to say more. Hostile inquisitors aren't really asking questions; they just want to say something. So let them.

The same strategy works to keep reactivity from escalating in everyday conversations. Here's how a friend used this advice to reduce the antagonism that was starting to poison his second marriage.

When Rob married Carla, they got along wonderfully well, except when it came to Rob's daughter. According to Carla, Rob spoiled Melanie, like "lending" her money that she didn't usually repay and letting her have the car whenever she wanted, even though she didn't always bring it back when she said she would. But whenever Carla raised any objection, Rob felt she was attacking his child, and so instead of hearing what she had to say, he fought back. Many second marriages are broken on this very issue.

When Rob realized the situation had reached the point of crisis, he resolved to at least listen to Carla the next time she complained about Melanie. Two days later he got his chance. Melanie promised to have the car back by eight so Carla could go shopping, but she didn't get home until nine-thirty, after the stores were closed. When Carla complained to Rob, he felt his stomach knotting and the counterarguments forming. But instead of getting defensive, he said what he'd prepared himself to say: "Tell me more."

Carla said that overindulgence wasn't doing Melanie any good. Rob, sticking to his resolve not to interrupt, kept listening, and Carla went on. She talked about feeling like an outsider in her own house. She knew that Rob and Melanie had a special relationship, and she respected that. She had no wish to play Melanie's mother or tell Rob what to do. She just wanted to be able to talk to him when she felt concerned. Having determined not to argue, Rob found it remarkably easy to listen—that is, after he checked the rising emotions that Carla's first few sentences triggered in him. He stopped hearing in Carla the overbearing voice of his ex-wife, who was always so critical of him and the children, and started hearing how left out his new wife was feeling. He was able to hear that Carla wasn't asking him to change anything, just asking him to listen to her point of view. After that, things changed. They didn't always agree about how to respond to Melanie, but now that Rob knew that he could listen to Carla's opinion without necessarily following it, their differences ceased to divide them.

Prepare for Tense Encounters

The best way to defuse reactivity is to avoid becoming reactive yourself, something more easily said than done. One thing that helps is planning, as Rob was able to do once he realized how serious his breach with Carla was becoming. You can predict many of the difficult conversations in your life. If you stop to think about what the boss or your teenager is likely to say to trigger your anxiety, you can prepare for it.

> Anticipation frees you from overreacting.
> Plan ahead of time how you'll respond instead.

One way to remain calm is by schooling yourself to ask questions instead of flaring up at the usual provocations. This is a variation of the "tell me more" strategy. Another way to tone down emotionality is to respond to rhetorical questions and sarcasm literally, instead of being provoked into a defensive retort.

"Don't you ever think about anything but sex?"
"No, it's kind of a hobby with me. Like woodworking."

"Must you pick on every little thing I say?"
"Yes, all in the service of helping you become the perfect person I know you're capable of being."

Another way to become calmer is to become curious about why you are getting hooked by this particular provocation. A mother who got punished severely for being disrespectful to her own parents may actually feel inordinately distressed when her son rolls his eyes at her. She bites her tongue, knowing it's not worth having a fight about a little "attitude," but the clench in her stomach is familiar, a sensation from long ago that unsettles her. Instead of becoming reactive, however, she reflects for a moment. She can then get unhooked. She takes a breath and remembers that he's basically a great kid. In her calm adult mind, she knows that eye rolling at a mom is just another part of being a teenager.

How to Understand a Speaker's Anger

When people start to cry, many of us feel an urge to comfort them so that they'll stop. We equate the crying with pain. In fact, crying isn't pain; it's the way people release their pain. The same can be true with expressions of anger (even if it's a little harder to keep that in mind).

I once watched a therapist interviewing a couple five years into a second marriage. They were having a hard time deciding how to balance their obligations to three sets of children and an even harder time keeping the discussion from turning into a shouting match. As the wife was saying her piece and starting to go on and on, rehashing the past and finding fault, her husband's foot started twitching ominously. Sitting behind the one-way mirror, I felt apprehensive. I could see an explosion coming but couldn't do anything about it.

Then the therapist, bless him, did exactly what needed to be done. He acknowledged what the wife had said and then let the husband speak— being careful to direct the husband to speak to the therapist who could listen, not to his wife, who at that point couldn't. Even so, the husband exploded. With hot emotion he refuted what his wife had said and explained the truth of things as he saw it. As he talked to the therapist—with his wife blocked from responding—he calmed down perceptibly. His jaw relaxed, the tension went out of his shoulders, and his foot stopped twitching. Not having a chance to express his anger made it build. Expressing it in a safe environment, *even in an angry way,* released the anger.

The hard part would be teaching this couple to listen to each other without flying off the handle in the future —without someone mediating and helping to diffuse the overwhelming feelings. It's one thing to understand that expressing anger sometimes helps detoxify it; it's another thing to be on the receiving end.

The wife in the couple I observed was angry because her husband questioned her motives. She thought one of the children, who happened to be her son, needed some financial assistance. Her husband was jealous of the attention she paid this son and felt she was neglecting him. "He's twenty-three years old. He can take care of himself." But it wasn't disagreeing that caused their problems; it was getting reactive and shouting at each other. If he would concentrate on understanding what she was *feeling* and not allow himself to react defensively, he'd understand that she was worried about her boy. She might or might not decide to give him some money; that was just an idea, a way of expressing her concern. Her husband wasn't really upset about the money but about not getting as much attention as he wished for. Unfortunately, instead of talking about his feelings, he blamed her for them.

Indeed, there was little in the exchange to suggest the husband even knew what his feelings were. For many people, the expression of anger can serve as a permissible and righteous stand-in for more vulnerable feelings. For example, the husband may have craved the comfort of her attention because he really felt jealous, ignored, frightened, worried, or lonely; he masked his vulnerability with rage. If he were able to give voice to these softer parts that the anger guarded like a junkyard dog, it's quite possible his wife would be better able to turn toward him in response.

· · · · · · · · · · · ·

When feelings of not being understood come out as anger,
hearing them, not shutting your ears or fighting back,
is the key to calming things down.

· · · · · · · · · · · ·

Lizzie had her driver's license and the use of her father's car as long as she followed his rules about it. She had to keep the tank full, let him know where she was and when she'd be home, and clean the Dunkin' cups out of it before handing back the keys. Lizzie was also a bit of a pushover about giving rides to friends; he had told her he worried that she was being used as a taxi service and she'd said she understood his concerns.

One day after school, she took her best friend, Gwendolyn, to a family planning clinic where she waited for three hours. She was late coming home and getting the car back. To protect Gwendolyn's privacy, she'd also intended, if need be, to lie about where she had been. Her father was angry and frustrated that she had not followed the rules. He had expected her home over an hour earlier. He was worried about her, and it came out as anger. Lizzie listened to his tirade, saying nothing other than "I'm really sorry, Dad; I should have texted" and "I was out with Gwendolyn" to reassure him she'd been with a friend. She didn't escalate matters by defending herself or making up lies or offering excuses. Her willingness to listen and apologize disarmed him, and his anger passed. After a few minutes, he was able to tell her that he had been really worried and they hugged and moved on.

Denise was backing out of a parking space when she felt the SUV smack into the right side of her car. When she opened her door, the woman in the SUV was screaming at her. "Why don't you look where you're going, you stupid bitch!" Denise struggled to stay calm while she exchanged insurance information, called AAA, and rode to the garage in the tow truck. When she finally got home and told her roommates what had happened, she started to cry.

"That woman had no right to scream at me!" she said with rising emotion.

"Calm down," Alysha said. "There's no reason to get upset. Just tell us what happened."

Monique piled on, adding, "You didn't get hurt, right? It's just a car, and you have insurance."

That's when Denise lost it. "Don't tell me to calm down!" she said. "You're not the ones whose car got smashed and then had to put up with that abuse!" At this point her anger shifted from that woman in the SUV to her housemates' lack of sympathy.

> Don't tell angry people to calm down.
> Doing so only makes them feel
> that you're denying their right to be upset.

If someone snaps at you in anger, how do you get beyond listening with a clenched mind? The obvious answer is to listen through the emotional static to what the person is trying to say. But that's easier said than done. When frustration and anger spill out into a relationship, our natural response is to become anxious and defensive. Listening to someone who assaults you with his feelings isn't easy. One thing that may help keep you from withdrawing into a defensive posture is hearing in the anxious speaker the voice of an unhappy child crying to be heard. Your empathy for her pain beneath the aggression can be the sympathy that keeps you present.

If, instead of dwelling on how difficult the speaker is, you can focus on your own efforts to listen and avoid overreacting, the anxiety in the relationship will begin to abate. Anxiety is electric. It requires conduction and amplification. If you listen and stay cool, the angry person will feel heard and begin to calm down.

In heated discussions, repeating the other person's position in your own words shows that you understand and interrupts your own defensive response. If the heat gets so intense that you start to seethe, try squeezing your thumb and index finger together and focus on your breathing. This momentary distraction (less hazardous to your health than "biting your tongue") may help you channel your tension in a way you can control.

If that doesn't work, or an emotionally reactive speaker is dumping on you and it's too upsetting, you may have to protest. Doing so before you get too upset, and without attacking, keeps your anger from boiling over: "I'm sorry, but I can't listen to this right now. I'm too upset. We'll have to talk later."

How to Take Criticism Without Overreacting

He says, "You're always late."

She says, "You're always rushing me."

One point for him. One point for her. Collective score: zero.

Allowing the other person to spell out her point of view before responding with yours is especially important—and especially difficult—when someone is criticizing you. If you start to react, ask yourself, Does the person have a sincere concern about this issue (even if she could work on her delivery)? If the answer is yes, keep listening. If she's right, step up and say so. Nothing stops a fight quite like acknowledging your responsibility in it.

If your partner complains about where you park in the driveway, you might consider that he has a legitimate stake in the matter. If, on the other hand, he criticizes how you talk to your boss, you might remember that how you decide to talk to your boss is your business. Come to think of it, remembering that might make it easier to listen without feeling the need to defend yourself.

If someone criticizes you, stay with that concern; don't switch to a different criticism of your own. Avoid cross-complaining.

> "Oh yeah? Well, what about you? You never take out the garbage when I ask you to."
>
> "I don't care if you don't like what's for supper. Maybe if you cleaned up your room once in a while like I asked, I'd feel more like cooking something you like."

After you allow your critic to spell out her complaint, agree with whatever you can, or at least acknowledge her concern.

> "Yes, I have been a little grouchy lately. I'm sorry."
>
> "So you think I've been favoring Cindy over Joshua?"
>
> "I know you are worrying about me."
>
> "Yes, I did run over your prize Pomeranian in the driveway. I'll get you a new one."

Okay, so I'm saying that when someone starts to criticize you, the thing to do is to hear him out and acknowledge his point of view before defending yourself. But isn't that a little like saying that to lose ten pounds all you have to do is cut out sweets? When someone starts in on you, especially someone close to you, it isn't easy to nod and say, "Oh, so you think I'm a selfish species of barnyard animal? I see. Please tell me more."

Listening to criticism is one of the hardest things we ever have to do. Unfortunately, getting defensive only makes things worse. To avoid doing so, train yourself to listen responsively—pay attention, appreciate what the other person is saying, and acknowledge it. This takes practice, but you can make it a habit. The active effort to listen helps prevent you from becoming reactive.

Focus on the issue. Try to hear in the criticism something the other person is asking you to do for him or her rather than a condemnation of yourself.

Sid and Nancy have a son who has a taste for exotic food. By the time he was twelve they had traveled all over the world, and Milo had sampled fried crickets and spicy curries. He can be annoying about what his parents, both working big jobs, manage to get on the table during the week. Nancy is trying to cut down on carbs even though when she gets home she's so hungry she'd eat a sleeve of crackers if that's all she could get her hands on. Sid doesn't much enjoy cooking but steps up when he has to.

Like tonight. It's already after six, so he makes spaghetti with a jar of sauce, which Milo greets with "Spaghetti again?" and Nancy sighs.

Sid is irritated. Where's the gratitude? He sulks for the duration of the meal, seemingly unaware that both Nancy and Milo have helped themselves to seconds. He finally sputters, "You guys are so critical. It makes me want to never cook dinner again." They look up at him in astonishment. What?

If Sid could take a moment and think about what just happened instead of only listening to his own hurt feelings, he might realize that Milo hadn't exactly been critiquing the meal and that Nancy's sigh might have indicated exhaustion and relief as much as disappointment.

Try to remember: expression *releases* resentment.

What if, despite all your efforts to be a good person and a patient listener, criticism (whether directly aimed or implicit as a sigh) comes out feeling like an attack?

If criticism is given in a nasty or offensive way, you have a right to object to the manner in which the message was expressed. But if you don't want to listen to someone who berates you in an assaultive way, simply state what put you off.

"I don't appreciate being called stupid" (or compared to my mother, or called a bitch or a son of one).

"I'll try to listen to your suggestion if you can say it in a less nasty way."

Actually, the word *nasty* is name-calling. Better to be concrete:

"I'll try to listen to your suggestion if you can say it without telling me how selfish I am"—or "if you give me some idea of what you want."

"It hurts my feelings when you talk to me that way; if your intention is to give me feedback here, can you try a nicer way to put it?"

Will kinder criticism calm things down and allow the two of you to understand each other? Probably not. But sometimes you have to let other people know what your limits are.

"Why Does He [or She] Have to Talk Everything to Death?"

DeMarcus wishes twenty-four hours would go by without Jada's complaining about how nobody appreciates her at the office. Sometimes he feels like screaming. If she weren't so preoccupied with her precious career, maybe she'd get a little more appreciation from him and the children. He doesn't say so, of course. She'd only get mad and sulk. So whenever Jada starts in on topic number one, DeMarcus just sits there in pained silence.

Maggie and Katie wish their mother would stop launching into a diatribe every time she feels overwhelmed by how much work it is raising them alone. They try to help, but they have school and activities. It isn't even that she doesn't have a right to complain; it's the way she goes on and on about everything. They try to be sympathetic and not to burden her with their problems, but it isn't easy. Cheryl knows they're actually pretty wonderful girls who help out as much as they could reasonably be expected to, but she still comes home and starts in about the house being a mess and the kids doing nothing useful with their time. The worst of it, as far as the kids are concerned, is that she's always complaining about the same things. "Katie left her clothes in the dryer." "Maggie, why hasn't the dog been fed?" "Who finished the milk and left the carton on the counter?" "You kids are going to be the death of me."

The issues that come up over and over again represent people's core concerns. (*Their* core concerns, not necessarily your greatest shortcomings.) The more understood and accepted people feel, the safer they feel to go deeper into these issues. The mechanical and repetitive feeling of some complaints stems partly from the fact that they rarely get a sympathetic hearing. Listening is the greatest gift you can give to help soothe a person's feelings. Jada's feeling that nobody appreciates her accomplishments, and Katie and Maggie's mother's worries about being able to take care of her children on her own will never be completely resolved. That's why they need to talk about these things from time to time.

When people bring up recurring issues, some of us get upset and say something like "How many times do we have to go through this?" Such retorts make sense if you feel that the speaker's complaints mean that you're responsible or that it's your job to solve whatever problem the person is complaining about. But is it really your job to resolve your partner's work stress or your mother's complaints about your sister? Once you understand that other people's talking about what's bothering them makes them feel better, you can relax, knowing that just listening without becoming reactive (or imagining there's a demand out there for you to fix something you can't) can make both of you feel better.

. . . .

Sharing problems makes people feel understood.
Listening is how we help them feel better
and how we build closer relationships.

. . . .

For those who can get beyond blaming others for "making" them upset, discovering what triggers their sensitivity leads to the question "Where does my emotional reactivity come from?"

Getting to the Root of Reactivity

Reactivity develops as a defense against personal attacks. The more our parents listened, took us seriously, and respected our opinions and feelings, the more secure and self-possessed we became. The less they listened, the more intolerant and critical they were, the more insecure and anxious we became. The more exposed we were to accusations and arguments, the more we learned to become defensive.

What happens in your family when people get anxious? Do they get into shouting matches? Stop talking and avoid each other? That's your legacy.

> **Back to the Past**
>
> Making peace with your parents means being in emotional contact with them, being yourself, and letting them be themselves. Changing your relationship to them doesn't mean changing them; it means changing the way you react to them. Notice what they do that drives you crazy. Notice how you respond. *That* you can change. The more you learn to resist the urge to flare up in the face of their provocations, the more self-possessed and unflappable you'll become in all the rest of your relationships (see Chapter 13). When it comes to emotional reactivity, your parents are the final exam.

Remember Peggy from Chapter 5? She was the woman whose mother's negativism provoked her into shouting matches. Peggy learned to see how her mother's negativism triggered her own rage—and how expecting it made her hypersensitive. Seeing this pattern was one thing; changing it was another.

When Peggy decided to stop trying to change her mother, she began to realize that her mother wasn't really a mean person, just someone who prized togetherness so much that she was threatened when people acted independently. This simple shift in Peggy's view of her mother made it a lot easier for her to listen the next time she heard her mother criticizing someone in the family for doing something different. However, she also found that simply remaining silent only made her seethe. So instead of just holding her tongue or criticizing her mother (for being critical!) she started to say, as calmly as possible, that she could see how her mother saw it but that she didn't agree.

At first Peggy's effort to clarify where she stood, rather than criticize her mother, was lost on her mother. "Oh, so you think I'm all wrong, do you?"

Much to Peggy's credit, she was able to maintain a calm, nonreactive position, even if her insides were churning. She listened until her mother was through and didn't contradict her or fight back.

When Peggy finally did speak, she said, "No, Mom, you're not hearing me. I'm not saying you're all wrong. I don't think that at all. You have a right to your opinion. I'm just saying that my opinion is different, that's all."

In the ensuing months, as Peggy continued to make an effort to speak up calmly when she disagreed with her mother's uncharitable opinions, she tried to make it clear that she was declaring her independence but not any lack of love or respect. On the contrary, as she learned to overcome her inability to tolerate her mother's criticism, the two women began to get closer. Peggy still occasionally slipped back into blaming and distancing, but not for long, and when this happened, instead of thinking of her mother as impossible and herself as helpless, she realized that she was just getting reactive again. That made it easier to control.

She and her mother still argued from time to time, but now Peggy spoke up before her annoyance reached the boiling point. That and the fact that instead of criticizing her mother she made a point of simply clarifying where she stood made the arguments much less toxic.

"I've Tried to Change Things with My Parents, but It Hasn't Worked."

Systems are tenacious and resistant to change; or to put it in more human terms, your parents have a long history of relating to you in a certain way. If you try to change that, you will be tense and their reaction will be intense. Have a plan when you visit. Remember that when you reenter the family's emotional force field, your ability to think about what's going on is impaired. So do your thinking beforehand. Formulate reasonable goals. When you try a new way of behaving, start with small steps.

The people close to us don't have any tricks up their sleeves. Their actions surprise us only because we keep looking for them to do what we wish they'd do. They do what they do. Once you learn this, you can stop being surprised and upset. You can let them be who they are. You might as well; they will anyway.[3]

---

[3]One of my patients once told me without irony that her father "could be a wonderful person, if only he were different."

A relationship matures when you can allow the other person to be who she is. If your mother criticizes everybody *and* you can't accept this, your life may be dominated by your attempt to stop her (and everybody else, for that matter) from criticizing anything or anyone. Once you can let your mother be a person who's critical—in other words, accept that she is who she is—you don't have to fight it or organize your life around it.

- - - - - - - - - - -

Once you accept that people are who they are,
you can stop trying to change them—
and stop overreacting when they do what they've always done.

- - - - - - - - - - -

Peggy's more relaxed approach didn't stop her mother from being critical, but it did make Peggy a whole lot less reactive—and to the other people in her life who touched the same raw nerves.

Why Emotional Reactivity Increases as Relationships Evolve

In the early stages, most relationships are fairly comfortable. People can talk and listen without too much tension; otherwise the relationship wouldn't get very far. Such harmony, however, is time limited. Relationships, like unstable chemical compounds, tend to deteriorate. Once a relationship becomes heated with emotional reactivity, it may have to be cooled down with emotional distance—avoidance of one another, or at least of potentially upsetting subjects. But if the two parties are closeted together or try to discuss emotionally charged issues, one or both of them may start spilling over with anxiety.

One person may act to preserve harmony by giving in and doing all the listening. The other person may be unaware of the disparity. But it takes two to preserve this inequality. The mistake the placater makes is to confuse self-denial with self-restraint. The latter strategy allows both people to win; the former makes losers of them both. But as long as one person is cowed by the other's emotionality, and the other continues to express himself in the same old way, both of them are preserving the unhappy equilibrium.

The emotional climate in a relationship varies from hot to cold, turbulent to stable, and safe to unsafe. The presence of unresolved conflict makes for storminess. For example, if Jack feels he plays second fiddle to Jill's hours of viola practice, whenever she goes to her studio or to rehearsals his anxiety will be triggered anew. That's their particular enactment of unresolved conflict. Most intimate partners engage in a particular "fight" that they haven't been able to finish that stands in for a core conflict between them.

> What is one conflict you have repeatedly with someone you are close to? What do you think underlies your emotional reactivity? How do you think you could respond to this underlying issue instead?

When someone opens up on you with a mean mouth or listens with only feigned interest, it's natural to blame personality. When someone erupts at something you say, it can be impossible not to blame this outburst on the other person. But reactivity, like everything else in a relationship, is interactional. The only part of the equation you can change is your part.

. . . .

Trying to avoid or control other people
doesn't resolve your reactivity.

. . . .

A listener's oversensitivity festers and flourishes when she is preoccupied about giving too much or getting too little.

Mim has a lifelong history of feeling like she gives more than she gets from people. Her sensitivity to rejection has created something of a self-fulfilling prophecy for her: she acts in ways that almost ensure the very abandonment she dreads. Mim's reactivity actually causes people to avoid her, increasing her sense of alienation and loneliness. Mim's insecurity leaves her feeling vulnerable. But she's stuck: she can't depend on other people to take care of her and doesn't really feel capable of meeting her own needs. Her anxious and unreasonable strategies for getting care and attention ultimately serve only to increase her reactivity and misery.

To cut down on reactivity, respect your right to be yourself
and other people's right to be themselves.

Self-possessed people aren't easily threatened by the loss of their own emotional integrity, and so their relationships are flexible. Periods of closeness and distance are tolerated. Both people are free to be close or pursue their own interests. Neither is threatened by the other's needs. Denying one's own emotional reactions, blaming those reactions on others, and avoiding or pursuing others to reduce anxiety are emotionally driven processes that rob relationships of flexibility. The point isn't to deny your feelings but to choose how to react to them.

Mature listeners are intentional about their own responses. Instead of thinking "So and so is impossible," they hear what is said, feel their reactions, and then decide how to respond.

"Hearing" someone who doesn't open up means recognizing that he doesn't want to say much. If the reticent person is someone you care about, you may feel shut out. But if you react to that feeling by pressuring the other person to open up, you are projecting your own anxiety and making him feel threatened.

Pressuring someone to open up isn't listening. You may really want to hear what's on her mind, you may think you can help, you may believe it would be good for her and the relationship if she talked more, but pressure is pressure.

The best way to approach emotionally reticent people is to make contact without pushing. Openness without pressure helps relax the assumption that it isn't safe to open up. Respecting the integrity of the emotional boundary that allows you to be yourself (someone who wants to get closer) and the other person to be herself (someone who wants to go slow) keeps anxiety from escalating. Sometimes listening to reticent people happens best without words at all.

Margaret grew up with a father who seemed most content on the outermost edges of family life. He engaged as little as possible with day-to-day matters. Like some other men of his generation, Margaret's dad had a very narrow emotional range; he was consistently disengaged. He sometimes took the kids on outings: bowling on a rainy Saturday, baseball games, the circus—that sort of special event. When she was little, he had taken all the kids fishing a few times, but only Margaret got hooked on it. She discovered that she could have her dad all to herself in the little rowboat, throwing a lure out, reeling it back in, untangling knotted lines, and eating soggy cream cheese and jelly sandwiches together. They hardly spoke at all, but even though she was otherwise a chatterbox of a little girl, Margaret had figured out how to be close to her reticent dad, accepting the love he had to offer, the way he could offer it.

> The self-possessed listener
> is not isolated or unfeeling but nonreactive.

How to Tone Down Your Message and Be Heard

You know how frustrating it is not to be listened to. But how often do you stop to consider that there might be something about the way you express yourself that makes others deaf to your concerns? Digital newcomers, slowly developing their texting skills, have stories to tell about misunderstandings due to inadequate punctuation, autocorrect, and adjusting expectations for the timeliness of the response they'll receive. One of the best stories I've heard involves the shorthand "LOL," which once meant "Lots of Love" and somehow morphed into "Laugh Out Loud" about a decade ago when no one was looking. A bereft son texts his father that his girlfriend has dumped him. The father, trying to be both hip and supportive, texts back "LOL." Later that evening, he finds out from his now doubly distraught son where he'd gone wrong.

The difficulty in interpreting emotions in text and email crosses the generations. Humor, sarcasm, concern, interest, anxiety, and a host of other, more nuanced emotional cues that color in-person communications can easily get misconstrued in writing no matter how young or old you are. The best advice about how to manage online reactivity is also probably useful when we are uncertain about someone's motivation in person: assume good intentions and control your emotions before you press "send." When in doubt, ask the sender for clarification before jumping to the worst possible conclusion. As the old bumper sticker says: Don't believe everything you think.

Several years ago my friend John tried to teach me how to tune up my temperamental English motorcycle. When he showed up on the appointed day and saw how nervous I was, he said, "The first thing you have to do is calm down." How do you calm down when you're about to take apart a fifteen-thousand-dollar piece of machinery on which you'll later be going over a hundred miles an hour? But he was right. The way my hands were shaking I'd never have been able to shim the diphthongs with the krenging hook. So we repaired to the kitchen for a beer. Later I had the satisfaction of knowing that it wasn't getting all wound up that made me unable to put the damn thing back together. It's just that I'm a natural born klutz.

Why is it that when it comes to relationship problems so few of us bother to follow my friend John's advice and calm down before we start?

As we've seen, one way speakers undermine their messages is to say things with such anger and upset that the listener becomes too anxious to really register—and therefore remember—the content of the speaker's message. All that gets communicated is the upset. Suppose, for example, that once every few months a man gets so tired of his roommate's always leaving the bathroom a mess that he blows up about it. It infuriates him that the roommate doesn't remember—even after he's told him again and again. All the roommate remembers is getting yelled at.

It's hard to listen when you feel attacked. That's why even though you may have complained about something for years, other people never really get it. You've told them a million times; still they don't understand. Anxiety is the enemy of listening.

One message sure to give someone's hackles a workout is pointing out financial extravagances. Here's the great humorist S. J. Perelman illustrating his technique:

> Weary of pub-crawling and eager to recapture the zest of courtship, we had stayed home to leaf over our library of bills, many of them first editions. As always, it was chock-full of delicious surprises: overdrafts, modistes' and milliners' statements my cosset had concealed from me,

charge accounts unpaid since the Crusades. If I felt any vexation, however, I was far too cunning to admit it. Instead, I turned my pockets inside out to feign insolvency, smote my forehead distractedly in the tradition of the Yiddish theater, and quoted terse abstracts from the bankruptcy laws. But fiendish feminine intuition was not slow to divine my true feelings. Just as I had uncovered a bill from Hattie Carnegie for a brocaded bungalow apron and was brandishing it under her nose, my wife suddenly turned pettish.

"Sixteen dollars!" I was screaming. "Gold lamé you need yet! Who do you think you are, Catherine of Aragon? Why don't you rip up the foyer and pave it in malachite?" With a single dramatic gesture, I rent open my shirt. "Go ahead!" I shouted. "Milk me—drain me dry! Marshalsea prison! A pauper's grave!"

"Ease off before you perforate your ulcer," she enjoined. "You're waking the children."

"You think sixteen dollars grows on trees?" I pleaded, seeking to arouse in her some elementary sense of shame.

Notice how Perelman employs his knowledge of psychology. Shaming someone is a sure way to get her attention.

But seriously, what can you do when someone becomes reactive? Perhaps whenever you say anything the least bit critical, a certain someone gets angry and shuts down. Try getting less invested in being heard but remain open to the relationship on the other person's terms. This can be done without compromising yourself. It's the difference between self-denial—caving in—and self-restraint—waiting for your turn.

Say, for example, that whenever Maria, now twenty-four and living back at home for the year, makes dinner for her parents, she also makes a huge mess of the kitchen. When her mom tells her, oh-so-nicely, that it really helps to "clean up as you go along," Maria gets a look of wounded petulance. The same thing happens when her dad reminds her not to "forget to take your laundry upstairs when you go," because he almost tripped over the basket. Maria glowers and sulks. She feels like they are on her case all the time. She made dinner. She did her laundry and cleaned out the lint trap. She's an adult! But if she can calm down enough to ask herself where their criticism comes from, she might discover that it stems, in part, from unrealistic expectations.

The people you live with have assets and limitations. If you pitch your expectations at their assets instead of their limitations, you stand a better chance of being heard. Coming to terms with the real person you're relating to, rather than agonizing over the fact that he or she isn't different, will do a lot to lower your reactivity.

Learn what makes people reactive and try to defuse it with preparatory comments.

> "I'm not saying it's your fault, but I'm tired of seeing the kids leave their toys all over the place."
>
> "I'm not sure how to say this . . ."

If you're trying to make a request, not an attack, say so. But maybe you should examine your motives a little more carefully. When you say the kids shouldn't leave their toys around, do you really feel that it's your partner's fault for allowing it? Is the inference that your partner reacts to accurate? Even if you don't make such criticisms explicit, they often come through.

If you want someone to hear what you have to say without getting into a snit, don't forget tone and timing. Do you bring things up at the wrong time? Do you allow a judgmental tone to creep into your voice? If you intend to bring up an upsetting subject, give a warning. What makes something traumatic is being overwhelmed. A person who isn't prepared is more easily overwhelmed, as borne out by John Gottman's research finding that the way a conversation starts almost always determines how it will end. The more reactivity you anticipate, the more important it is to set the scene. A note or phone call telling someone you need to talk to him about something might help him gird himself. So could a text or short email. If you can use these media to frame the anticipated discussion in constructive, nonblaming language—saying what you want and hope for, not what you don't want— you may set the tone for the outcome you want. Be appreciative; proofread for tone and content before you send it.

· · · · · · · · · · · ·

Although it may seem artificial, putting difficult messages
in texts or notes is an effective way to short-circuit reactivity.

· · · · · · · · · · · ·

Ultimately, of course, it isn't other people's overreaction that's your problem but how *you* react to that. You don't have to get upset when someone else does.

One thing to remember when emotional reactivity drowns out listening is that *it's always your move.* Waiting for other people to change—or hammering at them in hopes that they will—is understandable but unproductive. Sometimes it makes sense to write off unrewarding relationships that aren't central to your life. People who are so touchy that anything you say can trigger an angry response may be more trouble than they're worth. Unfortunately, some of us are more likely to give up on relationships that *are* central to our lives—spouses, parents, colleagues—because they're the hardest to manage.

"What's Wrong with Him?"

The next time someone overreacts to what you're saying, ask yourself, "Where does this emotional response come from?" "What sore spot must I have touched?", rather than "What's wrong with this jerk?"

The following remarks add fuel to the fire:

"You're such a baby!"

"Someone got up on the wrong side of the bed today!"

"Can't you take a simple suggestion?"

"You sound just like your mother."

"You're so immature."

"What's eating you? Every time I open my mouth you bite my head off."

According to Claire, her son Jeffrey is oversensitive. The least little thing she says to him can make him fly into a rage. One time she told him that his teacher probably wouldn't pick on him so much if he acted more mature in class, and he burst into tears and ran into his room. "He's always throwing tantrums," Claire said.

A child who bursts into tears and runs out of the room isn't throwing a tantrum. Kids aren't stupid. If they pitch a fit because they want to bend you to their wishes, they do it in front of you. (If you want to defuse a temper tantrum, remove the audience.)

The way to resolve reactivity is to understand it, not judge it. Imagine a little boy storming out of the room after his mother said something to him. Why would a child get so upset? Often it's because what she said made him feel shamed. When someone feels humiliated, he becomes foot-stompingly outraged; he thinks I-am-wronged! Injuries to self-respect are as bruising as muggings. If you asked him what was wrong, he'd probably say, "Mommy yelled at me" or perhaps "Nothing, leave me alone!"

Few of us, children least of all, label our experience as shame. Unfortunately, parents who don't recognize a shame reaction or can't tolerate a child's upset get into a tug of war that makes things worse. They demand to know what's wrong, as if a child (or anyone) convulsed with emotion could say.

Give a shamed person room to hide and lick his wounds. Shame is so painful that the child momentarily loses control of his feelings. He needs time to regain his composure. Let him have it. And then apologize for hurting him, even if that wasn't your intention.

If someone becomes enraged at something you said, think about how you might have offended his dignity. Did you treat him like a baby? Imply that his opinion was invalid? That his feelings aren't legitimate? The way to decode an "excessive" emotional response isn't to blame the other person—or yourself—but to consider what the exposed nerve might be.

Sometimes It's a Mistake to Try to Control Your Feelings

Some people are afraid to speak at funerals or weddings because they might start to cry—as if crying were a sign of weakness, not compassion. "But," one man protested when I tried to tell him there's nothing wrong with crying, "if I start to cry, I won't be able to finish what I want to say."

If you start to cry and tell yourself that's awful and try to stop, you may well have trouble speaking. It's hard to concentrate on two things at once. But if your heart moves and your feelings show, what's wrong with that?

A trick some people use to help them cope with their anxiety about public speaking is to accept rather than fight their nervousness. "Good morning. My name is so-and-so, and I'm a little nervous speaking in front of such a large group." Such candor makes listeners sympathetic. Most of us know what it feels like to be nervous speaking in public. Even more important, though, is the effort to accept your feelings as natural instead of trying to fight them.[4] There's an even more important way that trying to resist feelings leads to more reactivity. If you let someone know how angry you are by venting your bottled-up frustration in an emotional outburst, you're likely to come across as attacking. If the other person responds with angry counteraccusations or just walks out, you may conclude that it was a mistake to talk about your feelings. This conclusion leads to a control and release cycle. You hold everything in until you explode. The solution isn't more control but less.

. . . .

Speaking up sooner makes it easier to lower your voice.

. . . .

Instead of "You never do anything around here," try "I'm overloaded with housework. I need more help."

Don't turn discussions into a *zero-sum game*, in which one person wins (is right) only if the other loses (is wrong).

There is, however, a difference between expressing what you feel and dumping your emotions. Recently I got into an disagreement with a woman who was tired of her father-in-law's belittling comments and planned to tell him off. When I suggested she tone down her emotionality before talking to him, she blew up at me. "What's wrong with getting angry?" she demanded.

This woman had a reason to be angry. Her father-in-law's cutting remarks were hard to take. But if she allowed her upset to overwhelm her, her complaints wouldn't be voiced clearly and wouldn't be heard. Unloading her anger, rather than articulating her complaints, would allow her father-in-law to dismiss her as "oversensitive" or "having a bad day." I'm not advocating emotional detachment. Anger helps preserve our integrity and

---

[4]Thinking about "communicating with people" instead of "speaking in front of them" will shift your attention and help you calm down.

self-regard, but simply venting anger doesn't usually solve the problem it signals. The distinction I'm trying to draw isn't between emotion and reason but between impulsive and deliberate action. There's nothing wrong with emotion, and there's nothing wrong with telling someone off, if that's what you want to do. It's not responding with feeling that makes us feel childish and inept—it's losing control.

EXERCISES

1. For a week, keep track of the number of your communications that are (a) critical or instructional, (b) avoidant, or (c) affectionate or laudatory. To change the climate in a relationship, shift from (a) and (b) to (c) and see what happens. This deceptively simple exercise may be very difficult to do. But trying it may help you begin to think more about how you're coming across to the people you care about.

2. What kind of interactions make you lose your cool? Do you have trouble with anger? Do you start to cry when you talk about your feelings? Do you get flustered in arguments? Find a reasonably safe occasion in the next week or so when you can put yourself in a situation you usually become reactive in. For example, if you have teenagers, you can predict that they're likely to test the limits of house rules; if you have little ones, you can expect them to ask for treats. One of the easiest ways to identify situations that make you reactive is to think about what situations you habitually avoid. Don't expect too much of yourself; just concentrate on getting through the experience without losing your cool. (Hint: One way to avoid losing your cool is to focus on drawing the other person out.) And remember who the person is and the context of the struggle (e.g., a three-year-old at the end of a long, hot day; a lonely neighbor who has no one else to talk to).

3. The next time someone overreacts, consider where that reaction might be coming from. If you can do this during a confrontation, you're a better person than I am. But you can always think about a blowup later. You get an A+ on this assignment if you can use that sensitivity to express empathy for what the other person seems to be feeling. (Remember: you can always seek the person out and make amends later.)

4. Go back over the last five texts you've sent and the last five emails. Look at them for emotion and clarity, observing:

- How many misunderstandings can you detect between you and those with whom you are corresponding? How did you handle them?

- When you are texting or emailing with your intimate partner, child, or friend, how much emotional overload are you, perhaps unconsciously, piling on? (For example, are you asking how someone is and then adding a question mark, and then a heart emoji, and then, when there's no response in five minutes, adding another comment? Or doing something almost like that?)

- Are there things you communicated by text that might have been better to say or do in person (e.g., sharing health news, breaking up with someone, dredging up an old grudge, making a big apology)?

5. You probably know people who could use some of the suggestions in this chapter. Better them than you, right? Why not buy several additional copies of this book and leave them scattered around in strategic places?

PART FOUR

Listening in Context

10

"It Takes Two to Tango"

LISTENING BETWEEN INTIMATE PARTNERS

It started innocently enough. She met him at an office party, and all they did was talk. But when Maureen got home and her husband asked if she had a nice time, she found herself unwilling to mention Arthur, as though he were a secret she didn't want to lose by telling. The next day Arthur started texting. He invited her for lunch. One lunch followed another, and then there were drinks after work. They texted back and forth several times a day. The following week they drove up to Thatcher Park and talked as they watched the sun set over the valley below. Nothing happened, unless you count the brief moment when Maureen's glance left Arthur's eyes and dropped to his lips and a shiver ran through her.

It was at this point that Maureen consulted me. She felt on the brink of something. Arthur was everything her husband wasn't: successful, self-possessed, but most of all he really listened when they talked. Telling me this, Maureen was visibly nervous. Her eyes scanned mine, looking for understanding, expecting perhaps judgment, or maybe permission to do what she longed to.

When, I asked, did the passion in her marriage die? She looked away. Then she wiped her eyes and said that her husband was a good person; they'd just . . . grown apart. He never talked to her anymore.

My sympathies were with this woman. Life holds few choices as consequential as the one between satisfaction and security. Still, I'd seen too many stale marriages blamed on the other partner.

When I suggested she bring her husband to our second meeting, Maureen was reluctant. She wasn't looking for marital therapy, she said, and she was afraid of Raymond's finding out about Arthur. What finally overcame her hesitation was her hope that if I saw what Raymond was like, maybe I'd understand why she'd consider leaving him.

Raymond did come, and Maureen told him she was unhappy with their marriage. He seemed sympathetic, as though accustomed to obliging, but not really engaged. He listened but didn't say much. Only when I asked about his work did Raymond become animated. We talked for a few minutes until Maureen interrupted to complain that he never talked to her about these things. Why couldn't he share his hopes and fears about his job with her? Raymond didn't have a very good answer for that. Still, I was encouraged. Here was something to work on.

If two people can't talk, I said, something's wrong. Then I asked them to turn their chairs to face each other and asked Raymond to talk to Maureen about his work and what his concerns were. I told her to listen and help him bring out his feelings.

Raymond talked about the challenges of opening a new law practice in an unstable economy. Very little work was coming in, but he was convinced that if he could hang on for another year or so, things would start to turn around. Maureen broke in to say that things would never improve until he got rid of that idiot Ernie, his partner. They argued for a minute, and then Raymond shut up.

Here was one reason this couple didn't talk. When Raymond talked about what was on his mind, Maureen argued or advised; he protested feebly, then folded his tent. Perhaps she was comfortable with conversational give-and-take and he wasn't; she was trying to engage him in a more animated dialogue. Possibly, she was too anxious about their finances to give him the room he needed to speak on this topic. Maybe he couldn't listen to her opinions because he didn't believe in his own power to decide what to do or felt bad that he wasn't more successful. In any case, here was a concrete problem to address.

Before I could start to help these two sort out their relationship, I had to talk privately with Maureen. I would propose a trial nonseparation, a period of not seeing Arthur and putting her energy into improving the marriage, so she could find out if it could be improved.

Maureen was relieved that I'd met Raymond. "Now you see," she said, "how bad our relationship is. It's never going to change." (Maureen was a great believer in chemistry, that famous force of attraction with more power to excite than endure.) Nothing I said about postponing any decision until she'd waited a few weeks to see if the marriage could be improved made any impact. Maureen started seeing Arthur again that same week, and when Raymond found out the following week, the marriage devolved rapidly; it turned out neither was willing to work on it any longer.

Their divorce was finalized a year and a day after the one time I saw them together, eleven months after Maureen's affair with Arthur heated up—and eight months after it ended. Maureen had viewed her marriage as a predicament, an entity, something with a history, perhaps, but one that after a while takes on a life of its own. Most of us feel this way at times. But a relationship is not a thing, not a static state; it is a process of mutual influence. A relationship isn't something you have; it's something you do.

Couples who learn to listen to each other—
with understanding and tolerance—
often find that they don't need to change each other.

The impulse to change things, to make them better, is a natural and largely constructive one. But anyone who thinks of marriage as an infinitely improvable arrangement is making a mistake. The ideal of perfectibility breeds frustration. Many problems can be solved, but the problem of living with another person who doesn't always see things the way you do isn't one of them. Sometimes marriage isn't about resolving differences but learning to live together with them.

What Goes Around

When I was in the third grade, Miss Halloway used a stroboscope to show us how light affects what we see. Late one winter afternoon when the shadows were long, she took out a small fan with a metal blade and plugged it in. She turned on the switch, and the blade began to spin and then whir. Then she turned on the stroboscope. As she adjusted the rate of flash, the fan blade slowed down and then stopped. The blade looked so still and harmless! How easy it would be, I thought, to reach out and touch it.

The blade looks stationary, Miss Halloway explained, because the stroboscope illuminates only one point in the cycle. As I came to realize later, that is the same way we see our relationships.

The first thing to understand about couples is that *complementarity* is the governing principle of relationships. Behavior doesn't take place in a vacuum but in the context of relationships in which we act and react to each other. In any relationship, one person's behavior is functionally related to the other's. If at times we see only one point in the cycle—a friend's failure to call, for example, or a partner's lack of interest in what we have to say— that doesn't mean that relationships don't spin around in a circle.

The greatest impediment to understanding in intimate relationships is the injured feeling of unfairness that makes us look outside ourselves for the sources of our disappointment. We can't help wishing our mates would be a little more interested in what we have to say and a little less defensive about what we have to say about them. At about this time, the romantic vision of marriage gives way to melodrama—the story of villain and victim that unhappily married people tell themselves and, when things get bad enough, anyone else who will listen.

Many couples expect too much of each other and see their difficulties as more apocalyptic than they really are. The real tragedy of this tragic view is that our ability to see what's going on is compromised. Like Maureen, we fix on the hurtful things our partners do and think of our troubles as insoluble.

When all is said and done, intimate partnership and its famous complications can be illuminated by focusing on one thing: the basic pattern of interaction between two people. Start with the hurtful things your partner does—the avoidance or selfishness or irritability—but then ask yourself: What is the complementary other half of this pattern?

The Other Half

Whenever you have a problem with someone, note what the person does that bothers you; then consider what the other half of that pattern might be. Doing so might just give you the key to unlocking the problem.

Complaint	Complement
"He doesn't talk to me."	He doesn't like the way you listen.
"She's not very affectionate."	She has unspoken resentments.
"He's selfish."	He thinks you're selfish.
"He never asks me how my day went."	You never ask him how his day went.

The other half of the equation—your part—doesn't have to be something you do that causes the problem. It might just be your way of keeping it going.

What Annoys You	What Perpetuates It
"He touches me in a way I don't like."	You don't show him how you like to be touched.
He thinks "Here we go again."	He never lets you get to the heart of your concerns and never makes you feel that he understands.

Rhythms of Change in a Committed Relationship

Although the cycle of life may be orderly, it isn't a steady, continuous march. Periods of growth and change are followed by times of relative stability in which changes are consolidated. The good news is that life isn't one long uphill struggle; sometimes you reach a plateau and can coast. The bad news is that you can't stay forever in one place. Partnership too has its cycles and seasons.

Courtship—what a lovely, old-fashioned word—is a time of opening up and testing for compatibility. Enchanted by romance, the partners are absorbed and engaged with each other. Conversation flows, and listening comes easily. They find each other so novel and delightful. So attentive, so interesting, so *interested*. When together, they pay such close attention! When apart, their texts are frequent and unmistakably sweet. No one is too busy to respond to these early bids for attention and connection.

Fascination makes them overlook gaps in listening. Something puts her in mind of high school, and she asks him what it was like for him. He reminisces fondly about his experience, but when he doesn't reciprocate, doesn't ask her what it was like for her, she thinks it's an oversight. She'll get her turn later.

No matter the age we fall in love, we feel young again. We take such pleasure in each other's company that sober considerations give way to dictates of the heart. Falling in love is an act of imaginative creation. Romance is fueled by texts and emails; with enough time on those platforms, we can present ourselves as even more witty and attractive. Hearing the thrilling "bing" of a response and reading those love notes, we are all smiles. Later, our smiles may fade, our hearts may shrink, and with that our eagerness to listen. But that's later. Now, although we might be more compatible with partners more like ourselves, nature's urge to mix genes draws us to the otherness of the other.

> The great challenge of courtship
> is to come together and still be yourself.

With love at stake, we lie a little. We tell tender lies, a few self-protecting lies, and more than a few self-deluding lies. Looking back, we wish we'd been more honest, hadn't tried so hard to get our partners to like us.

Is falling in love the same as it always was? It seems that the rules for courtship among twentysomethings are changing; they are delaying that big step a few more years. In high school and college, they may not have dated much at all, hanging out in groups, hooking up now and then. Commitment doesn't seem as inevitable as it once did. So when courting couples eventually move in the direction of their intentions, trying to discover how far they can go together, it's usually two steps forward and one step back.

Marriage was once a "cornerstone" for couples in their early twenties—building adult life on the foundation of the partnership. It's now more of a "capstone" for young adults hovering around thirty years of age. Commitment follows accomplishment of individual tasks and personal goals. In some notable ways, the capstone approach may even make it harder to resolve differences in the partnership; it's hard to move from being your own person to being half of a couple, creating compatibility out of well-established lifestyles.

Over the years a dozen or so couples have sought me out for premarital counseling. What a good idea, I used to think. Unfortunately, these encounters often turn out to be quite frustrating. The people seeking help come not because they are amazingly cautious but because they are amazingly mismatched. Despite that, most of them have passed an emotional point of no return and intend to marry, no matter what. Among the obstacles they will overcome is their own good judgment.

· · · · · · · · · · · ·

If courtship were more conscious, people would
pay more attention to the quality of one another's listening.

· · · · · · · · · · · ·

Among the most important things to find in a mate is someone who's easy to talk to. Making friends and being able to listen to each other is a far more reliable guide than good looks, cleverness, or that dizzy feeling that people call "falling in love." (Try telling that to someone in love.)

He Needs Space; She Wants Closeness[5]

He wants to be left alone and she wants attention. So she gives him attention and he leaves her alone.

Jack and Samantha were a handsome couple in their midthirties.
"What brings you to therapy?" I asked, looking at both of them.
Jack answered first. "Well, I'm a little intolerant."
"What does Samantha do that's hard to tolerate?"
They exchanged looks. Samantha gave Jack a faint smile, and he turned back to me. "She yammers. She makes assumptions, and there's nothing I can do about it—about what she assumes—so I give up and go on about my business."
"You mean, you pull away?"
"Well . . . yes."

---

[5] In writing this revision, I noticed a Freudian slip here—he "needs" space, but she only "wants" closeness. Excuse me for a minute, my wife is trying to tell me something and I have to cover my ears and start humming.

He went on to describe himself as a man who isn't very emotional, married to a woman who is.

I turned to Samantha. "So, Jack is learning to be more tolerant and not react to you. What would you say you're learning?"

"I'm working real hard to identify and express my feelings to him. But he always wants an explanation of *why* I feel upset. Sometimes you don't know why; you just know that you are."

Jack's response to Samantha's distress took the familiar form of an obsessional person trying to comfort an emotional one: He barraged her with questions, all based on his own approach to emotion, which was to label and compartmentalize it.

Samantha felt things strongly without always being able to put them into words. At these moments her husband could have comforted her by just being there, and holding her perhaps, but certainly not demanding that she stop crying and explain herself. The truth was that when Samantha cried, Jack worried that it might be about him, so he felt accused. His comfort took the form of asking her to reassure him. "What's the matter?" really meant "Tell me you're not mad at me."

Jack went on to talk about Samantha's anger as the reason he didn't listen better. When Samantha approached Jack in an excitable way without any warning, he became anxious. He dealt with feeling emotionally overwhelmed by trying to be analytic or—if that failed—by distancing himself. His distance aggravated her emotionality, which then pushed him even further away. Their failure to listen to each other wasn't caused by Samantha's emotionality or by Jack's anxiety; it was the combination.

Jack thought Samantha could break the pattern by controlling her emotions. Samantha thought Jack should learn to be a little more tolerant of her feelings. Even as they talked, they played out the familiar progression. Samantha's rising pressure made Jack anxious and defensive—or, to look at the circular pattern from another angle, Jack's inability to tolerate what she was saying drove up her emotionality.

Finally I interrupted and told them the story of the North Wind. "One day the North Wind and the Sun were arguing about which was the most powerful force in nature. 'I can churn up the seas and drive a blizzard,' the North Wind said. 'Yes, but I can melt the snow and dry up a flood,' the Sun replied. Just then a man wearing a heavy overcoat happened by. 'I know how to settle this,' said the Sun. 'Let's see who can make that man take off his coat.' The

North Wind blew hard. But the harder he blew, the more the man bundled up. Finally the Sun said, 'My turn.' The sun shone down its warmth, and the man unbuttoned his coat. The Sun shone warmer, and the man took off his coat."

Samantha and Jack smiled broadly.

"Samantha, sometimes you come on like the North Wind. And I don't blame you, because it's frustrating to feel shut out. And out of that frustration, either you give up or out comes the North Wind."

"You're right. I never thought of it that way."

At this point Jack, feeling relieved, opened up and started to talk about needing space. He had a lot of pressure at work, and when he came home he needed time to decompress. Samantha was afraid to give him the breathing room he needed, the freedom to read or go for a walk or spend time with his friends.

"Jack," I said, "I could tell you understood the difference between Samantha being the North Wind and being the Sun. But you know, the guy wearing the coat is in the story too. It's both of them. The North Wind blows, and he bundles up, and so the North Wind blows more, and he bundles up more. He bundles up for a lot of good reasons—he has his moods, his job is stressful, he needs his space, he likes to read . . . I respect those things. But the bundling up is part of the problem."

"I understand that," Jack said. He went on to say that he's been making an effort. But, he admitted, "It's not the easiest thing for me, to be close."

By now, the atmosphere in the session had changed. Jack and Samantha had begun to see how they were locked into a pattern in which they pushed each other to respond in a way they didn't like.

Once Samantha learns to see that coming on strong only pushes Jack away, and *he* learns that keeping his distance only makes her more anxious and persistent, they can figure out how to break their halves of the cycle. Will that magically change everything? If you kiss a frog, will he turn into a prince? Maybe not right away.

Balancing Intimacy and Independence

In accommodating to each other, couples must negotiate the space between them as well as the space separating their couplehood from the rest of the world.

When you become intimate with someone, physically and emotionally, you open up the boundary around your private self to let the other in close. Being in love is to want no distance between you, but a wall of privacy protecting the two of you from outside intrusion. This closeness and privacy make conversation intimate, with the obvious rewards and risks.

Some couples don't move on from the symbiotic togetherness of early courtship. They have little tolerance for emotional or physical separation. Minimal self-reliance exists between two people when they text each other at work all the time, when neither has separate friends or independent interests, if they come to view themselves only as a pair rather than also as two individuals. "We loved the movie." "We don't think the cannoli at that place is worth the calories." Under such anxious pressure of togetherness, conversation is constrained by the threat of conflict. If you're alone with someone on a lifeboat, you'd better not argue.

In contrast, people who put independence over connection do little together, have their own rooms, take separate vacations, have few friends in common, are more invested in their careers or hobbies than in each other, and don't talk much. Listening is limited because they have so many distractions.

Most couples don't start out disengaged; the wall that grows up between them is a product of unresolved conflict. Often it's not specific transgressions so much as the not listening, the not hearing. They both feel as if the other doesn't care. That they do care very much but are too afraid of conflict to listen doesn't alter the feeling of being unappreciated. Some people pay too much for peace.

Typically, partners come from families with differing degrees of separateness and togetherness. Each partner tends to be more comfortable with the kind of relationship he or she grew up with. Since these expectations differ, a struggle ensues over how much to share and how much to keep to yourself. This may be the most difficult aspect of learning to listen to a new mate—developing sensitivity to a different conversational style. Even after many years together, we may still struggle with how we feel about revealing ourselves to our partners.

Notably too the line between private and public, sharing and avoiding is not nearly as clearly marked now as it was a generation or two ago, and that brings new confusion. Social media and the Internet have changed how we live our intimate lives.

I treated a young woman a couple years ago who had met a man on a dating site and was planning to have dinner with him in a few days. Of course, before they met, she had Googled him and knew a great deal about his life—where he had lived, how much he had paid for his house, talks he had given, and relationships he had been in. Partway through the evening, she noticed that she was getting angry about how he was answering her questions: she wondered why he wasn't telling her about his years in Berkeley or more about that Spanish woman he had dated for years.

She told me that she felt he hadn't been honest with her even on the first date and probably wouldn't see him again. We have always made assumptions about others based on inference and expectations; however, now we may also begin with quite a complicated backstory that our dates haven't told us directly—but will also shape how we see and understand them.

New relationships afford a special kind of attention we aren't likely to get elsewhere. That initial period of excitement and anticipation provides us a chance to see ourselves through someone else's devoted eyes and to feel, however briefly, that we might be wonderful in every way. Young lovers have long wanted to sing their rapture from the rooftops—now there's social media instead of a rooftop. And suddenly it's tougher to build the protective wall of privacy around a budding relationship as lovers post their romantic photos and story updates, garnering likes and comments and an enthusiastic audience. The intrusion of social media into our intimate lives has altered how we experience these new loves. Where we once had time to see ourselves through just each other's eyes, now we also view our relationships from the outside, along with our friends and followers. This element of performance creates an added tension to working out inevitable differences.

Tension in a couple can be resolved in one of three ways: working it out, triangulation, or distancing. When distancing between intimate partners is unchecked by a clear boundary around their relationship, the two often drift apart.

Brendan and Scott were very much in love when they were first a couple, also very young and unaware of how different their backgrounds were. Scott's was a large, close-knit family whose watchword was togetherness.

Brendan's was a small, fragmented family in which independence and personal achievement were the highest accomplishments.

In Brendan's opinion, Scott was addicted to attachment. He always wanted to talk. Even when they were watching TV or reading, he'd interrupt every few minutes to tell Brendan something that popped into his head. It broke Brendan's concentration and made him mad. This he tried to signal indirectly by sighing or saying "Yes?" with a weary note in his voice. But Scott didn't seem to get the message.

Scott took closeness for granted and found Brendan's "coldness" selfish and mean. Why did he have to shut Scott out all the time?

They each had their own point of view, at best sporadically sympathetic to the other one. It's a sad and familiar story. Two young people with too great a disparity in their expectations to fit together easily and too little experience to know how to work at it.

It wasn't really their differences that made the first few years together so painful; it was their inability to talk about them. Once a week or so, Scott would get fed up with Brendan's distance. At these times, Brendan was appalled by the meanness and exaggeration of Scott's accusations. The worst was "You don't give a damn about anybody but yourself!" *How could he say such things?* Brendan certainly couldn't listen to them. Feeling the frustration of not being heard, Scott would raise his voice, which only made Brendan shrink further into himself. Finally, Scott would break down in tears and sob, "Why are you so mean to me?" Brendan had the same question but only thought it, and never more than twice a day.

Like a lot of ill-matched couples, Brendan and Scott gradually did learn to live with each other. After a while they had children to cushion their couplehood. Gradually they learned to accommodate to each other. Scott got used to Brendan's silences and golfing with his friends. Brendan learned to spend more time with Scott and the kids. But what they never learned very well was how to talk to each other. Brendan didn't talk to Scott because he thought Scott was unreasonable in his expectations and didn't respect his right to his own preferences. Scott continued to express his disappointment with Brendan's lack of involvement from time to time, but Brendan never really did learn to listen. Scott made a tenuous peace with expecting less from Brendan than he'd hoped for and believed he deserved. He listened well enough to pacify Scott—"I'm sorry"; "Yes, dear"—but not enough to understand how Scott felt. He wished Scott were different, he wished he could escape, and these thoughts kept him from ever really understanding or coming to terms with the real person he had married. Like a prisoner who thinks of nothing but escape, he never really did adjust to the realities of his relationship.

Pursuers and Distancers

Pursuers want more connection, which makes distancers feel pressured. The more one pursues, the more the other distances; the more one distances, the more the other pursues. It's a game without end, though it does have interruptions.

When pursuers get fed up with being rebuffed, they withdraw in hurt and anger. But after a while they start to get lonely, and then they begin the cycle all over again.

If you're a pursuer, try backing off. Focus less on the other person for a few days. This planned distance isn't the same as reactive distance—getting fed up and giving your partner the cold shoulder. Snubbing isn't the same as giving someone space; it's an attempt to punish the person with silence, which of course doesn't lessen your preoccupation with your partner. Instead of being passive-aggressive, increase your emotional investment in other things.

When you stop pursuing, notice what happens. You'll probably find your anxiety rising. This is important. Consider how much of the pursuing is an attempt to cope with your own anxiety and lack of other avenues of satisfaction in your life.

Accept any forward movement on the part of a distancer—even if it's to complain. This is important. Pursuers say they want their partners to share feelings with them, but what they mean is positive feelings. A pursuer who experiments with shifting the pattern should avoid getting defensive about whatever the distancer does express. Distancers also want connection but often feel inadequate to meet the needs of their pursuing partner. They keep their feelings locked in tightly sealed compartments to keep peace and to soothe themselves. If a distancer does start expressing feelings, try to listen without getting reactive—he withdraws because he fears one or both of you will do just that.

"Why Won't You Talk to Me?"

How can you convince a distancer that you are open and receptive to what he or she might be thinking and feeling? How can you convince a distancer of your openness without creating more pressure?

The person who withdraws doubts that anything good will come of discussions. If you live with a distancer, you'll have to convince your partner that you're receptive to what he or she is feeling. Actually, you don't have to do that; you can just keep doing what you do, like most normal unhappily married people.

If you're a distancer, pursuers are hard to live with. They put you on the defensive. It's hard to stop running when someone is chasing you. The first thing to realize is that the chase can't occur without you; it's a pattern of pursuit and withdrawal. Instead of avoiding the pursuer, try initiating contact on your terms. Text your partner in the middle of the day; invite your partner to go for a walk. Say what's on your mind; ask what's on your partner's mind. Understand that your partner pursues to feel closer to you and doesn't know a better way make the connection.

Change Is a Three-Step Process

If you shift your part in a pursuer–distancer pattern for a week, you'll discover that change is a three-step process: First, you change. Second, your partner responds—usually in ways that are partly rewarding and partly annoying. Third, you respond to that response—either you change back, or you persist.

If a pursuer makes an effort to stop pursuing, the partner may not immediately respond by moving toward the pursuer. The resulting distance might make the pursuer feel even more alone and abandoned. The pursuer changed, but the distancer didn't. At that critical juncture—the third step in the change process—the pursuer would either revert to the old style or persist, making an effort to remain calm, develop other interests, and give the distancer space to discover a need for the pursuer.

Alternatively, if an emotional distancer decides to break the pattern by moving toward his partner, she might not immediately respond the way he wants her to. She might not, for example, be receptive to his opening up about things that are bothering him. She might be hurt and critical. If her response upsets him and he reverts to distancing, he might conclude, *I tried, but she'll never change.* But if he does change back, it wouldn't be because of how his partner responded; it would be because of how he responded to that response.

> At what point do you usually give up? What could you do to persist in your effort to make changes in your relationship? Try sticking with a small change and notice what happens—how *you* feel—when the other person tries to get you to change back. Remember: it isn't what others do but how we react to what they do that tends to defeat us.

Another reason the pursuer–distancer dynamic isn't so easily resolved is that pursuers and distancers tend to have constitutionally different operating styles dating back to experiences in their earliest relationships. Pursuers have an affinity for relationship time; distancers prefer time alone or activity together. (That's why some people are emotional distancers but sexual pursuers.) Pursuers tend to express their feelings; distancers avoid them. Pursuers have permeable boundaries and relate readily to a wide number of people. Distancers let down their defenses with only a select few.

Although each of us has a predominant operating style, the dynamics of complementarity trigger different roles in different relationships. A man may be a distancer with his mate and a pursuer with his mother or best friend. A woman may be a pursuer with her partner but a distancer from her younger sister.

If women are more often pursuers and men more often distancers, what happens when the relationship consists of two women or two men? A few years ago I did some research on the pursuer–distancer dynamic in gay and lesbian relationships. In about 70% of heterosexual couples, women are pursuers and men distancers. In gay male couples, the usual pattern is that both are distancers (in about 60% of cases), while in some of these couples one man is usually the pursuer and the other man a distancer. In about 70% of the lesbian couples I studied, both women were emotional pursuers. I studied only about 40 couples, so I hesitate to put too much stock in these percentages, but it does seem that gender influences but doesn't determine who pursues and who distances in a given relationship.

Distancers are unsure of themselves in relationships; they depend on privacy for protection. Pursuing only makes them feel hounded.

• • • • • • • • • • • •

To approach a distancer, don't push. Knock to enter.
Give the distancer time to anticipate company.

• • • • • • • • • • •

Distancers handle threatening issues by closing them off. Anxiety about these issues may not be acknowledged, but it is always present below the surface. The tension created by such unaddressed anxiety often triggers conflict in the relationship or the increased emotionality that distancers are trying to avoid. For their partners, such avoidance in the face of obvious distress feels like rejection and abandonment.

Emotional pursuers handle sensitive issues by talking about them over and over again, often in an agitated way. The issues never become closed off, and the emotionality surrounding them is never dealt with. For their partners, this repetitiousness is like salt poured on a wound.

Like most complementary patterns—overfunctioning/underfunctioning, strict/lenient, fast paced/slow paced—the pursuer–distancer dynamic isn't static. Very little about relationships is static.

Accommodating Differences

Intimate partnership is a process in which two individuals restructure their lives into a unit: The Couple. Friends invite The Couple over for dinner, the IRS taxes The Couple, The Couple accumulates belongings. The two separate personalities don't disappear, of course, but their relationship is now a system, their fates interwoven.

The first priority of intimate partnership is mutual accommodation to manage the details of everyday living. Each partner tries to organize the relationship along familiar lines, and pressures the other to accommodate. They must agree on the big things, like where to live and whether and when to have children; or what to do if they can't. Less obvious, but equally important, they must coordinate daily rituals, like what to binge on Netflix, what to eat for supper, when to go to bed, and what to do there. Unfortunately, there is a thin line between accommodation and capitulation.

Lynn was just nineteen when her mother died. After the worst of the grief gave way to emptiness, she decided to get out of New York and move to Montana. When she got off the plane, she was stunned by the intensity of the sunlight. The last of the snow was melting and the valley blossomed. Summer came, stretched, and yawned, and then it was early fall. That's when the loneliness set in, and Lynn started wondering what she was going to do with her life. Right about then she met Travis. After all the boys she'd known in New York who couldn't stop talking about themselves, Lynn took Travis's quietness for strength. She thought he was the real deal. So when he asked her to share his trailer with him, it seemed like the right thing to do.

A year later their relationship wasn't a lot better or a lot worse. Maybe a wedding would do the trick. So Lynn gave Travis an ultimatum: either they got married or she was moving out. But even walking down the aisle, she found herself thinking *This is never going to last.* Afterward she got drunk, hoping to numb this giant step into the unknown.

Lynn got pregnant on the honeymoon, and two weeks later Travis joined the Air Force. When Travis was posted to Korea, he went ahead to get settled, and Lynn moved in with his parents. It was not a happy time. And so, six weeks later, when she boarded the plane for Inchon, it was with as much relief as anxiety.

When the jet lag wore off and reality settled in, Lynn found herself alone all day with a baby in a tiny apartment. She'd written Travis about buying a car with an automatic transmission, because she couldn't drive a stick shift; but he hadn't listened. Not being able to drive sealed her isolation. When she tried to talk to Travis about it, he said, "You'll get the hang of it. Don't be such a baby." What could she say?

Unfortunately, Lynn neither insisted that Travis listen to how she was feeling nor asked how he was feeling. "I nagged," Lynn said. "I was angry and bitchy. Back then I wasn't very sure of what I was feeling, and so the frustration just built up and came out as attack. Instead of telling him how

I was feeling, I'd say things like 'We never do anything; you never take me anywhere.' He always put it back on me. 'What's the matter with you?' That was his answer to all my complaints." She didn't really remember Travis's complaints; all she remembered was that he didn't listen to hers.

Going into the marriage, Lynn thought that if she did all the right things, Travis could become the man she wanted—loving and affectionate. Losing her mother so early and yearning for the attention of her self-absorbed father, the question for her always had been *How do I keep people happy so they'll love me?* With Travis, she'd played the good wife, hoping for a payoff of affection and attention. But there was no affection; just sex. Lynn put up with not having her needs met because she wasn't sure how to put them into words.

When her frustration turned to bitterness, Lynn's conversations with Travis took on the form of combat. Each felt trapped and misunderstood, and both of them led with their defenses. After suffering so much neglect, Lynn was seized with rage when she tried to talk about her feelings. When she opened up on him with a mean mouth, his stomach knotted and he stopped listening. Once or twice, when she cornered him, he'd answer her accusations with an outburst of his own nursed resentment. Then they'd go back to avoiding each other.

The proximity forced on them in Korea may have kept them together longer than otherwise, or it may have put too much pressure on their shaky alliance. In any case, when Travis was posted back to the States and Lynn started school again, the marriage fell apart. With school and friends of her own, Lynn felt stronger and no longer willing to put up with a relationship that gave her so little satisfaction. Ironically, as Lynn started pulling away, Travis asked her to stay and, for the first time since the early days of the relationship, tried to listen to her. But it was too late.

Lynn said: "He wanted someone to mother him, to cook and clean and all that. I was willing to do it, and so he was happy. But when I wanted more from him, he couldn't deal with it, and he hated me. Then my independence gave him the room he needed, and so he started liking me again. But now I knew it had been a mistake to begin with." And so they ended it.

Travis and Lynn might have had an easier time adjusting to other mates. Maybe not. Second and third marriages don't fail because people keep picking the wrong partners; they fail because it's not differences that matter but how they're negotiated. Maybe Lynn did too much compromising. Maybe Travis did too little. He was a young man caught up in confirming his masculinity rather than achieving love, and perhaps he was afraid he'd lose himself by giving in. The trouble was neither of them dared to listen to the other's point of view.

Travis and Lynn might have found a way to talk about their differences if they'd managed to be less emotionally reactive to each other. Instead of holding her feelings in until they exploded, Lynn might have approached Travis calmly (it isn't necessary to *feel* calm to *speak* calmly), saying, perhaps, "Something's bothering me and I need to talk to you. Is this a good time?"

> The best way to tone down emotionality
> isn't to avoid talking about problems
> but to discuss them calmly—before the upset boils over.

Travis thought that if he didn't listen to Lynn's complaints, he wouldn't have to deal with them—and he could avoid the anxiety her accusations made him feel. But he found out that feelings are like any other form of energy: if they don't find direct expression, they come out in other ways.

The way to reduce defensiveness is to stay calm and stay open. Don't interrupt, contradict, qualify, or change the subject. If you don't understand something, ask for clarification. Otherwise, shut up and listen.

"Why Can't a Woman Be More Like a Man?"

Or maybe the question should be: Why can't a man be more like a woman? When the differences that attract turn out to be hard to live with, we may be tempted to think that a relationship might work best with a person as similar to us as possible. Actually, that's not true. With very similar partners there is the possibility for weaknesses to combine and create exaggerated, even destructive, imbalances. Two people with explosive tempers or who are both financially irresponsible often form disastrous unions.

Lynn told herself she had married the wrong person. Travis was good-looking and smart, but he didn't know how to trust people with the truth about his feelings. A man dedicated to autonomy, married to a woman who prized togetherness. Travis too thought his mistake was choosing the wrong mate. He never suspected that the desirable woman he fell in love with would turn out to be so needy.

"I Heard You the First Time!"

Few complaints are more common from men than that the women in their lives nag. Whenever someone is perceived as nagging, it probably means she hasn't received a fair hearing for her concerns in a long time. When our feelings are listened to sympathetically, we experience a sense of understanding and release. If no one listens, we feel alone with our feelings.

· · · · · · · · · · · ·

Nagging is in the ear of the beholder.

· · · · · · · · · · · ·

"He never notices how much I do around here. I never get any help without having to beg for it."

Not being listened to makes people resentful. No wonder they come across as nagging.

"She acts like she's my mother. Doesn't she know I always get my share of the chores done?"

Lloyd *hates* Cathy's nagging.

Stop leaving the bedroom window open; don't turn the heat up any higher than sixty-eight degrees. Do this, do that. She's always bitching about something. This he says to himself, and he gets no argument.

Cathy hates that Lloyd never listens to her. "Why do I have to tell you the same things over and over again? Why can't you listen to a simple request?" This she says to him often. To her friend Annie she complains, "I try to tell him something, and he just goes underground, with no warning—and I'm left there, all alone."

If You're Considered a Nag

In a series of conversations, each encounter bears the fruits and burdens of earlier ones. Persistent criticism creates a negative atmosphere and eventually results in the other person tuning the nagger out. It's like the Gary Larson cartoon in which a man is explaining something to his dog and all the dog hears is "blah-blah-blah."

The nagger becomes a nuisance. But what do you do if your repeated pleas to put dirty clothes in the hamper or clean up the mess in the bathroom go unheeded?

You're caught in the role of nag if, even though you know somebody isn't going to remember to do something, you keep bugging him anyway; you never ask for anything just once; you come at the other person in a critical or complaining way; you get annoyed by lots of things the other person does *and* you keep letting him know it; you appeal to what "should" be done rather than what you want; and the other person flinches when you make your request. You may not think of yourself as nagging, but if that's how the other person feels, he isn't likely to listen.

· · · · · · · · · · · · · · ·

If women are doing the majority of nagging,
it probably has something to do with the fact
that they are still doing about 70% of the housework.

· · · · · · · · · · · · · · ·

> **"Why Is Everything Always My Fault?"**
>
> Cut down on the number of things you ask people to do and the number of times you remind them. No fair, you say? You have a right to gripe? True, but asking less results in getting more.
>
> Pick out your most important concerns, make your requests clearly, and make them sound like requests.
>
> Devote more time to establishing and agreeing on the tasks that need doing, who will do them, how and when will they do them, and how each person will be accountable for this process.

Listening is hard because it involves a loss of control, and if you're afraid of what you might hear, it may not feel safe to listen. Among the things that someone who feels nagged (even though he didn't listen the first twelve times) doesn't want to hear are blame and requests he doesn't think merit this much discussion.

In all our communications we struggle to maintain our independence, to resist being controlled by others without sacrificing our involvement or losing their love. If someone hears your requests or complaints as implying power over him, he may resist—not because he's unwilling to do what you ask but because he's unwilling to accept the metamessage (implied or inferred) that you're the boss.

To avoid sounding overbearing, add "What do you think?" after making a request or a suggestion. This helps keep the airways open. Emphasize how important the request is to you and be sure to understand the other person's perspective—"What do you think?" Then make sure that an agreement is really an agreement. If you aren't willing to accept "no," you can't trust "yes."

People other than our intimates are more likely to listen to us airing our frustrations because they know it isn't their fault. If you want to get heard more around the house, try telling your partner, "I know it's not your fault" or "I'm not blaming you." Then if he does listen, let him know you appreciate it: "I feel relieved that I can talk about this. Thanks for listening."

> Make lots of room for gratitude every single day. Notice the cleanup of dishes after dinner, the cup of coffee in the morning. Appreciation is the opposite of nagging.
>
> This goes for listening too: Saying "I really appreciate your listening to my feelings; it means a lot to me" encourages people to listen more.

Finally, if you want to get out of the role of a nag, try listening to the recalcitrant other's side of things. Maybe the husband who makes a large purchase without consulting his wife feels that he has a right to do so if he wants. Perhaps the wife who won't see a doctor about her dizzy spells might be too fearful to make the appointment. Or, when the compost is piling up in the bucket by the sink, perhaps each believes it is the other's turn.

Even if you don't agree with someone's reasons for not complying with your requests, the other person will feel a whole lot more like compromising if you listen to and acknowledge that point of view.

> **Should You Say "No" More Often?**
>
> Those who feel nagged are often people who have trouble saying "no." If a woman asks her husband to take out the garbage and it doesn't get done, probably there was a false sense of agreement to do it in the first place. Some people should say "no" more often.

How to Complain Without Starting a Fight

Directly related to nagging is complaining. The problem is that your expectations, often quite legitimate, that things should be different may provoke unwanted flare-ups if the other person feels attacked by what you say.

First decide whether what the other person does has a direct effect on you. Leaving dirty dishes around the house does, especially if you're the one who has to clean them up; your partner's ten extra pounds doesn't (unless you happen to own his or her body).

Consider your relationship to the person you're criticizing. It's one thing to tell your twelve-year-old that you want the lawn mowed more than twice a month. Saying the same thing to your husband may make him think *Who does she think she is, my mother?*

Partners who expect to be treated like adults may not take kindly to being told how to fold the laundry, load the dishwasher, or park the car. If you want these things done differently, maybe you should do them yourself.

If you decide you have a right to complain, consider whether or not the person is likely to change. Most of the annoying habits we have won't cease simply to please someone else. Research has proven that, if properly motivated, people can learn to put dirty dishes in the sink. But few people lose weight or start exercising because someone else thinks they should.

If you've had to ask your partner a thousand times not to leave dirty dishes in the living room, maybe you should let it go. Maybe it's better to give up on some things—even if it's not fair—than to play the role of constant critic, a voice against which people learn to deafen themselves.

How to Complain

Do you have a tendency to hold your complaints in until you get fed up and then unload on the other person? Can you see how the consequences of such confrontations might reinforce your tendency to avoid complaining until you once again get good and mad?

How to complain? Start gently.

How you express criticism is important. Alert the person that you want to talk.

"Something is bugging me, and I need to talk to you. How about tonight after work?"

"I have a problem, and I need to discuss it with you. Can we go for a walk after supper?"

Advance notice allows people to realize that something's coming and they'd better be prepared. Be sensitive to time and place. The best time to talk about difficult issues is when both of you are calm and relaxed. And alone. Remember: the best predictor of how a conversation ends is how it begins. A gentle start-up won't ensure things go well, but it can certainly help.

That criticism is best given in private may seem obvious, but many people infuriate their partners by bringing up their faults in front of their friends or children. Another version of the same mistake is criticizing your partner's family or friends. It's okay for her to complain about her mother, but when you do it you're crossing the line. Some people take advantage of being out with another couple to criticize their partners. Often they make a joke out of their comments. It isn't funny.

. . . .

If you have something to say to someone, tell him or her.
If you have something to say about someone's friends
or family, keep it to yourself.

. . . .

Telling someone "I have a problem" and "I need your help," even if your problem is about something he or she is doing, is more likely to be heard than direct criticism. Least likely to be heard is criticism framed as blame, put-downs, moralizing, or invidious comparisons.

"Why must you always . . . ?"

"You never. . . ."

"You should. . . ."

"Why can't you be more like . . . ?"

Emphasize your feelings, not the other person's shortcomings: "I wish you'd get dressed up when we go out. I feel more special when you wear your good clothes." This works better than "Why do you always have to be so grungy?"

Describe how the situation is affecting you rather than being accusatory. Stick to behavior and make it clear that you're talking about what you like and don't like, not what's right or wrong. Focus on how the other person can help rather than on what he or she is doing wrong.

Even if you're the one with the complaint, remember to give the other person a turn. Mention your concern, but before elaborating, ask her how she feels about it. Don't get reactive if the other person gets defensive. Remember, you've just told her there's something wrong with what she's doing.

If you ask someone to make a change, and he agrees without saying much, he's less likely to follow through than if you inquire and acknowledge why he may not want to change or why changing might be hard for him.

Henry told Benita that he needed more help chauffeuring the kids to their activities. Benita agreed. But Henry went further and said, "I know you don't feel like it; otherwise you'd volunteer more often. When do you feel *least* like driving?"

Benita really appreciated this consideration of her feelings. (Feeling like it's okay to say no made it a lot easier to say yes.) She said she didn't mind taking the kids places on weekends or early in the evening, but, because she started work early, she hated going out after nine on week nights. She also mentioned that it's easier for her if she knows a day in advance that she has to drive them somewhere.

Then Henry went one step further and asked, "Anything else?"

Benita paused. Then she said, "Yes, there is. Frankly, I think you drive them far too many places. I don't think we should drive them wherever and whenever they want to go."

Henry, who hadn't known Benita felt this way, said that the next time Benita disagreed she should say something. If Henry's willing to take them anyway, even if Benita isn't, he'll do the driving. "But," he added, "maybe you're right. Maybe I do drive them around too much."

On the way out of the movie theater, Tiffany turned to Carmen and said, "Wow, that was a little lame, wasn't it?" She went on to describe how a good story was ruined by Melissa McCarthy's overacting and the director's heavy-handed approach to comedy.

Carmen didn't say anything. She had enjoyed the movie. She loved Melissa McCarthy. Tiffany's running the picture down was ruining it for her.

Since Carmen was the one who wanted to see this picture, she felt that Tiffany was criticizing her taste and that while she was enjoying herself, her partner had been having a lousy time.

In fact, Tiffany hadn't thought of this movie as Carmen's choice. She may have mentioned it first, but Tiffany had wanted to see it. And Tiffany hadn't had a lousy time. Far from it. She enjoyed laughing at parts of the movie, and she enjoyed laughing at some of its excesses.

What should you say on your way out of a movie you didn't like when you're with someone who apparently did? Nothing.

If two people both hate a movie or concert, their saying so brings them together. Shared experience, shared sensibilities. But if you enjoyed the performance, hearing someone else pick it apart spoils your fun.

Criticism of the movie or restaurant we liked feels like criticism of our taste. If you thought the food was lousy or the play was boring but sense that your companion liked it, let your partner savor the enjoyment. Save your criticism for later. Much later.

You Say To-May-To, I Say To-Mah-To

Your partner doesn't have the power to say what is and forever shall be or who's right and who's wrong. Even the person who puts things that way doesn't have the power to make it so; *you* give him that power if you react as though he did.

> You don't have to agree
> in order to acknowledge that someone has a point.

The simple act of omission involved in not acknowledging what the other person is saying before countering with your own opinion may be the single greatest impediment to shared understanding. If we don't know that we've been heard, we're not about to hear what the other person is saying. Instead, we turn away or raise our voices. Maybe if we scream at her, she'll hear.

Emotional discussions should be kept as brief as possible. Don't unload everything. Doing so only makes the listener feel inundated, nailed to the wall, with just two choices: fight or flight.

If you know the discussion will be emotional, set your intention ahead of time. Say, "I have something important to talk about, and this is what I hope we can get to at the end." Setting the intention helps both of you stay focused on the task and headed in the right direction. It keeps you from raising all kinds of other complaints and reduces your partner's anxiety about what's going to happen next.

Nowhere to turn. That's the way a lot of unhappy people feel about their relationships—trapped in the space of a relationship with someone who has some pretty stubborn ways. Accommodation means finding a way to fit together, but many people mistake fitting together as an all-or-nothing proposition.

A couple who were celebrating their sixtieth wedding anniversary were asked the secret to their success. Without hesitation, they concurred: "Look the other way some of the time; you don't have to react to every little thing."

Wise couples accept their differences and accommodate. But accommodating doesn't mean they must become two peas in a pod. Maybe she'll never be interested in politics. Maybe he'll never really get to like her parents. Rather than battle over these differences, or be untrue to themselves by giving in entirely, sensible partners avoid dwelling on subjects about which they don't agree.

But instead of drifting apart or insulating themselves from each other, they search for alternative avenues of connection.

Adjusting to each other's realities requires tolerance and selective coming together. Mates may tire of hearing about each other's jobs, but they owe each other a few minutes of listening at the end of the day. (Asking questions may make familiar stories more interesting.) But couples must also figure out which subjects are most rewarding to talk about together. The same balance applies to activities other than talking.

When Dennis returned from a run on Sunday morning, Lorraine was still in bed, so he took off his clothes and crawled in beside her. When he kissed her awake, she gave him a dubious look. It wasn't what he'd hoped for, but over the years he'd learned the difference between a red light and a yellow one. When they were first married, Dennis expected Lorraine to be ready for sex on demand. When she tried to slow him down and later said no, he felt rejected and avoided her altogether. Now he read her look as saying that she was happy to see him but not really in the mood to make love. They did a lot of talking with their eyes, but he made himself say, "Let's just hug a little." They did, and after a while Lorraine relaxed enough to become more affectionate. In the end they did make gentle love.

After lunch Dennis mentioned that he was going to watch football for a while. Once he'd expected to watch football all day on Sunday, and Lorraine, who came from a family that didn't follow the national obsession, would get angry. For years they'd alternate between his watching and her fuming and his not watching and feeling resentful. This day he watched the first half while she had a long phone conversation with a friend, read the paper, and occasionally looked up when the crowd roared. At halftime she asked if he wanted to go to the movies. He did. Movies were one thing they never had to compromise about. They went to see *Iron Man 27* but didn't go shopping afterward, as he knew she would have liked and she knew he would not have. After supper, they watched television together for a while, until Lorraine went upstairs to read and Dennis watched the second half of the game he'd recorded. It was a nice day.

As this example illustrates, listening, in its full sense, means taking each other into account. Dennis listened to Lorraine signaling her mood; later she listened to his wish to watch football, and between them they found a balance between separateness and togetherness.

In spite of the large emotions involved, long-term commitment isn't about monumental issues; it's about little things, about everydayness, about knowing that tomorrow morning you'll wake up with a new chance to work at it, to get it a bit more wrong or right.

Getting Beyond Bitterness

Although couples who survive the break-in period tend to mellow, they still go through cycles of closeness and distance. Some conflicts are resolved, others are avoided, and some keep cropping up from time to time. Arguments still occur, but the nature of these quarrels should change over time. They become less bitter and less acrimonious. There is less blaming and a greater feeling that both of you are in the same boat. If arguments don't become less frequent, less intense, and shorter, partners would do well to see what they're doing to keep resentment present and listening absent.

Successful couples learn that attempting to induce unilateral change using emotional manipulation—complaining, cajoling, sweet-talking, nagging, guilt-tripping, getting angry—doesn't work very well.

When empathy doesn't come easily, successful partners work at it—making themselves listen even when it's hard. (You don't have to *feel* sympathetic to listen. Sometimes showing concern works from the outside in, the way smiling can put you in a good mood.)

Problems arise when partners keep too many secrets, say yes when they don't mean it, or withhold the truth of their feelings because they're afraid of arguments. The broken promises that result from being afraid to say no are too great a price to pay for avoiding honest argument. Learning to say no enables you to say yes and mean it. If you're wishing that your partner would realize this, ask yourself, why would someone lie to you?

Trust allows people to relax into themselves. Being honest is central to establishing this trust, as is being open, listening to and acknowledging the hard things your partner says. Love that grows out of self-respect is love for ourselves as we are, not for a partial and carefully selected portion. The person who hesitates to speak wonders if it's safe to broach certain subjects. The person who struggles to open up to you may have already decided.

If you want the truth from people,
you must make it safe for them to tell it.

Unfortunately, even with the best of intentions, some couples reach a point where they get bogged down in bitterness. Pursuers get sick of pursuing and distancers get tired of the pressure, until one or both of them pulls back behind a wall of indifference. Pursuers can burn out and stop trying. Anger builds to resentment, and two people who once thrilled to each other now give up on each other. Retreating to an island of bitterness is cold comfort. But even loneliness sometimes feels better than constant conflict.

Mates bogged down in bitterness can take a step toward releasing themselves from frozen hopes by taking a hard look at those hopes. If you're willing to let go of blaming and look for a way back together, examine your expectations. Are your conflicts based on a desire for a partner who is fundamentally different from the one you committed to? If you're irritated with your partner for being who he or she is, rather than about some particular behavior, then you are in the wrong relationship. The only things worth fighting about are the things that can be changed.

People come to intimate partnership with a self-contradictory pair of expectations. They expect their partners to duplicate the good aspects of their own families and make up for the bad. To make matters worse, these expectations are often directed at a partner's limitations rather than his or her strengths. ("I know he could be a more sociable person, if he only tried.")

Don't judge your partner by measuring him against your strengths; measure him by his strengths. We all want to be appreciated for who we are.

No one benefits when weaknesses or shortcomings
become the principal focus of attention in a relationship.

To move away from bitterness, concentrate on your partner's virtues. See if some of the things you find objectionable are actually the downside of attributes you appreciate, that may have attracted you in the first place. He's late a lot, but when he gets there he's fully engaged, and you don't mind that he loses track of time when it's with you. She's willing to have six teenagers and all their noise and appetites come sleep over on a Saturday night, but that's because she's got a big heart. That sort of thing. If your partner were different in ways you'd like, she would also be different in ways you wouldn't like. Request changes of certain behavior, but don't punish your partner for what is really minor misbehavior or transient disappointment. Find your way to acceptance. Tenderness will follow.

With maturity, the human quest moves to greater acknowledgment of our interdependence, from prioritizing individual pursuits to being effectively dependent—to be who we are and to be connected with others. Looking for love that will simultaneously recreate and undo the past, we latch on to someone and hope for the best.

New couples are ripe with possibility. Over time they become structured into a system, organized by the demands of living together and perhaps raising a family. As we've seen, the process that transforms two people into a pair is based on accommodation and boundary making.

At first, patterns of behavior in a couple are free to vary; later they become entrenched. But even then, change is possible. The key is complementarity. Those who would remake their own luck must learn to see the annoying things their partners do as one part of a pattern, a pattern that connects two people together in cycles of action and reaction. Look to your part.

• • •

What I've tried to show in this chapter is how a better understanding of the joys and sorrows of intimate partnership comes from looking beyond personalities to the patterns of interaction between them. Problems, it turns out, are more likely to be resolved not by trying to change what your partner does, but by changing how you respond to it. Once you discover that the more you do X, the more he does Y—or he realizes that the more he does Y, the more you do X—either one of you can change the pattern by altering your own input. But when a twosome becomes a threesome, or, with remarriage, even a four-five-six-some, things get a lot more complicated.

As I'll explain in the next chapter, to understand what goes on in families, it's necessary to look beyond the dynamics of interaction between two people to the overall organization of the whole group. I hope these considerations will prove useful to you in understanding what goes on between you and every other member of your family.

EXERCISES

1. Identify three negative assumptions about your partner. During the next week, look for evidence contrary to any of those negative assumptions. (Hint: Consider motivation, not just behavior.)

2. Look back over the last few days and try to list three or four times when your partner did something good for the relationship and you failed to let him or her know that you appreciated it. It's never too late; express appreciation now.

3. In your relationship, are you more of a pursuer or a distancer? Why do you do that? Are you afraid of change? Afraid of feeling alone and abandoned? Afraid of conflict? What are you seeking when you pursue? Are you looking for mutual benefit or for changes that would mainly benefit you? What do you distance yourself from? Why does what you're avoiding make you anxious? What would you gain by shifting from avoidance to approach once in a while? If your partner is a distancer, what do you think he or she is avoiding? What can you do to reassure your partner that what he or she is afraid of isn't going to happen? If your partner is a pursuer, what does he or she want from you? How can you initiate giving more of what he or she wants in a way that doesn't make you feel like a victim?

4. A friend is someone with whom you can relax and be yourself. You can ask a friend for a favor. A friend is someone you can count on. A friend is someone you can talk to, whether it's over a meal or during a shared activity, walking side by side, or in the parked car on FaceTime. What would happen if you went out of your way to be a friend to your partner for a few days? Why don't you try it and see?

5. Make a list of your differences from your partner that he or she has trouble accepting. For each one, how would it affect your relationship if he or she were to become more accepting? Make a list of your partner's differences that you have trouble accepting. For each one, how would it affect your relationship if you made an effort to become more accepting?

6. The next time there is a "nagging situation" in your home, try to sit down when things are calm and compare your different views of what happened. What combination of what she was asking for and what he was willing to do produced the accusation of nagging? Try not to bring up a lot of past dirt; keep the conversation on this one instance. Sort out each of your contributions. Is this a task he just doesn't want to do? Did she make it sound like it wasn't that important? Would it be better to have asked in writing on a "honey-do" list? At a different time? Was he even listening the first time she asked? Did it sound like she was blaming him? How might this work better in the future? How do we get rid of the word "nagging" once and for all and have it be a reasonable request for help instead—no matter who asks?

11

"Nobody Around Here Ever Listens to Me!"

HOW TO LISTEN AND BE HEARD WITHIN THE FAMILY

As we've seen, the quality of understanding between people isn't fixed in character but depends on the *process* of their interaction. The advantage of seeing the process of relationships is flexibility. What can be recognized as a pattern of mutual influence can be changed. But there's a catch. Once children arrive on the scene, the dynamics of couplehood are no longer sufficient to explain what goes on in the family.

And when parents become the sole or primary caregivers through choice or circumstance, the family relationships shift in still other new directions. Now add to this: divorce and remarriage, step- and half-siblings, LGBTQ+ families, extended multigenerational cohabiting families, grandparents raising grandchildren, foster and adoptive families—and all the other sorts of contemporary family arrangements—and we see remarkable diversity and complexity in the structure and functioning of the American family. Indeed, fewer than half (46%) of U.S. kids younger than eighteen years of age are living in a home with two married heterosexual parents in their first marriage. So if you thought communication between two married people was complicated, imagine all the challenges our diverse families bring to the literal and figurative table.

Now, it isn't just how two people interact that can lead to problems in understanding, but how the overall organization of the family affects every single individual and combination of family members. Patterns of communication in families are hard to change because they're embedded in powerful but unseen structures.

Family Structure

Families, like other groups, have rich possibilities for satisfaction. (Don't we marry and bring children into the world with clear and simple hopes for happiness?) Walt Whitman said, "I contain multitudes." The same could be said of family relationships, though, sadly, many congeal into limited and limiting molds.

. . . .

Listening is an art that requires openness
to each other's uniqueness and tolerance of differences.

. . . .

As they are repeated, family transactions foster expectations that establish enduring patterns. Once these patterns are established, family members use only a fraction of the full range of behavior available to them. The first time the baby cries or the in-laws come to visit, it's not certain who will do what. Will the load be shared? Will there be a quarrel? Will one person get stuck with all the work? Soon patterns are set, roles assigned, and things take on a sameness and predictability.

When a father tells his son to put away his toys and the boy ignores him until his mother says he must, an interactional pattern is initiated. If it's repeated, it creates a structure in which the mother becomes the final authority and the father is marginalized.

. . . .

Family members tend to have reciprocal
and complementary functions; the more one parent does
for the children, the less the other is likely to do.

. . . .

The Possibilities in Every Pair

A family system differentiates and carries out its functions through *subsystems*. Every individual is a subsystem, and dyads (such as husband–wife or mother–child), as well as larger groups, make up other subsystems, determined by generation, gender, and function.

Individuals, subsystems, and whole families are demarcated by interpersonal *boundaries*, emotional barriers that regulate the amount of contact with others. Boundaries protect the autonomy of the family and its subsystems. A rule forbidding cell phone use at dinnertime establishes a boundary that insulates the family from outside intrusion. When children are permitted to freely interrupt their parents' conversations, the boundary separating the adults from the children is blurred.

Subsystems inadequately shielded by boundaries limit the potential of these subgroups. If parents always step in to settle their arguments, children won't learn to fight their own battles. Similarly, when in-laws are too actively involved in a couple's affairs, the couple will be slow to develop their own resources and allegiances.

These days when work and after-school activities consume so much of our lives, we have limited time for ourselves and less time for our families. In the few hours we do have with our families, many of us are reluctant to exclude some members of the family so that others can do things together— such as a father taking a daughter to a basketball game or a mother and son taking in a movie together. This is unfortunate.

Time alone together allows every pair in the family
a chance to talk and freedom to listen.

The most obvious example of a relationship that suffers without time alone together is the subsystem of the couple.

Lewis felt that he'd lost his wife to the new baby. Once Iris had been his friend and lover as well as his wife. Deciding to have kids and the pregnancy and birth and those first few wonderful, exhausting months of babyhood brought them closer together. Then, as Lewis saw it, Iris pulled motherhood over her head like a blanket. They were still friends, sort of, but they were more parents than anything else. They rarely listened to each other because they rarely talked. When Lewis decided to move beyond cursing fate and casting blame, he found that the simple act of spending time alone together with Iris was the first step in revitalizing their marriage. (In the process he discovered that two people who aren't spending time together aren't just busy, they're also dissatisfied with the listening they're getting.)

Parents also need time alone with each of their children. One of the best ways for parents to listen to their children is to arrange little outings with each one. Once a week isn't too much to aim for. Even if a child has a good relationship with a parent, conversation and intimacy are easier away from everyday distractions. The time a parent spends taking a child out to dinner or for a hike or to a museum may well be the best time in both of their lives. Every pair has its possibilities.

And the time spent getting to know your children can also be good for your marriage: when Lewis started taking the baby in the backpack carrier on special Daddy outings, he became more of a parenting partner for Iris—who felt closer to him as a result.

Now let's look at how some familiar structural flaws create problems in listening.

When Boundaries Are Blurred

The two biggest mistakes parents make in listening to their children both involve blurred boundaries: failing to establish control over their children's behavior and interfering too much in their lives.

The most important point to keep in mind when listening to children is the difference between allowing them to *say* what they want and letting them *do* what they want. A child who says "I don't want to go to bed" is expressing a feeling and making a request. A wise parent distinguishes between the two and acknowledges the feeling before ruling on the request.

Of course children don't want to go to bed! They might miss something. Staying awake is their way of clutching at life. Parents who blur the distinction between expression and action get into foolish debates with their children. They say, "I don't care what you want; you're going to bed anyway." Or they try to convince children that they're tired, as though obeying the rules depended on agreeing with them.

Parents who confuse love with leniency often fail to enforce their rules. Mistaking permissiveness for understanding and democracy for respect, such parents confuse their children about who's in charge and end up too anxious about controlling the children's behavior to be able to listen to their feelings. The dichotomy between authority and understanding is a false one; actually, they go hand in hand.

The most common alternative to effective discipline is nagging. Constant bickering with children wounds their pride and does more to engender insecurity than to establish parental authority. Effective parents take control early in their children's lives and use it sparingly. They are clear in their own minds about the difference between "No" as a complete response to something that is nonnegotiable and matters that might be open to more discussion.

A tired child wants to stay up later. Mom says, "I know you really want to read another chapter now, but it's time to turn out the light." That's not open to debate. But on the weekend, the child asks to go on a bike ride. They can talk together about when they'll go, where they'll ride to, and how long an outing it can be. They can figure out when chores and homework get done and think about what else is happening on the weekend to make sure that the adventure fits with everyone's plans. Establishing the difference between a firm "no" and a conversation means that boundaries are clear and children feel safe knowing what to expect.

. . . .

Children learn from the consequences of their behavior.
If the consequence of every third or fourth thing they do
is that their parents nag them, children learn that their parents
are nags and that they themselves are a nuisance.

. . . .

The boundary that makes it easier for parents to listen to their children because they are in charge is related to one of the crucial elements in listening: acknowledging what the other person says before responding with what you have to say.

Remember Tommy, the boy whose stepfather lectured him on the evils of anger? If only he had first acknowledged what Tommy was feeling, the boy might have been more open to that message. Seeing Tommy storm upstairs and slam his door, his stepfather might have said, "It's frustrating when the mower doesn't work, isn't it?" or "Sounds like you had a bad time."

Being a parent in charge doesn't make you a good listener, but it does release you from some of the anxiety about control that gets in the way of listening.

Suppose a little girl runs into the kitchen saying, "Look, I caught a caterpillar!" The mother who responds with "Go wash your dirty hands!" is obviously deflating the child's enthusiasm. Saying, "Yes, that's nice, but go and wash your hands" isn't very responsive either.

. . . .

"Yes, but . . ." is never enough. The but drowns out the yes.

. . . .

"Yes, but . . ." isn't a real acknowledgment. Like adults, children need to feel heard before they're open to a new thought. If a mother were to take a minute to acknowledge her child's enthusiasm, she might say, "What a pretty caterpillar," or "Hey, wow! Good for you!" The little girl, feeling heard and appreciated, might then wash her hands without needing to be told, especially if she knows that's the rule.

> If children suffer when the boundary between them and their parents is too diffuse, so do the parents. Parents too actively involved in their children's lives tend to be less actively involved with each other. This may not be obvious to some parents because they do so many things together. But how many things do they do together without the children?

Emotional Triangles

When he came downstairs, Marshall was surprised to see his teenage daughter sitting at the breakfast table sipping hot chocolate. Before he could ask why she was still home, Paula jumped up and threw her arms around his neck: "No school!" Looking out the window, Marshall saw the yard blanketed in white.

Assuming the driving would be bad, Marshall decided to wait until after nine before going to work. By that time the roads would be clear and the worst of the traffic would be gone. While he boiled water and ground the beans for coffee, Paula built a fire in the fireplace. When the coffee was ready and the fire blazing, they sat on the couch to watch the flames and share something that had lately gone out of their relationship: time alone together.

Just then the front door flew open, and in walked Paula's boyfriend. "Guess what? School's canceled!"

"Hi, Jerry," Marshall said, none too enthusiastically. Then he went upstairs to his study. He didn't exactly slam the door, but he didn't close it very gently either.

Paula and her father, who had been so close, were growing farther apart in this, her last year of high school. As Marshall sat there brooding about how Paula seemed to drop everything, including her homework, when Jerry was around, he knew he was wrong. Daughters grew up and had boyfriends; a father had to accept these things. He knew he was wrong to be so resentful of Jerry, and now he had that bitterness as well to swallow.

When Paula was born, Marshall vowed never to be one of those fathers who said, "I'll play with you tomorrow." What a remarkable thing it was to be a daddy, gifted and burdened with the power to bestow moments of total joy. As Paula grew older, they still did special things together, but he noticed that her pleasure in his company was no longer entirely spontaneous; he knew that at least part of the time they spent together now was only to please him.

Two weeks later Jerry broke up with Paula. She cried but showed no sign of real grief. These things happen. Marshall didn't feel he should pressure her by asking too much about it. Also, he couldn't help being secretly relieved and said so to his wife, Elaine.

On Monday Paula said she couldn't face going to school. Couldn't she stay home, just for one day? It seemed little enough to ask. That afternoon Elaine decided to come home early and cheer Paula up with a little shopping expedition. Finding Paula asleep in her room, still in her nightgown, was no great surprise. After all, it wasn't easy being seventeen and having your heart broken. Elaine never knew what made her go into the hall bathroom, where she found the empty bottle of aspirin in the wastebasket.

Paula spent two weeks on the adolescent unit of the local psychiatric hospital, where she learned the importance of giving voice to her feelings. When she discovered her anger, she started raging at her mother for always wanting everything to be "nice" and for thinking that shopping could be the answer to her problems. Her mother then did a surprising thing: she listened. But when Paula directed her anger at Marshall, telling him that he'd been unfair to blame her for growing up and having a boyfriend, Marshall got defensive. Nothing hurts like the truth.

During the last week of Paula's stay in the hospital, Jerry came to visit her, and after she was discharged, they started seeing each other again. Marshall was not happy.

Aside from his earlier objections about Jerry, he didn't think it was a good idea for Paula to put herself back into a vulnerable position so soon. His mind filled with bitter thoughts—about this callow boy who'd hurt his daughter, and might do so again, and about Paula's unforgiving anger at *him*. Well, maybe bitter thoughts were easier than wondering how a father stays connected with his daughter who is no longer a little girl.

Now when Jerry came around, Marshall was barely civil. He wanted to talk to Paula about not becoming dependent, about the importance of having many friends, but he was afraid of her anger and his own. So he started complaining to Elaine.

Paula too complained to her mother. "Why is Daddy so unfair?"

Time passed, and the crisis—that's what Marshall called it; he couldn't bring himself to say "suicide attempt"—began to seem unreal and long ago. Routine reasserted itself, and the only truly tense moments were occasions in which Paula wanted to go somewhere with Jerry and Marshall looked grim and said nothing. If Paula pressed him, he said sarcastically, "Ask your mother." He felt angry and bereft, but increasingly less so.

Winter passed, and then it was spring. After graduation Paula broke off with Jerry, saying she wanted to have her last summer at home free to be with her friends. Men, she had learned, can be pretty jealous and possessive.

In D. H. Lawrence's *Sons and Lovers*, Paul Morel, the young artist, doesn't feel free to become his own person until his adored mother releases him from her jealous love by dying. In the last scene, when Paul's sweetheart,

Miriam, asks if he is now free to marry, he says no. He's become free to go his own way.

One of the great themes of literature is the oedipal conflict—a child's passionate attachment to one parent and rivalry with the other. In real families, children fall in and out of love with both parents many times. We expect fathers to become antagonistic to their sons—and hope they will grow out of it. But when a father becomes alienated from his daughter, as Marshall did, we seek explanations in character and circumstance. Maybe Marshall was too attached to his daughter to tolerate a rival. Maybe he was too self-pitying to be empathic to her suffering. Or perhaps we can be more generous and say that it was only natural for him to worry about Paula's relationship with Jerry, considering what happened.

The trouble with these explanations is that they may account for the conflict but not why it wasn't resolved. Most family conflicts eventually get worked out—*if* the individuals involved are willing to listen to each other.

The Cotherapist in Family Therapy

Families, as you may have noticed, sometimes get stuck in ruts. Their problems are reinforced by the interlocking actions of more than one person. That's why the first family therapists described families as homeostatic systems that resist efforts to change them. Over many years of practice, I learned to look in every family for a cotherapist—one person willing to set aside blaming and take the first step toward transforming family patterns by changing his or her own contribution. It takes more than one person to make a family what it is, but one person can initiate change. Could you be that person in your family?

When Paula felt the innocent indignation of being misunderstood by her father, it seemed only natural to turn to her mother. Likewise, when Marshall worried about Paula's seeing Jerry again, it seemed reasonable to complain to his wife. In turning away from each other and detouring their dispute through Elaine, Paula and her father created a triangle, one of the great roadblocks to listening.

Take a minute to think about your most difficult relationship in your family. Chances are you thought of your spouse, or maybe one of your parents, or a child, or perhaps one of your in-laws. Actually, the relationship you thought of is almost certainly between you and that person and one or more other parties.

Virtually all emotionally significant relationships
between two people are shadowed by a third—
a relative, a friend, even a memory.

Triangles form across and within generations. Stressed couples usually have no shortage of people to bring in as a third party to their struggles. Libbey and her grandmother have always had a tight connection. Whenever she and her partner have a fight, she tells her grandmother all about it.

Some triangles seem so innocent that we hardly notice their destructive effect. Many parents can't seem to resist complaining once in a while to their children about their mates. "Your mother's *always* late!" "Your father *never* lets anyone else drive." These interchanges seem harmless enough. If you're really upset about something, you need to talk about it, right?

If something's really bothering you about someone and you're afraid to talk about it—afraid you won't be listened to—the urge to confide in someone else is almost overwhelming. The trouble with triangles isn't that seeking sympathy is wrong. The problem is that triangles can become chronic diversions that corrupt and undermine listening in family relationships.

Parents also create triangles when they complain to children about their siblings. "Your sister is such a slob." "Wow, can you believe Sean ate all the pie and didn't leave any for us?" Sometimes the irritation is spread evenly, but at other times a parent is, no doubt about it, playing favorites. Favoritism of a particular child will inevitably spark conflict and rivalry among siblings; this too interferes with the structure and functioning of the family.

Children are ever on the lookout for signs of love distributed unevenly and see it everywhere: "You gave him the bigger cookie!" "She always gets to sit in the front seat!" One family I know celebrates by going out to a special restaurant when their children get straight As. However, of the three children, only their conscientious middle son delivers a perfect report card. Can you blame his little sister for pitching a fit when it's time to go out to eat?

Perhaps more subtly, parents may also dole out their listening and engagement in imbalanced ways. This favoritism can be even more resented. It happens in all kinds of families, but it's more often an issue if there is one child who is particularly demanding, has some special needs, or just seems to connect more with a parent. A squeaky wheel needs more grease, but this can be frustrating for the less squeaky siblings. And the favored child doesn't necessarily have it easy either. Imagine being resented by your siblings and feeling more singled out than a child ought to. When parents play favorites, no one benefits.

Amelia has never been a good sleeper, and her bedtime routine lasts an hour or more. By the time her mom gets her tucked in and settled, she doesn't have much energy left over for Amelia's easygoing twin brother.

Django is his dad's mini-me and the only boy in the family. Django's sisters resent how much they are missing a comparable relationship with their father and do all they can to torment Django when the adults aren't looking.

Such favoritism can also include a preference for a particular beloved son or daughter over the spouse, creating a particularly toxic triangle.

When Marv proposed to Bethanie, he already had a couple of grown kids. This was Bethanie's first marriage, and she badly wanted a child of her own. Nathan was born a year later, and she was over the moon. Marv never had much of a chance after that. He tried to find his way back into the partnership. They argued and negotiated and went to couples therapy. He was Nathan's father, but he felt like an afterthought in his own home. Bethanie was so focused on Nathan, she simply lost interest in Marv. In addition to the troubled marriage, this enmeshment placed a heavy burden on Nathan. (The child is not supposed to win the oedipal conflict.) When the time came, Nathan applied only to colleges on the other side of the country. He needed boundaries and found a way to establish them when his mother would not. The marriage, long neglected, needed life support by the time Nathan was out of the house.

When you hear a story in which one person is a victim and the other is a villain, you're being invited into a triangle.

Triangles form across three generations, too. Mary was a twenty-six-year-old single mother who came to the clinic because she was having trouble controlling her rambunctious three-year-old, Tamara. She also said that her mother, who lived in the apartment next door, was making it harder because she spoiled Tamara and undermined the limits Mary tried to set. After she'd been describing her life to me for about forty minutes, Mary confessed that she got so angry when Tamara wouldn't listen that she was afraid she might hurt the baby. I offered to help her with parenting skills, and Mary brought Tamara to the next session.

Mary, who lived alone and had few friends, often related to her little daughter like a playmate. For example, when the baby was building a tower with blocks, Mary grabbed away some of the blocks to make her own tower, insisting that Tamara "share." Later in the session, when I was trying to ask Mary about her life as a single mom and Tamara started throwing blocks, Mary yelled at her—"Quiet down, okay? I'm talking to the doctor"—but didn't follow up. Tamara looked up for a minute and then continued throwing blocks.

Over the next two sessions I listened closely to Mary's concerns: her insecurity about what to do, her difficulty standing up to her mother, and figuring out reasonable expectations for what she might ask of a three-year-old.

I then helped Mary understand what it means to be a mother-in-charge. Parents take charge by being parental, which consists of two things: nurture and control. (The latter makes the former easier.) Mary learned that she could follow Tamara in play—this was a kind of listening. She didn't have to control everything the baby did. However, when she did need to enforce a rule, she had to speak clearly and directly and then follow through with consequences: "It's time to clean up the toys. When we are done, we can have a snack." "It's bath time. Put your clothes in the basket, and I will dump the duckies in when you are sitting in the tub." Becoming more confident of her authority made it easier for her to be more tolerant of Tamara. The language of small children is a language of action; "listening" to them means letting them take the lead in play and responding in a safe and supportive manner.

Mary had been feeling isolated and full of doubt. It's hard to parent alone. With my support and encouragement, she began enjoying Tamara more, setting clearer limits, and feeling less overwhelmed. They started getting along better; but in the fifth session, Mary reported that she was still having trouble with Tamara at home. For example, when she tried to get Tamara to clean up her toys, she'd say, "NO!" and then run down the hall to her grandmother's apartment. Instead of supporting her daughter's authority, Mary's mother tried to comfort Tamara by telling her not to worry, "Grandma loves you."

The grandmother's interference with her daughter's discipline may strike you as too obviously misguided to be of much relevance to the problems of listening in your own life. But aren't you playing the same game whenever you take one person's side against another?

Most family problems are triangular. Changing one part of the system sometimes causes the other parts to change. If you stop needing to have the last word in a fight with your ten-year-old, the argument will end sooner. But the triangle is a sturdy shape. Getting better at setting limits with the ten-year-old may not resolve the marital problem that led you to become over-involved with the boy as a result of your husband's emotional distance—or that caused your husband to disengage as a result of your maternal preoc-cupation. You might be a more effective parent, but the problems in your marriage probably won't go away immediately as a result of just this first effort. You and your husband will still have to speak directly with each other for that to happen.

Are triangles always a problem? No. Sometimes you just *have to* talk to someone other than your partner. For example, when I complain to my friends that my wife expects me to do my own laundry, it's because my wife doesn't understand that I don't always feel like doing it. Besides, if I tried to discuss this directly with her, we might get into tedious and unnecessary issues, like fairness and inequality and so on.

When Rigid Boundaries Keep People Apart

Some people establish rigid boundaries, so restrictive that they permit too little contact, resulting in *disengagement*. Disengaged people are independent but isolated. On the positive side, this fosters autonomy. If parents don't hover over their children, telling them what to do and refereeing their battles, the children will be forced to develop their own resources. On the other hand, disengagement limits affection and nurture. One of the paradoxes of modern life is the simultaneous fear that parents are hovering too much but are also too distracted and busy to pay sufficient attention to their children.

The disengagement may not necessarily reflect a parent's rigidity but instead his difficulty managing the overwhelming, simultaneous demands on his attention. His toddler is whiny and hungry at the end of the day, and he hears the ping of an urgent email. Glancing at it, he determines that it will just take a minute but he should deal with it right away. With the screeching child wrapped around his leg, Daddy first attends to the screen. By the time he switches his focus, the little boy is in full meltdown mode. It would have been better to prioritize the child, but that's hard for many of us jugglers to do now that work emails follow us home this way. Being listened to by their parents is how children build confidence in their powers of communication. Parents may not always listen but, in general, a parent has been a child's best chance to get someone to focus just on her. Once they start day care or preschool, other children will be competing for the adult attention. The undistracted loving gaze of a caregiver gives sustenance; however, it's evidently becoming rarer all the time. Many recent studies suggest that, from a very young age, children are competing with screens—as well as jobs, siblings, household chores, and other people—for their parents' attention.

MIT psychology professor Sherry Turkle, who studies the impact of technology on relationships, calls this "the flight from conversation in family life." She writes, "When adults listen during conversations, they show children how listening works. In family conversation, children learn that it is comforting and pleasurable to be heard and understood . . . to give children these rewards, adults have to show up, put their phones away, look at children, and listen. And then, repeat."

Sometimes if parents spend a few hours in their child's classroom, they can see how urgent it is that they listen more. They can see the world

through their child's eyes. They may gain insight into the multiple challenges for their dear small one navigating such a busy, noisy environment.
They may realize that teachers in most schools do a lot more talking than
the kids. This observation might lead to a renewed commitment to giving
children the gift of their undivided listening.

Spending relaxed, nondemand time in conversation with your
children—without turning everything into a struggle for control—helps
them traverse their own stressful days away in the world. Your loving engagement is the best antidote to peer pressure and schools' sometimes stifling
expectations for conformity and compliance. Make time. Shut those screens
and hold firm to an expectation that your kids will also give you their undivided attention for a few minutes. Convey in words, tone, and body that you
are ready to listen. Do this again tomorrow, and the next day too.

> The way to help children figure out who they are
> is to listen to them.

Disengagement is a behavioral description for lack of involvement—
spending time together, sharing activities, talking. People who are disengaged aren't necessarily uncaring, even if they do seem to spend a lot of time
pursuing their own interests. Often these individuals are using distance and
displacement to insulate their own sensitivities.

I had a family session with a smart, straight-talking fifteen-year-old
named Casey and her stepdad, Will. She came into my office on the verge of
tears, reporting that on their half-hour ride to my office, he took a business
call instead of focusing on her. Will travels for work at least half of every
month, so she'd been looking forward to this afternoon together with him
in the car and in therapy. She then went on to say, in no uncertain terms,
that she was really upset with him and she wanted to use the therapy hour
to help him "at least act interested" in her.

Will had taken on three young stepchildren when he married their
mother ten years ago. He was doing the best he could. And the last thing he
would have wanted from his own abusive and neglectful parents was more
attention; he truly had no idea what was happening here. By now, though,

tears were streaming down Casey's face, and she was hammering away with these demands. Gamely, Will pulled himself together and protested—carefully—that he *had* tried to talk to her before taking the call. His version of events included the fact that when they got in the car, he'd actually asked about what she was reading in English class. In his recounting, Casey just mentioned the name of the book and then stopped speaking entirely. He reported that, "to get the conversation going," he had said a couple things about how he'd loved that book in school, but she'd continued to be non-responsive. When the phone rang, he figured they were done, so he moved on and answered it.

Although we had discussed her desire for a better relationship with him on a couple previous occasions, Casey's version of what happened was still genuinely surprising to him. She said he just used that opening question about school "to talk about himself." Her monosyllabic answer to Will's inquiry absolutely did *not* mean he should stop asking questions and get on the phone. It meant—on the contrary—he needed to work a little harder. He might do better if he would ask her a follow-up question or two and then (this is a critical element) *wait* for her to come up with a response.

Disengaged relationships don't exist in a vacuum. To close the distance between you and someone you love, keep two things in mind: You catch more flies with honey than with vinegar. And if you want to close the distance in a disengaged relationship, be prepared to hear some complaints. Disengagement isn't just distance; it's protective distance.

When Closeness Smothers Intimacy

Sometimes the boundary separating family members from the rest of the world is so rigid that family relationships become enmeshed, offering closeness at the expense of autonomy. Isolation—from conversation, broadly speaking, with the rest of the world—puts too much pressure on any relationship. Intimacy grows with time together and time apart.

Some people are togetherness oriented. They value closeness and connection, but these values can actually reduce intimacy if they result in pressure to conform. To achieve genuine closeness, you must respect every family member's sovereign individual experience, their right to their own feelings and their own point of view.

Enmeshed relationships can comfort like a warm coat on a cold day or chafe like a wool blanket on a hot night. Children enmeshed with their parents become dependent. They're less comfortable by themselves and may have trouble relating to people outside the family.

We usually assume that parental involvement with children is a good thing: if children are having problems, their parents must not be sufficiently engaged. In some cases, this is true. But sometimes the problem is parental overinvolvement, robbing children of room to be themselves—to have problems, make mistakes, and learn to chart their own course.

A clear boundary between the generations puts parents in charge, allows them to claim their own rights and privacy, and helps them respect the children's autonomy within their own orbit.

When family therapists encounter mothers enmeshed with their children, they certainly don't blame mothers for this arrangement (as though a family's structure were the unilateral doing of one of its members). Oh, no, they would never do that!

Enmeshment, unfortunately, *is* usually blamed on mothers. Who else? They're the ones responsible for the primary—if not sole—care of their children, aren't they?[6] Blaming mothers for a family structure that leaves them unsupported by their partners and feeling totally responsible for their children is like saying that a car without spark plugs won't go because the pistons don't fire. Even infants and mothers engulfed in the blissful intimacy of baby love need the involvement of fathers and extended family. They need a supporter and a confidant, not a frustrated competitor.

. . . .

Children need attachment? So do their parents.

. . . .

Some of the overidentification of mothers with their children may be due to their being wedded to their traditional gender roles as nurturers. Critics often suggest that enmeshed mothers should have more of a life of their own. Many of them would like that too. But one in four mothers are raising children with little or no help from a partner. And even in two-parent households where both parents have full-time jobs, the lion's share of the

---

[6]Most people still harbor ancient grudges against the hand that rocked the cradle.

child care and logistics still falls on the mothers. They feel exhausted and stretched too thin. They love their families, but this arrangement causes them to harbor resentment for their partners. A recent poll conducted by *Forbes Woman* found that 63% of working mothers agree with the statement "Sometimes I feel like a married single mom." They would like more concrete support and the experience of being listened to and empathized with. It's getting the help and the listening you need that makes you strong, not having to go it alone.

Single parents particularly need to find other adults with whom to discuss their adult lives, or they may rely too heavily on their children for emotional support.

Kim and her adolescent daughter Allegra are both dating. It's a little crazy in the apartment on Saturday nights as they prepare to go out. Kim has been seeing her girlfriend, Melanie, for six months, and they are planning to move in together. Allegra likes Melanie but is not enthusiastic about having her invade their space. Her mom is her best friend, and she likes it when it's just the two of them at home, exchanging clothes, doing jigsaw puzzles, watching movies, eating ice cream late at night. They come to therapy to discuss Kim's plan to have Melanie move in; they want help with deciding how much of a vote Allegra should get in the decision. Melanie, who doesn't come with them, says to tell me she thinks it shouldn't be up to Allegra—but then she hasn't been a single mom with a daughter for a companion all these years.

In single-parent homes, the primary relationship is often cross-generational; the oldest daughter frequently takes on additional functions that would be more expected in an adult partnership—confidante, coparent for younger siblings if there are any. The bond can be deep and complex and difficult to rearrange. But family structures need to change with development. In this case, it's a new partnership, and again there may be more change in another couple years, when Allegra graduates from high school.

In one way, though, being a single parent can be easier than having to share in decision making, too, since parents may disagree on important issues and can have debilitating conflict around how to raise the kids. Single parenting is lonely, sure, but there's no one to contradict you in the living room. Parents need to try to be united. But most parents have different opinions on at least some issues involving their children. What should they do? They should talk about their opinions and listen to each other. Then they can decide how to act.

Forming a United Front

To forge an alliance that works, both parents must yield on some issues to gain in unity. *Accommodation* is the process by which people adjust their differences to come together. It is the mechanism of compromise, sometimes a deliberate result of negotiation, sometimes the result of instinctive adjustments. Unified family leadership is based on communication and compromise between parents and then presented to the children as one policy. Most parents eventually discover how important it is to accommodate their differences in order to present a united front.

True, this is complicated with step- and blended families; the biological parent may feel she is entitled to make decisions on her own. Similarly, as many people eventually discover, regardless of the family constellation, it's learning to accept each other, not trying to improve your partner, that preserves family harmony and makes couples last.

. . . .

When children continue to misbehave,
you can bet that one parent isn't backing the other up.

. . . .

If you don't feel supported by your partner in parenting, if you get stuck with all the driving or always have to be the one to enforce the rules, don't put all the blame on your partner. Maybe he or she disagrees with what you're doing. Try asking.

"I get the feeling you don't really agree with my way of handling this. Maybe you don't think I'm interested in your opinion—but I am. I'd really like to hear what you think."

Parenting is also an excellent place to observe the other side of complementarity—polarization. Instead of coming together on certain issues, parents push each other further apart. If one is too strict, the other may become too lenient. The more one harps at the children, the more the other tries to compensate by being indulgent.

Polarization is what happens when the controls on your electric blanket get switched. The first attempt by either of you to make it warmer or colder will set off a cycle of mutual maladjustment.

Small differences can drive couples to antagonistic opposites. A mother whose threshold for telling the kids to quiet down is only slightly higher than her partner's may never get the chance to discipline them if he always shushes them before she feels the need. Every time he reprimands the kids, she'll feel he's being too harsh. If she complains about his impatience, he'll get angry. Family life then becomes a battleground, where instead of sticking together, two parents become adversaries in a game where everybody loses.

Why do couples accommodate on some issues and polarize on others? Because we compromise where we're able but polarize in response to our own inner conflicts.

The engine that drives conflicts within us to become conflicts between us is projection. This dynamic comes into play when an ambivalent balance between pairs of conflicting impulses (dependence–independence, emotional expression–restraint, desire–anxiety, privacy–companionship) is resolved by projecting one's own motivation onto the other person. A man (or woman) who's afraid of anger may express it through passive control that provokes his (or her) partner. When they fight, she gets angry and he gets hurt. The man who feels only hurt may be seething with rage but remains unaware of those feelings as long as he has an obliging mate to act out his anger for him. In the process, the partner who shows anger may be able to avoid facing inner feelings of helplessness.

When children are in the home, they are watching this dynamic closely; they are learning how to love, fight, apologize, and repair from how their parents do these things. Children who can be manipulative in getting people to do what they want may well have learned this at home from a parent who communicates obliquely. Children who are ready to admit when they made a mistake or violated a rule also likely have at least one parent who takes responsibility for his or her behavior. Our children don't know it's projection; they just think this is how things are done. Even when we are not speaking to them, our children are still listening to us—with their eyes and their minds, as well as their ears. A teenager lurking about with headphones on or with a face on a screen is likely hearing just enough of the tone of things, if not the content, to know if tension is brewing.

Polarized mates fight in each other
what they can't accept in themselves.

Luckily, parents don't have to agree on absolutely everything—and if you pretend it is so, rest assured that your kids are probably remarkably attuned to the vulnerabilities in that facade of unity. What's more important than faux agreement is that adults in the home have skills to listen to each other. They are setting a lifelong example for how differences get managed and settled, how people consider others' viewpoints without toxic levels of criticism or contempt in the way of a productive conversation.

When parents have become so polarized that they've separated and divorced, it's common that, at least for a little while, communication and effective problem solving about the kids go out the window. After a few months, when the emotionality and hurt subside, at least a little, most couples start moving forward again. This is not to suggest that all the polarization that led to the separation gets resolved, but just that most couples learn a strategy for coparenting in two homes and, if the acrimony diffuses somewhat, all involved are likely to survive this upheaval.

Some parents even do better as exes. For example, Marv and his first wife became good friends over time; indeed, she often joined Marv and Bethanie for holidays when the two grown kids were back in town. It had gotten easier to coparent without the other's constant scrutiny and judgment; anxious tension had dissipated further when the children were old enough to speak for themselves.

A few families come apart intentionally and carefully. Those parents are often good listeners to begin with. My friend, Jon, for example, had one of the least acrimonious divorces I'd ever seen. When I asked him his secret, he said that when he started getting riled up he "kept his eyes on his girls" and then he did right by them. He listened better, compromised more willingly, and treated their mom as kindly as he could, for them. Try with all your might to avoid pulling your children into a toxic triangle with your ex-partner. Don't ask them to take sides; remember they get to love both of their imperfect adults.

The biggest factor in how well kids do after divorce is how well their parents get along. Keeping respectful and clear channels of communication open can make a huge difference, reducing the distress in your kids. And, if you are separated and trying, in vain, to maintain consistency between the homes, take heart. Kids are astonishingly flexible. In no time at all, they'll figure out how to manage going back and forth, adapting to two sets of rules and expectations.

Hearing their parents work through different viewpoints, listen to one another, and focus on a solution that is in the child's best interest teaches kids that important questions can take a lot of time to figure out—and that the people who love them most in the world are willing to take that time to speak and listen to one another all the way through—even when the conversation proves to be difficult. In the future, these kids will then be able to expect that when they are struggling with a tough problem, there will be people nearby who will listen to *them* and take all the time that's needed to help them sort it out.

EXERCISES

1. Make a commitment to listen to everyone in your family for five minutes this week, without distraction or another agenda. If parents make a conscious effort to engage in one-on-one conversation with their children and each other, the tone in the home might start to change. Do you see yourself differently when you are listening on purpose? Are you curious about how much or how little people have to say when you open up space for them and ask them to talk to you?

2. Make a list of three annoying things someone in your family does on a regular basis. Next, for each one of these things, write down how you think that person would prefer to be seen. See if you can direct yourself to the person's preferred view in your next encounter. In other words, try to treat the family member as his or her best self.

3. Identify one boundary in your family that you don't like—for example, your wife is too involved with the children, or your daughter is too secretive. Remembering that boundaries are reciprocal (enmeshment in one place is related to disengagement in another), try to identify the part you play in perpetuating the boundary you don't like. Don't be in a rush to change anything; just observe.

4. Try to identify two or three triangles you participate in. If there is a triangle where you are on the uncomfortable outside, try moving not to the person you want to be closer to but to the person or activity on the other pole. For example, if you're still competing with your favored older sister for your mother's attention, even now as adults, reach out to your sister.

5. If you haven't tried having a couple of screen-free family hours a week, establish a plan ahead of time to do just that. Have a nice meal, play board games or charades, take a family walk, or just hang out together doing nothing. See what that's like—what's fun about it and what's hard or boring. Listen to your kids talk about how they miss their screens and tell them how you feel.

12

"I Knew *You'd* Understand"

BEING ABLE TO HEAR FRIENDS AND COLLEAGUES

Friends make the best listeners. They may not love us quite as much as our families do, but then they don't need quite as much from us either, and that frees them to listen better. No matter how close we are to our friends, we retain a certain independence, which enables us to listen with less need to control them or protect ourselves.

Why Friends Make the Best Listeners

Sandy had just come from a workshop on counseling high school students when she met her friend Roberta for lunch. If she didn't trust Roberta's support so completely, Sandy might have hesitated to tell her that she was thinking about doing something that would mean an end to their lunches. The two of them had been teaching at the same school for nine years, and now Sandy had decided to go back and get a master's in guidance counseling. It was a big decision, scary and exciting, and she needed someone to talk it over with.

Roberta was taken aback by Sandy's plan. Giving up tenure and going back to school seemed risky. How did Sandy know she would like counseling? Wasn't she taking a big chance? Besides, Roberta couldn't imagine getting along at work without her friend. Sandy was the only sane person in the place. It would be awful if she left. But Roberta didn't say any of this. No matter how much she questioned Sandy's plan, it was her decision, and Roberta could see how excited she was by this new dream of hers. So she just listened.

It took Sandy two more days to get up the nerve to mention going back to school to her husband. "I can't believe you'd even think of such a thing!" Gordon said. "Are you crazy? You've got a perfectly good job. How are we going to pay for you to go to school?" Sandy started to protest, but she was too hurt to bother, and they finished supper in silence.

Roberta's ability to listen to Sandy was the mirror opposite of her husband's inability. Roberta could listen because she wasn't threatened—or at least not *as* threatened.

Clearly Gordon had a stake in whether or not Sandy went back to school. He had a right to his concerns. At some point the decision might become a joint one. But his inability to even listen to Sandy's plan not only deprived her of the chance to think out loud, but also made her less likely to consider his feelings in the final decision.

Whether it's money, the kids, or in-laws, there are unsafe subjects in every family. A woman doesn't talk to her Catholic relatives about having an abortion. The same woman might not risk telling her husband that she might be able to sleep better if they got separate beds if she was afraid he'd be too offended even to entertain the possibility. He might not tell her about a problem he's having at work if he was afraid she'd respond with unwanted advice. He might not want to burden her with financial worries (or share the decision making). It's not necessarily a question of keeping secrets, though most family members have a few. Rather, it's just hard to tell the people you live with everything. With friends, few subjects are off limits.

In conversations between friends, little misunderstandings can be passed over or forgotten between breaks in contact. Disagreements between people who live together are harder to forget.

The relationship between friends is voluntary; you can leave if you want to, and therefore it's safer to be honest. You can talk over painful or embarrassing subjects, reveal self-doubts, try out different sides of yourself, and be who you are.

People show caring and respect through the quality of their listening. Friends who listen make us feel interesting, and their interest inspires us to say more interesting things. Their receptivity is transformative: by listening intently to us, our friends make us larger, more alive. That's the glory of friendship.

> ### A Good Friend Is a Good Listener
>
> Most people think more about what they want to say than about what is being said to them. To be a good friend, learn to listen better. Once in a while, try approaching a friend with the intention of finding out what's on his or her mind and listening for an extended period of time. If he switches the subject to you, tell him you'll get a turn later; you want to hear from him now.

A friend is someone with whom you can talk about almost anything. With such friends we take turns submerging ourselves for a time, being there without strings for our friend. Friendship grows with mutual disclosure. So do we. The compassion friends offer when they listen to our triumphs and worries deepens us; their understanding keeps us from feeling alone—and helps us understand ourselves.

Friendship deepens us; it also broadens us. Friendships expand our definition of ourselves and awaken unrealized possibilities, possibilities that aren't part of the scripted roles we play in our families. With many friends we can express many sides of ourselves. The intimacy of friendship, the function of being there for someone else, strengthens us. Mutuality, the sharing function, stretches us.

> ### "I Wish I Had More Friends."
>
> Write down the five most important things on your agenda for the next seven days.
>
> Was spending time with a friend on the list? Was trying to strike up a friendship with someone at work or the gym on the list? Was strengthening an already established friendship by expressing your affection on the list?

Social media have made sustaining casual friendships easier and can enrich our close friendship ties. We can "friend" and "follow" people we've known forever, keeping up with their accomplishments and sorrows even if we don't see them more than every five or ten years at school reunions. But social networking has expanded the idea of "friends" to encompass both people we have never met—friends of friends—and those we have cared for since playing together on the playground. We may wish these people happy birthday because Facebook reminds us to (and there is no way we would have known or remembered otherwise) and enjoy seeing pictures of their activities, their pets, or their kids and grandkids growing up.

We can be connected to our friends in ways unimaginable a generation ago. There's some real satisfaction in being part of our own web on the Web; belonging makes us feel a little warmer (even if sometimes there's a little too much trivia). For most of us, virtual friendships aren't everything, but we're all crazy busy, and they are surely better than nothing. Friends who can't find the time to see one another in person can text a few times a week, FaceTime a flu-ridden buddy while waiting for the bus, or make an appointment to chat on the phone with a best friend far away in Tucson next weekend. For many of us, it's got to be good enough because it seems like the best we can do.

On the down side of the screen, however, is the techno-crowding of already precious free time as emails sent all evening blur the line between work and home. Too many of us are back on a device after getting home from a long work day, hacking away at the correspondence we didn't get to yet—perhaps during just that hour we might once have spent catching up by phone with a friend. We have to schedule phone dates, because otherwise one of us might call at an inconvenient time—and the resulting phone tag is a drag. And we may prefer to text instead of calling anyway, because we don't want to interrupt people who are also crazy busy. In crowded and hurried lives, competing obligations squeeze out anything optional, like spending time with friends. But even though many of us may be busy and preoccupied these days, it's more than lack of time that undermines friendships.

When Friends Take Sides

After her divorce Maggie turned to her friends. They saw her through the shock of separation and the months that followed. Though she felt adrift, at least she wasn't alone.

Maggie's friend Liz was also divorced and disillusioned; she understood what it was to be single again, having to start all over, the indignities and misunderstandings of online dating almost the only way to meet anyone now. The two women had known each other for nine years, ever since they met at a workshop (ever since, in fact, they both skipped the afternoon session and ran into each other at a local art gallery).

Liz made friends easily. She embraced Maggie with her warmth and held her with her intelligence and keen eye for the pretentious and foolish. They met often for lunch or for a drink after work, enjoying conversations about their jobs, families, friends, what they were reading, how they felt—if any subject was off limits, they hadn't come to it yet.

Maggie met Dominic three years after her divorce. As chance would have it, she met him in the lobby of Liz's building where they ran into each other several times before he acknowledged her. She found him attractive but couldn't imagine speaking to him; he was busy getting his mail and heading for the elevators the first couple times they crossed paths. He seemed unapproachable. It came as a surprise, therefore, when he started talking to her one Saturday afternoon as she waited for Liz to come home—and, after no more than five minutes, he asked her out. To her equal surprise, she found herself accepting.

If opposites attract, they were a perfect match. Maggie had the ruddy complexion and emotional reserve of her Scottish ancestors, while Dominic was Greek, with dark hair and olive skin and an openly expressive nature. She liked the way his mind worked, all intuition and confidence. What a relief after all those pale, shadow men the Internet dating sites had produced!

The passion Maggie felt with Dominic was thrilling. Unfortunately, as she soon found out, the price to be paid was a series of equally passionate quarrels. Dominic was jealous of her time, her friends, and just about everything else. Though he might sometimes be busy for days, he expected her to be available whenever he wanted to see her. When she wasn't, there were storms of jealousy.

When Maggie told her other friends about all the trouble she was having with Dominic, they were sympathetic. Liz got angry. She considered Dominic's possessive jealousy abusive and thought Maggie was wrong to put up with it. "I'd never let a man treat *me* that way," she said.

After one particularly violent outburst, Maggie decided not to see Dominic for a while. As long as they'd been going out together, Liz had held back the worst of her criticism, but now that Maggie was considering ending the relationship, Liz broke a cardinal rule of friendship and served up judgment. She spoke strongly against Dominic. Maggie would be better off without him, she said. In this opinion, Liz was not alone. All of Maggie's friends felt the same way: If Dominic was causing her so much unhappiness, she should dump him.

Unfortunately, sympathy can get in the way of empathy. Unable to suspend their own emotional impulse, which was to rescue Maggie from the grief she shared with them, her friends urged her to put an end to what was making her so unhappy. That's what friends often do when we complain about someone: they take our side and push us to retaliate.

It's one thing to honor a friend's right to happiness, but far more difficult to respect her right to put up with unhappiness if she decides to go to war for love.

Maggie was buoyed by the sympathy of her friends but felt pressured by their urging her to break up with Dominic. While it's comforting to have someone to share your feelings with, it's not always comforting to be told what to do about them. People have a right to their ambivalence.

After a while Maggie stopped talking to her friends about Dominic. She wasn't only angry at Dominic; she also loved him. While it's okay for us to criticize our own loved ones, it's a mistake for friends to agree. Our griping expresses just one side of our ambivalence—and leaves us free to do whatever we decide about the relationship. But a friend's agreeing that someone we're close to is a terrible person is a boundary violation that disregards the fact that our griping only expresses one side of our ambivalence.

There is no formula for an empathic response, but it may help to remember that there are two sides to every conflict—even when it's an internal conflict. Understanding—empathy—therefore often means acknowledging uncertainty. If a person hasn't acted to resolve a problem, there's probably a reason.

Liz might have said something like "You sound pretty unhappy, but I guess you're not sure what to do." Instead she said, "Dominic's not good enough for you. If you go back to him now, you'll hate yourself for it."

. . . .

There are things that have no place in friendship,
and judgment is one of them.

. . . .

Showing empathy to friends doesn't mean just caring about them; it means listening to their point of view, whether or not you agree with it. Friendship doesn't require neutrality or total acceptance; but before they disagree or give advice, real friends listen.

Here is an example of a friend struggling to be empathic from Paul Auster's novel *Leviathan*. Peter's friend Sachs is telling him about the accident in which he fell off a four-story fire escape, trying to explain that he feels responsible because he wouldn't have been out there if he hadn't been flirting with a woman:

> There were questions I wanted to ask him then, but I didn't interrupt. Sachs was having trouble getting the story out, talking in a trance of hesitations and awkward silences, and I was afraid that a sudden word from me would throw him off course. To be honest, I didn't quite understand what he was trying to say. There was no question that the fall had been a ghastly experience, but I was confused by how much effort he put into describing the small events that had preceded it. The business with Maria struck me as trivial, of no genuine importance, a trite comedy of manners not worth talking about. In Sachs's mind, however, there was a direct connection. The one thing had caused the other, which meant that he didn't see the fall as an accident or a piece of bad luck so much as some grotesque form of punishment. I wanted to tell him that he was wrong, that he was being overly hard on himself—but I didn't. I just sat there and listened to him as he went on analyzing his own behavior.

To be with other people authentically—that is, to respond to them as they are, not as we want them to be—is no easy feat. This ability depends on an awareness of ourselves as self-contained individuals who relate by listening to and accepting other separate and autonomous individuals.

Maggie and Liz's attachment was built on shared interests and understanding. When Maggie began to feel judged unfairly, the friendship waned.

The two friends didn't know how to tolerate the differences that were emerging between them. Maggie felt she was betraying Liz whenever she was happy; she then didn't feel she could rely on Liz when she was miserable. Neither of them knew how to talk about the feelings they were experiencing. Liz felt abandoned by Maggie. Their differences and their inability to talk about them formed a widening gulf. As in so many situations where differences between friends can't be talked about, the friends drifted apart.

When Maggie eventually worked things out with Dominic, she stopped seeing Liz altogether. Years later she would say to someone offhandedly, "Oh, we just lost touch."

Resolving Conflicts with Friends

Why, if Maggie was able to work things out with her jealous and demanding boyfriend, wasn't she able to resolve the conflict with her like-minded and appreciative friend? Here's the irony of listening in friendship:

The same elective quality of relationship that enables friends to speak freely about so many subjects makes them less likely to speak openly about problems between them.

The binding nature of family ties makes it more urgent to speak up about our unhappiness in those relationships. While friends do sometimes voice complaints to each other, they are less likely to talk about serious problems between them, like envy, jealousy, or resentment. Because the ties of friendship aren't as obligatory as those of family, there's a greater fear that friends will abandon us if we voice complaints to them. Sadly, when such feelings are strong, friends often drift apart.

Friends who are struggling to resolve a difference may resort to the less emotionally vulnerable strategy of just texting. On the one hand, it's possible to stay connected this way, perhaps to cool off and see how things unfold until the next time they are together. On the other hand, it's much easier to drop a text conversation when it gets tough and then differences don't get resolved. And feelings can get hurt even more when one friend "ghosts" the other by not responding at all. If a friend goes into gentle breakup mode by writing brief, bland, or noncommittal texts, or taking a longer than usual time to respond, she is probably uncomfortable with the conflict and fearful of addressing it directly. A friend breakup that doesn't require us to see the hurt and disappointment in the other may seem more antiseptic, but it will feel disrespectful and unkind to the person being dismissed this way.

> If you have a gripe about someone and the relationship is optional, let it go. But if you have a grievance about someone you care about, find a way to say something.

People who hesitate to speak when something is bothering them often imagine that those brave souls who do simply have more confidence in themselves. Perhaps. But most of the people I've known to tell friends that something is bothering them were just as worried about saying so as those who keep silent. What enabled them to take the risk wasn't only respect for themselves and their right to their feelings, but also respect for the relationship—and for their friends.

The longer you avoid telling a friend that something's bothering you—say, that you wish your friend wouldn't make a habit of bringing along a third person when you get together—the more preoccupied you become with your grievance. In your internal debate about whether or not to complain, you probably imagine phrasing your complaint in such a convincing way that your friend will have to hear you. In fact, the most effective way to address an impasse between friends is to take into account what you imagine your friend's position to be.

> Acknowledging your friend's position releases him or her from brooding about it and opens him or her to hearing your side.

Let's say that you always seem to be the one to contact a certain friend about getting together. You're not the sort of person to keep score, but his never inviting you to do anything together troubles you. You're starting to wonder if he really likes you. You hesitate to say anything because he might feel attacked. What to do? Tell him all of that. Use your ability to empathize to anticipate how your friend might feel about what you have to say. "Something's been bothering me, but I've hesitated to bring it up because I didn't want you to think I was blaming you. Actually, this may have to do with my own insecurity . . ."

. . . .

**Sometimes an honest complaint
can save a friendship.**

. . . .

Ian got tired of Arlene's constant complaining—about her jerk of a boss, her numerous aches and pains, and her rich repertoire of boyfriend troubles. But he didn't want to say anything. He didn't want to hurt Arlene's feelings. (Isn't that what we tell ourselves when we don't want someone to get mad at us?) So instead of saying anything, he just stopped being available when Arlene called, and the friendship withered and died.

When friends don't speak up about what's bothering them, grievances gnaw at the relationship. Even if it doesn't completely resolve the conflict, hearing each other's position makes a big difference. The best place to start to address an impasse between friends is not to state your position but to consider what your friend might be feeling and try to acknowledge that in a way that invites him or her to elaborate.

Few friendships last long if all one person does is complain about things. We all have troubles in mind, but remember that listening, especially to complaints, is a burden. If you have a friend who takes advantage of your willingness to listen without reciprocating, you can accept this burden until you get fed up—like collecting enough frequent-flyer miles to trade in for the right to walk out on the friendship. Or you can say something.

If you only have one or two friends, you may be unwilling to allow the friendship to end. It's hard to walk away if you believe that lopsided listening is better than none at all. And in a long-term friendship, keeping this kind of ledger might not be such a big problem anyway. If you have a friend you've known your whole life and see infrequently, you just step up if you are needed. It's easier, of course, if we have enough community of other friends and support from a variety of places that we don't have to rely so heavily on a single friend for our own listening.

When Adam had rotator-cuff surgery, followed two weeks later by his son getting arrested for underage drinking, and then a month later by needing to move his mother to a nursing home, his friend Martin checked in every few days. Martin would first quickly say things were fine at his end to switch the focus to his lifelong friend. He felt no resentment, only sympathy, when he encouraged Adam to "tell me the latest." Martin didn't need to have his turn because they had been friends for forty years and he had already had plenty of turns.

A running friend of mine used to complain about all the trouble he was having with his stepson. I'd listen sympathetically and occasionally offer advice (it's okay, I have a license). But if my friend talked for more than a few minutes, he'd get self-conscious (maybe partly *because* I have a license) and apologize. I'd remind him that in our relationship complaining was a two-way street. I didn't mind hearing about his problems because I was grateful for the time he spent listening to mine.

When two people are locked in silent grievance, the best way to open the subject is to ask about the other person's feelings. This applies especially to mutual misunderstandings. Don't be too quick to tell your side. In cases of major misunderstandings, concentrate first on listening to the other person. Save your feelings for later. But if your friend has hurt you and doesn't know it, eventually saying something about how you feel may be the only way to keep your resentment from poisoning the relationship.

Alice and her husband were both independent and regularly did things like go out to dinner or to the movies separately. Alice's friend Marie, on the other hand, didn't feel comfortable socializing without her husband. So the two friends sometimes got together alone, but more often they did things as couples, as Marie preferred. They both understood their different situations, but each came to feel that she was doing more of the accommodating. Gradually, they saw less and less of each other.

Marie was hurt. She was disappointed that Alice wasn't more sympathetic to her situation. The less they saw of each other, the more Marie brooded over how hurt she felt; and the more she brooded, the more she imagined confronting Alice. Could Alice's feelings conceivably mirror her own? It was a possibility she hadn't considered, but she decided to take a risk in the interest of preserving the friendship.

Marie called and said she imagined Alice must be frustrated by her having trouble getting together except as couples. Alice, relieved to have her feelings acknowledged, said yes that was true, but deep down she worried that Marie didn't really like her enough to want to do things alone together.

Once Marie had broken the ice by showing concern for Alice's feelings, the two friends were able to talk about their misunderstanding and resentment—feelings that often seem too threatening to talk about. The basic conflict didn't disappear—Alice still preferred to get together alone with Marie, and Marie still had trouble going out without her husband—but it no longer festered. The two friends now understood each other, and their friendship endured.

Friendships can get stressed by different expectations for responsiveness when someone texts. There is an on-call quality that comes with the device; we can "be there" for our friends in a new way; we can also disappoint them if we are insufficiently responsive.

Dante has a stressful job that he mostly hates. He's in a cubicle in a huge room of cubicles, and he has no privacy. His boss wanders the room and makes sure people stay on task. Dante's good friend Sammy works from home and has a lot of flexibility about how he gets his job done. Although Dante has told him repeatedly, Sammy seems not to appreciate that Dante can't respond to him online from the office. Sammy texts and calls whenever he gets the urge. Sammy says Dante is uptight about his boss; Dante is increasingly frustrated that Sammy doesn't respect his limits. Sammy's free time and casual attitude make Dante resent his job and his friend in equal proportion.

Clear conversations and defined boundaries can help friends navigate these different expectations about how available they can be to one another. Technology has had a seismic impact on our expectations for the length of time friends can take before responding to a text. If we are accustomed to hearing back immediately from someone, it's natural that's what we'll want the next time we press send. So anything less than on-call availability—our personal limits—need to be established . . . . preferably in person.

How to Offer Constructive Criticism to a Friend

There are times when just listening to a friend you think is making a mistake is less than honest. However, if you feel like offering advice, it's a good idea to first ask if your friend wants to hear it.

"Would you like to hear what I think?"

Advice implies criticism, and even well-intended criticism can backfire. If you suggest that a friend change something he or she isn't interested in changing (or likely to change), your comments, however well-meaning, can leave the friend feeling resentful.

Sometimes when we give our opinion, we feel rejected if our friend doesn't follow it.

"Why did you ask for my advice if you weren't going to take it?"

Taking advice means considering it, not necessarily following it. The best kind of advice has no strings attached. A good listener allows friends to accept or reject suggestions without acting slighted.

· · · · · · · · · · · ·

The time to press your point of view is when you disagree
with a friend about what you should do,
not the other way around.

· · · · · · · · · · · ·

If you're not sure how your friend feels about your advice, ask.

"What do you think?" If friends give even one reason why they probably won't do what you suggest, drop it.

Do Friends Outgrow Each Other
or Just Forget How to Listen?

For all too many people the story of friendships is a history of broken connections. The loss of friends may not be as wrenching as that of people who live together and share destinies, but the process is similar. We make friends in one set of circumstances—in college, say, or starting a new job or, like Maggie and Liz, as veterans of divorce. Then one or both of us changes; we move on, and the connection becomes harder to sustain.

The reasons we marry at twenty or thirty aren't the same reasons we stay married at forty or sixty, but friends, who have fewer ties to bind them, are less likely to do the maintenance it takes to sustain a relationship through major life changes. A lot of that work involves respecting each other's differences over the years and learning to listen when it doesn't come easily.

Gil and Roy were friends in high school. Both were basketball players and good students, and they gravitated together naturally. It was a friendship based on shared interests and the kind of wisecracking teenage boys use to test themselves. Their listening to each other, if you can call it that, took the form of taking turns showing off.

As they grew older, Gil found Roy's constant ribbing exasperating but often invigorating, too. Others just found it annoying. Eventually Gil too got tired of Roy's aggressive wisecracking. When he finally said so, Roy got upset, and the two friends stopped speaking to each other.

A couple of years later Roy called Gil, and the friendship was renewed, only now it seemed more superficial, at least to Gil. Roy still seemed so adolescent. He was always posturing, looking for an angle, a spin, a take.

Together the two friends attended their twentieth high school reunion. Gil remembered how the waves of emotion and memory washed over him but that Roy remained his old wisecracking self. Afterward the two of them went out for a drink with Gil's old girlfriend.

Janice, who was still sensationally pretty, brought out the old competitive edge between the two friends, who spent an hour in the bar tossing barbed comments back and forth. Gil didn't think Janice was very impressed by their performance, and later he felt a little embarrassed.

Much later Gil learned that Roy had taken Janice home that night and the two of them had begun seeing each other. The way he found out was that Roy called him, all upset, to tell him that Janice had broken it off with him. Gil was furious. It seemed like such a devious thing for Roy to have done—not just to score a conquest with his old girlfriend, but to keep it secret. Why, if there was nothing sneaky in what Roy had done, hadn't he said anything about it? Still, when Roy turned to Gil to nurse him through his hurt, Gil was forgiving, the way friends are.

The next time the two friends got together was when Gil invited Roy to his annual company picnic. Roy, who'd again had a few beers, started making jokes about private things Gil had said to him about various members of the company. Gil was embarrassed and tried to shut Roy up but wasn't very successful. The following week, Gil wrote an email to Roy saying that he didn't trust him anymore, that he didn't plan to see him again, and that he didn't want Roy to contact him.

Gil found this act—deliberately severing a tie that had become a burden—quite liberating. It felt like a declaration of self-respect. Thinking about the end of the friendship, he remembered a Herman Hesse quote from college days: "Some of us think holding on makes us strong, but sometimes it is letting go."

But it's not always easy to know when to give up on an old friendship. As we get older, these connections become more precious and rare; we know that it takes effort over time and distance to sustain our attachments. Maybe when we're kids friendship comes easily, but as we get older we may have to work at it. The idea of working at making friends and keeping them may go against the grain, but that's true of a lot of things worth doing. Gil's friendship with Roy may have become one of those relationships that persist out of habit even though they are fundamentally unrewarding. But many friendships, even based on a more solid connection, may require repair from time to time. For friendships to grow with you, you may have to put in some effort.

One important ingredient in getting the listening you deserve is cultivating relationships based on mutual exchange. This means remaining open enough to form new relationships and selective enough to drop those that aren't worth the effort. Deepening relationships requires a balance between self-disclosure and listening. But then, inevitably, many of us find ourselves stuck in relationships with people who have trouble listening. Instead of remaining bitter or fatalistic, it's possible to teach them to listen—by setting an example and, if necessary, asking for reciprocation.

Having friends means making time for them. If friends come second, if you're too busy working to be with your friends, what are you working for? For friendship to flourish the relationship must be given priority. Keeping friends means being willing to work at it. Not all the time certainly, but listening sometimes when it's hard and speaking up sometimes when it's necessary.

Finding and Making Time to Listen to Friends On- and Off-Line

When Tessa gets home from the office, it's almost seven and she's still on the move. She wants to go to the gym, but she's hungry and a dozen work emails await her response. Tessa is standing at her kitchen counter gnawing on a rotisserie chicken leg when her phone buzzes. She glances at the screen: it's her lifelong friend Amber with just this text: "Well, I think it's over." In an instant, Tessa considers her options for how to respond: Pretend to have missed the text? Worried emoji? Text back? Call later when I get back from the gym? What would Amber want me to do? What do I want to do? Although Tessa knew Amber's relationship with her partner had its problems, she'd never read a text as dramatic as this.

With a rueful sense that her evening plans just changed drastically, she opted for the most all-in solution short of a five-hour drive to Amber's apartment: video chatting on FaceTime. When Amber appeared on the screen, tears streaming down her face, Tessa murmured, "Tell me everything" and got ready to listen.

> When a friend sends a text that conveys some underlying urgency, how do you respond?

With so many ways to stay in contact with friends, we may have an easier time touching base but be less motivated to carve out the time for more in-depth conversation. This may not seem like a big problem. We can be in daily or weekly conversations with many people, so we may be having ongoing conversations with several friends, in little bits over a long period of time. Texting is also both efficient and seductive; few among us can resist glancing at a text message when the phone beeps. Many people have a variety of individual and group chats going on continuously. Yet, arguably, one of the great paradoxes of our time is that we can be so "connected" and feel so isolated at the same time.

Our hearts and minds need that actual human contact more than we may realize. We didn't evolve to "listen" to a text; if we feel distressed or anxious, we need the comfort of the human voice, the actual presence of a supportive friend. Notably, though, one of the most frustrating elements of social media is simply how tantalizing it can be. It *almost* works to fill our fundamental need to be seen, heard, and felt. *Almost.*

Texting and posting keep us in touch with our friends. Yet for a lonely soul, these disembodied messages may also feel more like eating potato chips on the couch than sitting down to a real meal. Research suggests that online connections really do supplement face-to-face engagement, but the real empathy that sustains deep friendship requires felt presence—and tearful emojis don't cut it when what we crave is good listening.

> Listening to friends comfortably across modalities of text, email, social media, video chat, telephone, and in person is a generational thing. If the phone rings and you feel an obligation to answer it, chances are you are a digital novice: Gen X or older. Younger digital veterans are amphibious and don't make such a distinction between connection to friends on- and off-line. For them, it's their life: all one platform for keeping in touch.

Tish flew out to the Midwest to be with her father who became ill unexpectedly in his fifties and was deteriorating rapidly. She texted from his bedside over the week with her best friend, Diya, exchanging lines just now and then. They never spoke, but Diya was there for her friend. Diya wrote a few times a day, sending love and asking for updates—just checking in. She also maintained a group text with their other friends for Tish, updating them on how Tish was doing. It meant a lot to Tish that her friends were thinking about her.

Reflecting later on her experience, Tish noted that texting worked particularly well in that situation. With a line of communication always open, she could know that Diya "was just listening to me in a back-of-the-mind, low-level way all the time." After Tish's father died, Diya got on a plane and Tish picked her up from the airport. Then Diya was there, in person, for her dear, grieving friend.

The greatest advantage of technology—the opportunity for continuous contact—is also the source of its greatest challenge. When we make ourselves available to others so much of the time, we lose some of the perspective required to decide what is most important to attend to. Balancing our need to connect and to establish boundaries around the relentless pace of online communication is hard work. And just as there are more ways to sustain engagement with friends, so these platforms offer many more possibilities for misunderstanding, hurt feelings, and confusion.

If you find yourself struggling to be heard through texts and posts, remember this: Human beings evolved to live in an actual community, not a virtual one. If the demands on your time and resource are causing your metaphoric battery to drain even faster than a smartphone, try taking a break from it for an hour or two. Commit to a renewed effort to be with your friends IRL (In Real Life).

Technology has also changed our relationship to the workday—and with the people there—because we may feel an expectation (real or imagined) to stay on top of work even if it means emailing with colleagues into the night. Indeed, it is quite possible that you are spending more time reading emails and listening to bosses and colleagues than to your partner or friends. If your place of employment doesn't offer support for turning off email after work, your inbox may be like a newborn baby, crying for help at all hours. Sadly, the time seems long past when most of us feel entitled to maintain a firm boundary between our personal and work lives.

And this is not all bad. Work friendships can help us get out of bed on a cold, bleak Monday morning; electronic contact with coworkers keeps a group project humming along. Our need for affiliation and attachment doesn't magically end when we get to the jobsite. We may imagine that, at work, there are more important things than special camaraderie. But, almost invariably, we're trying to belong, connect, and feel seen and heard in our working relationships too.

Getting Your Point of View Across at the Office

Marshall and Steve were thoroughly charming to Marianne when she applied for a job at the small publishing firm where they were respectively publisher and senior editor. They asked the usual questions about her training and experience, but spent more time talking about what a great place it was to work and how she'd be right in the middle of where all the editorial decisions were made. Marianne needed little convincing. Any small publisher, she felt, would be better than the huge conglomerates where editors were drowning in profit-and-loss statements and where books of substance were considered with suspicion and irony. And here she stood to learn how to make acquisition decisions and negotiate contracts, aspects of publishing she had been far removed from at the large firm where she'd been an assistant. When she was offered the job, she was thrilled and couldn't wait to be mentored by veterans like Marshall and Steve.

Marshall and Steve seemed happy to have Marianne around. But she soon discovered that they considered themselves a team and her an appendage. Their mentoring seemed perfunctory, and the conversations she had imagined, about authors they had known and what they'd learned from their successes and failures, never materialized—at least not with Marianne involved.

Over her first few months at the company, Marianne watched from the outside while Marshall and Steve formed lasting, loyal relationships with their authors, agents, and publicists. She was perplexed by their response when she approached them about the manuscripts she was having problems with. Marshall and Steve made a pretense of listening, their brows furrowed in concern like bureaucrats on autopilot, but they asked no questions. When she was done, they told her just to continue to do her own good work.

Eventually she opened up about her frustrations to a coworker who was becoming a friend and found out that the firm's board of directors had forced them to hire a woman editor and that Marshall and Steve resented this intrusion into what they considered their fiefdom.

Now Marianne felt humiliated. She hadn't been hired with the intention of molding her into their rising new star editor but simply to increase the staff's diversity. And she wasn't getting the support she needed to develop her skills even though she was willing and able to do much of it on her own. More than advice, she needed collegiality, that comforting sense of shared enterprise that had sustained her through the hard years of school and publishing apprenticeship.

Denied that, Marianne became cold and hostile. But Marshall and Steve barely noticed she had retreated; they may have even been relieved to have to deal with her less. But the atmosphere in the office became so unpleasant that in her most frustrated moments Marianne thought about quitting, a luxury she, a single mother, didn't have. So she sought counsel with some of the women who had worked at the firm for a number of years. They laughed knowingly at Marianne's complaints and shared their own experiences of being excluded from the Marshall-and-Steve boys' club. Most had accommodated to the prevailing culture—but not by giving in to the bosses' style. As they talked, Marianne heard one theme rise to the surface: they asked for what they wanted directly, with as little animus as they could manage.

The atmosphere changed at work when Marianne stopped fuming silently at her employers and started rethinking how she could get the support she wanted and the respect she knew she deserved. Her new tack started when Marshall, who was filling out her annual review, rated her attitude "Below Expectations," Marianne refused to sign it. Taking a deep breath to calm her ire, she said, "I want to talk about this," and when Marshall said he didn't have time, she insisted. "You *have to* talk to me. Make time." He sighed theatrically but agreed.

"You *know* I deserve a good evaluation," Marianne told him when they finally met. "What's the problem?"

"I call it as I see it," Marshall said, getting up to leave.

"Please sit down," Marianne said. "We have to talk about this."

And talk they did. Marianne acknowledged that she may have expected too much when she arrived, but she also pointed out that she'd been treated like a second-class citizen and she was tired of it. She spoke with dignity, but also with intensity.

When Marianne finished saying what was on her mind, Marshall apologized. He changed the evaluation, and after that both he and Steve started treating her with more respect. In return, Marianne dropped the icy silence, and when her bosses reverted to dismissing her requests for input, stood her ground and calmly made it clear that she was no longer willing to put up with not being listened to.

Why were Marianne's bosses so unresponsive for so long, and why now all of a sudden did they start to listen to her? Could it really be that all she had to do was speak up?

Marshall and Steve had allowed their resentment about being pressured to hire a woman to turn into a grudge. Unwilling to confront *their* bosses, they took out their frustration on Marianne, shutting her out and treating her as someone to be seen but not heard. What they didn't realize was that grudges have no place at the office.

· · · · · · · · · · ·

Holding on to resentment of people you have to work with
punishes you as much as it does them.

· · · · · · · · · · · ·

It may be a cliché, but people who work together are a team, and sometimes it's necessary to get past personal feelings that interfere with the functioning of the group.

Although Marianne had tried to complain, her expectations of instant camaraderie got in the way. Like many of us, she wanted to be liked and had a reasonable hope that Marshall and Steve would be as warmly welcoming as they had seemed in her job interview. When that didn't happen, she let her disappointment take priority over asserting her right to be treated fairly.

The problem was that she didn't really know how to speak up to people in power. She had assumed they were offering her a spot on the team, but then she began to wonder whether she had been presumptuous. Had she misunderstood them at her interview? Instead of being treated like a valued new colleague, she felt like she was getting treated in a paternalistic way. How could she modify the dynamic between her and her bosses without inviting further disdain?

Marianne came up with a plan that allowed her to gather the confidence to speak more directly and carefully on her own behalf. She would push resentment about how she'd been treated into the back of her mind and address specific problems when they arose. When she needed guidance on acquiring a new book and was brushed off, she said firmly that she needed Marshall's more experienced opinion to know how to make her decision. When she was at a loss for how to deal with an author who needed hand-holding, she told Steve she simply needed some guidance into how much of an editor's time spent with authors should be considered profitable for the company. *She* wasn't asking for hand-holding; she wanted to contribute as much as she could to the firm's success. Presented with these concrete parameters, Marshall and Steve started to listen to Marianne, and it wasn't long before they started to come to her to offer the kind of mentoring she had been hoping for.

Marianne now realized that she was entitled to be listened to, and when important issues arose, she insisted on it. Knowing she could fight back effectively made her more relaxed, and so there was less often a need for it. No longer anxious for Marshall and Steve's approval and acceptance, as though she were the new kid in a club, Marianne lost her need to please. The company, as usual, published some very good books that year, and an author Marianne had brought in had a great success, both critical and commercial. She and Marshall and Steve had a wonderful celebration with him one evening, and their gratification was genuine and shared.

Marianne's unhappy experience at the office is instructive for two reasons. First, her colleagues' lack of consideration illustrates one of the greatest mistakes senior people make in work settings: not listening to their subordinates. Second, that insensitivity placed Marianne in the kind of situation that tempts us to feel like victims, wearing our suffering as a rebuke to the villains we hold responsible. The fact that Marianne was a woman striving for acceptance and inclusion in some of the male camaraderie of her office also offers an example of how difficult it can still be for women to speak on their own behalf and be treated as equals in a male-dominated workplace. There are so many different types of management structures today, and Marianne's experience won't reflect everyone's experience, but listening to one another seems to be ever more important to employers and employees in all kinds of work environments.

A Good Manager Is a Good Listener

Managers are expected to lead the people under them. Unfortunately, people get promoted because they were good at the jobs they were doing, not because they've proven themselves as managers. In fact, according to the Peter Principle, people tend to advance until they reach their level of incompetence. As a result, many managers pay more attention to the product than to the people producing it—to the detriment of both.

> **"Yes, Master."**
>
> The more powerful and admired the boss, the more people tend to hold back their opinions rather than risk angering the person in charge.[7] Good managers make it safe for everyone to offer their ideas and opinions—even ideas that appear to

---

[7] That's one reason presidents make a mess of things: they fail to correct misguided policies because their advisors trip over themselves to agree with the boss. If agreement equals access, bad choices are unlikely to be challenged (think about the wars in Vietnam, Iraq, and Afghanistan).

be wrong or at odds with their own beliefs. This openness accomplishes two things: it adds to the pool of information, which makes for more informed decisions, and it makes people feel included in the decision-making process. The larger the pool of ideas, the better the final decision is likely to turn out. And the more people feel they have participated in the decision making, the more willingly they are likely to act on the decisions that get made.

Effective managers are proactive listeners. They don't wait for members of their staff to come to them; they make an active effort to find out what people think and feel by asking them.

The manager who meets frequently with staff members stays informed and, even more important, communicates interest in the people themselves.

An open-door policy allows access, but it doesn't substitute for an active effort to reach out and listen to people. The manager who doesn't ask questions communicates that he or she doesn't care. And if he or she doesn't listen, the message is "I'm not there for you." Even if a manager decides not to follow a subordinate's suggestion or not to give someone a raise, listening with sincere interest conveys respect and makes the employee feel appreciated.

When Marshall and Steve hired Marianne, they were impressed by her maturity. They thought of her as a self-sufficient person who would come in on day one and be able to share the load. You might think that as experienced people they would have been more sensitive to a new colleague's need for support. But the truth is, Marshall and Steve did their best work outside the office. When they sat down to court an author or negotiate with an agent, they were very sensitive.

Marshall and Steve didn't offer Marianne any formal supervision because *they* never got any. What didn't occur to them was that their friendship had sustained their own need for support. The mistake they made in dealing with Marianne was thinking about her only as a worker and not as a person. Interest in peers may come easily; but, even if it doesn't come naturally, senior people must take an interest in junior people. They're the ones who get the work done.

. . . .
Communicating by email doesn't substitute
for personal contact because it closes off the chance to listen.
. . . .

Simply going through the motions of meeting with people doesn't work. The fake listener doesn't fool anyone. Poor eye contact, shuffling feet, busy hands, and disingenuous replies, like "That's interesting" and "Is that right?" give them away. The insincere supervisor's lack of interest in the conversation betrays a larger problem: lack of interest in the person.

Failure to listen isn't necessarily a product of meanness or insensitivity. Anxiety, preoccupation, and pressure can undermine the skills of even a good listener. The point is, really, that at work, as in every other arena of life, listening requires a little effort.

Effective managers develop a routine in which communication time is an integral part. They meet with their staff and ask questions. They don't react before gathering all the facts. If they don't know what their people are thinking and feeling, they ask—and they listen.

Listening to Empower

A family therapy institute invited six leaders in the field to serve as a board of advisors. At their initial meeting each of the first five experts made suggestions about how the institute could improve their programs. The sixth member of the board took an entirely different approach. He asked everyone on the staff to talk about what they most wanted to accomplish and how they thought he could support them in doing that. It was a remarkably productive way to bring out the best of people's ideas.

What If Your Boss Doesn't Listen?

If at this point we were to leave the subject of listening at the workplace, we would have fallen into the easy habit of reducing a complex subject to a simple formula: thoughtful managers listen to what their employees have to say. Where does that leave those who don't get listened to?

When we don't feel heard by our superiors, few of us give up right away. We write memos, we ask to meet with them, we try to communicate our needs and convey our point of view. Then we give up. Eventually we do what Marianne did: complain to other people.

Once Marianne came to the conclusion that her bosses were uninterested and unavailable, she started griping to one of the other women at the office. Marianne may have imagined she'd find a natural ally in another female employee, but there are many reasons why friendships that are formed this way contribute to a toxic culture at work.

Gossip is a form of consciousness lowering. The rules of the game are simple: players are free to run down anybody who's not in the room. (Hint: If you play this game, don't leave the room.)

Triangulation—ventilating feelings of frustration to third parties rather than addressing conflicts at their source—takes on epidemic proportions in work settings. Letting off steam by complaining about other people is a perfectly human thing to do. The problem is that habitual complaining about superiors locks us into passivity and resentment. We may have given up trying to get through to the sons of bitches but, by God, we don't mind saying what we think of them—as long as they aren't within earshot. Fortunately for Marianne, her new friend at the office knew what she was up against with Marshall and Steve and was able to help her find camaraderie and constructive advice among the other women at the office, rather than fueling an us-against-them resistance.

I once worked in a clinic with five other therapists, where everyone except the director went out to lunch together every day. Guess what the main topic of conversation was? The director and what a rigid guy he was. And guess what the group did about it? Complained regularly among themselves, as though they were a resistible force and he were an immovable object.[8]

---

[8]When I became the director of an outpatient psychiatry department, I remembered this lesson. I scheduled weekly staff meetings, the first half of which was devoted to discussing patients, and the second half was for the staff to bring up anything they were unhappy about, any suggestions they had, or anything they could think of that would make their jobs more rewarding. The result was a pretty cohesive unit.

But, some of you might be thinking, my boss *really is* insensitive! I've *tried* to talk to her; she just doesn't listen!

I don't doubt it. People aren't promoted because they're good listeners. They get promoted because they're good workers, or maybe good talkers. Moreover, positions of authority encourage the directive side of human nature, often at the expense of receptivity. The mistake people make in trying to get through to unreceptive superiors is the same mistake most of us make in dealing with the difficult people in our lives: We try to change them. And when that doesn't work, we give up.

> You don't improve relationships
> by trying to change other people,
> but by changing yourself in relation to them.

Start by examining your expectations. What do you want, and how do you expect to go about getting it? Are you, as Marianne was, expecting to have your personal needs met at the office? Do you work hard and wait patiently for the boss to tell you that you're doing a great job, like a good little boy or girl? Have you learned to seek a reaction by being clever rather than competent or by being pleasing rather than productive?

The workplace isn't a family. Yet many of us relate to our bosses as though they were our parents. If we work long hours and have little actual family, we may come to depend on work relationships to get more of our emotional needs met than is advisable or realistic. The alternative is to think of yourselves as two self-respecting adults who happen to occupy different positions at the office. Marianne wanted Marshall and Steve to take her seriously, but by not speaking to them as a capable adult, she may have unwittingly invited them to treat her like an errant child.

The paternal, white-haired chairman of the department of psychiatry once complained to me that certain faculty members responded to him as though he were their father. I had to laugh.

One of the things that comes with a position of responsibility is becoming the object of people's attitudes toward authority. Supervisors should remember this when they meet with their subordinates.

When you think about all the bosses you've had in your career, when did you treat one like a parent? How did that work out? Have you had bosses who treated you like a child? How did you handle that?

When employees are summoned to meet with the boss, they may expect a reprimand—why else would the boss call you in?—rather than an open forum. Supervisors must break through this anxiety by asking questions that show interest. And listening to the answers.

Listening to Colleagues and Getting Them to Listen to You

Because we spend so much of our lives at work, it shouldn't be surprising that interpersonal dynamics can sometimes take up as much energy as the job itself. In the following five vignettes, imagine what you would want to say and do if you were that employee. Think about how you might listen to the other person and the kind of response that a coworker might give that would let you know you've been heard too.

Melody works as part of a team on a construction crew. As a woman and a relatively new hire, she doesn't expect that her team leader, Arturo, should go out of his way to hear her ideas. But at the morning meeting before they head out for the day, he asks if anyone has thoughts about how to proceed. The few times she speaks up with a suggestion, she gets talked over by Dom, who fundamentally just paraphrases *her* comments. Arturo says. "I agree with Dom," and she feels resentful and invisible. She debates whether she should speak to Arturo, Dom, both of them, or the HR person back at the office. She imagines she should just suck it up and keep plugging along, but for how much longer before she should say something?

Nick is a rising star in a medium-sized law office. His immediate superior is a smart, demanding female partner who wants him to stay late and work closely with her. He thinks she's flirting with him, but he isn't sure and he doesn't want anything to interfere with his path to partner in the firm.

He thinks about making excuses for having to leave earlier, saying casually that he's in a relationship if an opening arises, or gently confronting her with the suggestion that he doesn't feel comfortable with their after-hours interactions. He worries that things might escalate if he remains silent.

Kira is a social worker in a child protection agency. She likes most of the other people in her office and tries to stay focused and professional. She sees herself as a team player and is willing to do more when necessary to support her colleagues when they are feeling overwhelmed and buried in paperwork. But recently she has felt increasingly frustrated by having to pick up the slack for Lexi, who struggles with problems at home and doesn't attend to the details this kind of work requires. When Lexi's clients arrive in distress at the office, Kira feels she needs to intervene to keep volatile situations from escalating, but, on a regular basis, this is surely not her job. She has tried to talk to Lexi about working more efficiently and getting personal help, but Lexi has been dismissive and defensive. Kira is debating about whether to try again to have a productive conversation or to speak with Lexi's supervisor, potentially creating unwanted conflict between Lexi and Kira. She worries that vulnerable children and families are getting inferior care and that something terrible might happen if she keeps quiet.

Tyler has a great job doing sales with a tech start-up. The staff fridge is full of snacks, and there is a pool table in the community room. He can come and go as he pleases as long as he gets his work done. People drop in to chat with each other over the course of the day. He especially enjoys the casual time with Fiona, a coworker with a dry sense of humor. Recently Tyler has started thinking about Fiona as more than a colleague. He's well aware of possible repercussions should she reject him or, worse, they try to take it to the next level and it doesn't work out. The company doesn't have a formal policy about dating among coworkers, so there are no rules he'd be violating if they were both into it. Even as he sees the downside, Tyler can't wait for the midafternoon when he will drop in and flirt with Fiona. He contemplates waiting to see if she makes the first move, putting his cards on the table, or, looking together with her at the possible negative repercussions, telling her somehow that he's feeling a need to set clearer limits on their work relationship. But what if it's all in his head and such a conversation will make for an awkward office interaction?

Leslie was sympathetic when her administrative assistant told her about the problems she was having at home. But once Donna discovered what a willing listener Leslie was, she started taking up more and more time talking about her problems. Donna's troubles were beginning to interfere with work getting done, and Leslie was getting annoyed. She wanted to be understanding, but she didn't want to be Donna's mother. What to do?

Setting Limits at Work

In all of these scenarios, the lines between respectful work relationships and personal needs are blurred. There are plenty of good reasons to be a team player and to accommodate some kinds of neediness, slights, and idiosyncratic behavior among coworkers to get through the day in one piece. But for most of us, work is hard enough without having to endure treatment that feels unfair, burdensome, distracting, or downright harassing.

If you identify with any of these situations, or are facing your own work-relationship dilemma with a colleague or peer, here are three ideas about how to approach difficult work conversations:

Begin with curiosity and the intent to listen. When you raise the issue, be prepared to hear what the other person sees is happening. How does Arturo view Melody's contributions—to the morning meeting and her part of the construction project? Does Lexi want more support than she's getting, not necessarily from Kira, but from her supervisor and others in the agency?

Be prepared to hear how people feel (even if that's different from how you feel) and take time to sort out your own feelings first. What's it like for Donna to feel heard by Leslie? Are Nick's feelings valid? Does Fiona feel differently about Tyler than he imagines?

Take time to understand what the situation means to you—and to your coworkers. Does Melody's resentment mean to her that she's incompetent or an inferior person? Why do Kira and Leslie feel so responsible for the emotional lives of other people in their offices? What does Nick think it says about him as a man to feel uncomfortable and harassed?

. . . .

To be able to assert clearly what we need
from a work relationship, we must be able to hear
what others have to say, to understand why speaking up
is important to us, and to be up front about how the blurring
of boundaries makes us think and feel about ourselves.

. . . .

If you have a good relationship with someone at work and find the boundaries between you blurring, your willingness to take one for the team, go along, and listen helps lighten the burden. But some people are so full of their problems and concerns for status that they take advantage of anyone willing to listen.

Once you have made space to listen, considered everyone's feelings, and grappled with what the issue says to you about who you are as a person, you might not even need to set more limits, because the air between you will be clearer. But go ahead: maintain gentle and meaningful boundaries for yourself and see how that further detoxifies the office for you.

For example, when personal conversations start keeping you from your work, cut them off gently but firmly.

"I'd like to hear more, but I have to get back to work."

"This all sounds pretty painful. I hope you have somebody to talk to about these things?"

"I hope that we can work on this project later this afternoon; I need to get home by six tonight."

Listening is important at work because it enables people to understand each other, get along, and get the job done. *But*: Don't get too personal. Don't let your compassion (or desire to be appreciated) allow someone's agenda, talking about her problems, or his neediness to interfere with work. This may be happening if you're the only person he talks to or if she uses your sympathy as more than an occasional excuse for not getting things accomplished.

Listening to the people you work with isn't the same as becoming friends with them. Many people worry that if they allow themselves to get personal at the office, things might get sticky. But those who think that effective teamwork isn't also about listening (it's just about getting things done) are wrong. Without being heard we are diminished, as workers and as people. Our work relationships require care and attention too. They matter and shape who we are just as all of our other sustained connections do.

EXERCISES

1. In your next conversation with a friend, note any tendency to drift away while the other person is talking. How much effort would it take to concentrate on listening for exactly two more minutes? How much effort is this friendship worth?

2. Make a list of friends you'd like to be closer to. Then note things you know those people like to do. Pick a friend and try to arrange doing that activity together.

3. Become a proactive listener. If you are a supervisor, manager, teacher, therapist, parent, or otherwise in a position of authority, find a time in the coming week to ask a subordinate what ideas or feelings about your mutual enterprise he or she might have but has not had a chance to tell you about. Be sure to make that person feel appreciated for opening up to you. If the person says nothing, say that's fine; if anything comes to mind later, you'd be glad to hear about it.

4. Think of a difficult colleague or supervisor. How do your interactions with that person usually go? What do you do? For the next time you meet with that person, plan to concentrate on listening and drawing out his or her point of view. Notice what your feelings about this interaction say about you as a person. Afterward, evaluate your listening and its impact on the relationship.

5. If you are maintaining friendships and work relationships almost entirely through online communication, take a few minutes to evaluate the pluses and minuses of this approach. If your stress level and feeling of loneliness are high, consider the growing body of research suggesting that *more* voice and face-to-face contact with people you love is a good way to reduce these problems.

13

"I'm Not Wasting My Time Talking to *That* Person!"

HOW TO LISTEN TO PEOPLE IT'S IMPOSSIBLE TO AGREE WITH

Why are some people so hard to listen to? As the previous chapters suggest, the answer is complicated. And as you know by now, in our most significant relationships both parties contribute to the struggle to be heard and to listen well—although some people are harder to listen to than others.

But we often need to talk with friends and relatives we won't ever agree with. And it's difficult to imagine a time in history when it's been harder to engage in respectful conversations across ever-widening political, cultural, and generational divides—or when it's been more urgently needed.

There are plenty of reasons not to bother. Maybe some people are just too wrongheaded and self-absorbed—or just plain pigheaded—to waste your time on. It's easier to tune them out than to let them get you all worked up for nothing. With casual acquaintances, colleagues at work, or the chatty fellow on the train, there's no need to get too invested. But it matters that you stay connected with the infuriating people in your life who mean something to you—whether it's your mother, your uncle, the woman who's dating your brother, or the guy you have to collaborate with on a project—even when their view of the world makes them almost impossible to listen to. An indicator of how much it matters is how worked up or distressed you get just thinking about the conversation. Are you:

- Having angry dialogues in your head, playing both parts?
- Avoiding or writing off someone you used to be closer to so you don't have to argue?
- Recruiting people to be on your side in judging the person?
- Making rules about what is acceptable to talk about even if the tolerable topics turn the relationship dull and superficial?
- Feeling sad that you can't share your lives with each other anymore?
- Dreading family or social gatherings that could become tense and uncomfortable?
- Dwelling on all the reasons that person is impossible to listen to?

If you answered yes to any of these questions, here's your answer: It matters. *A lot.*

> It's important to sustain connections to friends and family
> even when it's hard to do so. When we give up
> on relationships that matter, our lives are diminished.

When Celeste came home from college for Thanksgiving, she was, like many politically engaged young adults, full of passionate ideas. Accustomed to being taken seriously by her father and stepmother, and surrounded by like-minded people at college, Celeste wasn't used to listening to perspectives opposed to her own. Although she enjoyed an intellectual debate, her preference—as is true for most of us—was to be able to leave the interaction with the conviction that she'd been right all along.

Celeste's sparring partner for the afternoon was her uncle Jim, whom she saw just once a year at this gathering. His conservative views had been formed over decades working for the government in the Middle East. Her early memories of him were pleasant enough. He was family. Last year, though, he'd held forth on something to do with immigration policy—and she'd strongly disagreed with what he said, but she hadn't been well informed enough at that time to challenge him.

Uncle Jim was the only conservative she'd ever actually spent time with, so when she started to develop her own, more liberal ideas this past semester, she'd argued successfully against an imaginary version of him. She never lost those imaginary arguments. This year, Celeste could be more comfortable engaging with him in conversation while they feasted on her dad's specially brined turkey.

Once everyone had settled down to the meal, Celeste began to tell Uncle Jim a bit about what she was learning in her international relations class. Before she'd finished, he talked a little about an experience he'd had in one of the countries she'd been studying. He may have created some heat by cutting her off and pointing out her ignorance of recent events there. Perhaps she then added fuel to the fire by suggesting that he actually had gotten a couple details wrong—and saying that her professor was a real expert.

When political disagreements heat up, they get personal so fast that it can be hard to say who struck the match.

After just a few minutes trying again to stake out her position, Celeste's heart started racing and she couldn't think logically any longer. When Uncle Jim rolled his eyes and reached for the cranberry sauce, she fled the room on the verge of tears.

What caused this conversation to devolve so quickly?

Was it Uncle Jim, who was an impossible know-it-all, or his contrary political views? Did she get all worked up because he went on and on with tangential explanations, or because he had so little interest in what *she* had to say? Perhaps his dismissive attitude triggered insecurities in Celeste that could best explain her escalating distress.

When righteous indignation takes over, we may fail to distinguish between a person and his or her opinions. It's true that Uncle Jim had been patronizing to Celeste, and she a bit bratty to him, but cooler heads would have been able to chalk that up to simple differences of age and experience. People in families disagree all the time, but not like this. When social and political differences are involved, divergent opinions can make it impossible to hear anything the other person is saying.

Suki is a health-conscious vegan. She and her boyfriend, Jaden, were in couples therapy because Suki refused to speak to his brother, Logan; Jaden thought Suki was making him choose between his family and his girlfriend. Three years ago, she got into a yelling match with Logan, who has a hunting license and is an avid meat eater. She was so upset by Logan's viewpoint that, to this day, she can't stand to be in the same room when the brothers FaceTime and she has to hear his "annoying voice."

After Artie had been a widower for a year, he fell for Marina, a woman who treated him deferentially, eager to anticipate his every need. In turn, he overlooked her contempt toward the immigrants who had settled in their town. He dismissed the criticisms of his grown sons about her bigotry as unnecessary meddling and saw less of them. Marina's daughter was more appalled by the relationship; she tried to see her mom when Artie wasn't around so she could lecture her about diversity. It's possible that those middle-aged children couldn't handle thinking about their parents dating in later life. But they experienced those choices as personal rebukes to their liberal world views. Caught up in their judgments, they had trouble hearing how happy Artie and Marina were.

Wanda and Natasha have worked for the same start-up for three years. The office is designed as an open collaborative space, and people are expected to get along. They have chatted over lunch about intimate topics—relationships, family problems, health concerns—and so they are friends as well as coworkers. But when Natasha started talking about her support for a local candidate with a mixed record on the environment, Wanda was appalled. She said, "Are you really canvassing for that corporate hack?" Natasha backed away, saying, "I'm entitled to my opinions." How can it be that these two women, who weeks before had been able to talk about their sex lives, can't bear to listen to each other's ideas about environmental policy?

For all of these people, opposing opinions somehow morphed into indictments of the other person's worth. People won't listen when they feel you are trying to judge, convert, or silence them. The kind of openness and tolerance that would get all of these combatants to slow down and understand each other better is in short supply these days.

WHY SHOULD YOU GET BETTER AT LISTENING TO PEOPLE YOU DISAGREE WITH?

- Difficult conversations become easier with practice.
- You will become a better listener across the board—with your partner, kids, parents, and friends.
- You will experience a heightened sense of control in contentious situations.

- By learning to communicate with respect, curiosity, and openness, you are more likely to elicit the same consideration from the other person.
- You will increase your confidence and self-respect.
- You will strengthen that important relationship when you navigate successfully to the other side of a difficult conversation. Like a fractured bone that heals stronger, repairing ruptures fortifies connection.
- You will be part of a growing movement of people who believe that we will be closer to finding peace if we are able to engage in dialogue with people who have different perspectives from us.

In recent years, a growing social, political, and cultural divide has opened fault lines everywhere. When people stop listening to each other, the damage becomes more entrenched. Of course, disagreements about fundamental beliefs have always existed, but there's plenty of evidence that the divisions are getting worse and, consequently, people are feeling more alienated and antagonistic.

Your emotional investment in your side of these divisions lets you know that it's not just your ideas and values that feel under attack but your very being. As such, an intense disagreement about what you believe in is also painfully personal.

The animosity tears at the very fabric of family and community life, disrupting routines and rituals—those holidays, special events, and other gatherings that hold generations together. Celeste isn't the first person to disrupt a Thanksgiving meal, and she won't be the last. But in a time when people feel particularly isolated, this fracturing of family and social identity has immediate and enduring costs.

> On the right, guns are freedom and abortion is murder;
> on the left, abortion is freedom and guns are murder.
> —JILL LEPORE

Of course, it's not just politics that divide families and friends these days, but an entire range of social issues. Family arguments about guns and abortion may serve as convenient shorthand for the culture wars on all the other fronts too—religion, gender and marriage, civil liberties, climate change, economic systems, identity, and power. We're fighting about (or avoiding) the big issues that can chafe and erode goodwill to the breaking point—and make the usual, day-to-day misunderstandings even more intolerable.

Once triggered, our polarized opinions take us down one of two unhappy paths: angry conflict and rupture or opting not to talk to people we disagree with. Instead of learning how to have difficult conversations, we hit the boiling point or duck for cover—and, as a result, come to feel a little more anxious and misunderstood. How our beliefs about the person we're trying to listen to (or trying not to listen to) produce feelings that in turn morph into lasting conclusions about that individual is shown in the following box.

How Do You View Those on the Other Side of an Issue? (They probably see you that way too.)

I Believe	I Feel	I Conclude
She's the enemy.	Hate/Fear	She wants to harm the country/me.
He's an idiot.	Contempt/ Mistrust	He should know better/ waste of time.
She's been duped.	Pity	She's well-meaning but clueless.
He might have a point.	Basic respect	That gets me thinking in new ways.
She has some good ideas.	Respect, appreciation	I can see where she's coming from.

Though it can also be challenging, it may be easier to disagree with someone you don't know well or have weaker ties with; conflict with someone you care about can feel like disloyalty and betrayal. Our reactivity and emotionality tell us how high stakes the conversation may be: more than just being right is clearly on the line.

Listening When It Feels Impossible

When Responsive Listening Isn't Enough

Four generations of the Rizzo family live in the same area, and they gather to celebrate birthdays and anniversaries all year round. People don't exactly listen to each other. In fact, there is seldom a time that just one person is speaking without being interrupted. Family members are used to gatherings being loud and contentious. So when someone says something that is blunt or hurtful, others will usually rally to persuade the wounded party to let it go. Some families, like the Rizzos, value blood ties above individual needs.

When Harper Rizzo was twenty-three, he moved in with his boyfriend, Manuel, who had heard for a couple years about the raucous Rizzo cookouts but had never been invited. Manuel felt it was time for Harper to include him. Harper worried that his grandmother would be inhospitable. While he hadn't hidden the fact that he was gay, he had been careful to avoid overt confrontations with the older generation. But he also wanted Manuel to be included, so despite his trepidation, he agreed he'd at least try to build this bridge with her. Harper understood that he might be very disappointed by the outcome. And with Manuel's encouragement, he also went into the conversation fortified by the belief that just listening to Nana respectfully and calmly would be an accomplishment in its own right.

When we decide it is time to have a hot-button conversation like this, we may need to call on more than responsive listening skills. Discussions about diversity and culture are often inflammatory and hard to extinguish once they ignite. Harper had avoided this conflict with his grandmother for many years—really, for as long as he could. Even in a family as close as his, the potential for rupture was still high. To have an honest and respectful exchange with his grandmother, Harper would need to be able to listen across the vast divide of gender, age, and education. This exchange would be a tightrope walk.

He would need to be able to hear Nana as she talked about beliefs she held that were deeply painful and even enraging for him. And even if he managed to remain calm, there was only a remote chance she would listen much to what *he* had to say. And whatever happened, the whole family would certainly hear all about it within twenty-four hours, probably questioning why he'd upset Nana. But how would things get better if he didn't talk to her? It was worth a try.

. . . .

To have a difficult conversation with someone you love,
just listening may not be enough. You need
to treat the other person's opinion with respect.

. . . .

> **How Prepared Are You
> to Listen to Someone Who's Hard to Listen To?**
>
> Rate yourself 0–5 on these following qualities. Lower scores suggest areas for self-exploration and development of new skills:
>
> ____ Tolerating conflict
> ____ Managing disagreement in relationships
> ____ Regulating strong emotions such as anger and fear
> ____ Self-reflection
> ____ Patience
> ____ Compassion for others
> ____ Respect for yourself
> ____ Being a good listener
> ____ Genuine curiosity

Being a good listener will definitely help you handle a difficult conversation, but it's not always enough. Be intentional and pay attention, speak carefully with I-statements, check an impulse to argue or interrupt, and try to clarify what you hear. All of this is necessary—but not sufficient. These strategies have to be backed up by an authentic interest in finding out what the other person believes.

Are you curious? Do you actually care about what the person has to say?

If the answer is "No" or "Not sure," then you might not be ready to converse—listening as well as speaking— about something that matters deeply to you.

People who take the risk to have these hard discussions with you don't just want to be heard; they want to *feel* understood.

Acknowledging the Other Person's Position

Acknowledgment (which, remember doesn't mean you agree, just that you are listening well) can't be a rote performance. True acknowledgment lets people know that you understand their feelings, that their feelings matter to you, that you can understand them. If you are only pretending to be interested, the way you might when hearing about your spouse's meeting at work, that won't cut it. You actually have to *be* curious and really listen.

Can you imagine yourself in the other person's story, thinking and believing as she does?

If you aren't sure how curious you are—or have a voice in your head saying that you are right and the other person is so wrong —you may be able to negotiate with yourself to make that needed attitude adjustment. It might help, for example, to remind yourself that you could actually learn a thing or two if you became more open and receptive. Indeed, it's a lot easier to stay in your own bunker than to venture forth and be brave in not knowing. That voice that says it's hopeless may be keeping you safe, but, make no mistake, it's the voice of fear.

Don't forget that understanding another person's world is always harder than it seems. And, not to be too harsh here, but if you think you already understand how someone else feels or know what he's going to say, it might be time to get over yourself. There is always more to learn. And remember: you have a much greater chance of understanding someone than of converting him.

. . . .

Telling people to change
makes it less likely they will.

. . . .

Setting Your Intentions

Even if things don't always go according to plan, it helps you stay focused if, ahead of time, you set some goals for yourself, noticing what you have control of and what you'll do in the event that things escalate. Setting the intention to remain open and receptive will help you stay focused.

- **What do you hope to accomplish?** "At the end of the conversation we will. . . ."
- **Are your goals attainable?** "I'd love to learn about how you have come to these conclusions. Would that be something you'd be willing to discuss with me?"
- **What would be a good outcome?**

  Good: I can learn about the perspectives, feelings, and experiences of someone I care about who differs from me socially and politically.

  Not Good: I will teach that ignoramus what's right.
- **What are my values?** When you think about and set your intentions, you'll have an easier time sticking to them if they really align with your values and enable you to behave in ways that feel genuine. Here are some examples of listening intentions that may help you stay motivated through a difficult conversation:
  - I can listen in a way that the person is heard and feels understood (value of respect).
  - I can be open and kind (value of kindness).
  - I can set and maintain a constructive tone and handle difficult moments (value of self-restraint).
  - I can feel effective if I can convey my perspectives, feelings, and experiences with calm and compassion and in a way the person can hear (value of intentionality).
  - I will try to find similarities and commonalities in values and concerns (value of bridging differences).
  - I will remember that this is someone I care about (value of love).
  - Even though this will be hard, it is important for me not to give up (value of courage).

Managing your internal voice and staying curious
are at the heart of good listening.

Demonstrating an Open Mind

When you are entering into a prickly discussion, you may be tempted to pretend to listen, while silently keeping a closed mind. Sarcastic questions don't help: "So you don't care that we're destroying the planet?" "So Republicans are wrong and Democrats are always right?" "Oh, people should be allowed to carry as many guns as they want?" To avoid this, try the following:

- **Make curious overtures:** "What do you think we should do about rising sea levels?" "Can you tell me how you understand the president's views on women?"
- **Ask permission to pose questions instead of launching into a frontal assault:** "Can I ask you about your views on immigration?"
- **Ask open-ended questions:** "Tell me more." "Help me understand better." "Can you say a little more about how you see things?"
- **Ask for concrete information:** "How would that work?" "Can you give me an example?"
- **Ask real follow-up questions, not loaded questions:** Try to ask just to learn; if you are listening for opportunities to shoot holes in his argument, you won't end up learning much at all.
- **Listen for her underlying values and aspirations and acknowledge them:** "I hear that, for you, fairness is a big issue when it comes to immigration. Can you tell me about that?"
- **Note where her value is similar to your own (e.g., fairness):** "It sounds like we both worry about fairness in immigration policy."
- **Note where you agree on a topic:** "We both want kids to be safe from school shootings."
- **If you have strong feelings, you can certainly say so:** If you disagree fully, you can let him know and still encourage him to go on: "I care a lot about this, and I am very curious about your perspective."
- **See if you can remain calm and focused on a topic when others**

come slip-sliding along: Keeping to a simple issue is hard to do when the issues all seem interconnected, but this constraint makes a challenging conversation a lot more manageable. Remember: every time you can refrain from escalating a debate via witty (but not helpful) snarkiness you are living out your better intentions.

. . . .

Name it to tame it: If you are having trouble listening, say so.
That can actually help you listen.

. . . .

Shifting from Being Right to Being Curious

To make the shift toward curiosity, realize that every difficult conversation takes place on three levels at once: The Topic, Big Feelings, and Identity. Discussions across the social and political divide are challenging because all three of these elements invariably operate together, even when you imagine you're "just" arguing, for example, about climate change or health care or the second amendment.

. . . .

Social and political conversations across deep divides
are especially contentious because they are never, ever
just about the topic at hand.

. . . .

Level One: The Topic

As much as some of us may wish otherwise, difficult conversations don't run on information and data. They are about conflicting perceptions, interpretations, and values. Letting go of your single-minded version of the truth can enable you to shift your purpose from delivering messages and toward asking questions, exploring how the other person makes sense of the world. It's better to offer your views as just that: your own observations and beliefs—and not as The Truth.

We may disagree vehemently about a specific social or political issue because we understand it to be of unquestionable importance to us (and, if others were more enlightened, it would matter to them too). But polarized conversations with our relatives and loved ones are never just about the topic itself. Whatever the contentious issue may be, you'll see it more clearly if you begin with these five questions:

- What is the topic? (Try to keep just one in mind.)
- Why is this so important to me?
- What do I want the other person to understand about it?
- What can I learn about his or her experience that will help me understand him or her better?
- What are my intentions? That is, at the end of the conversation, what do I hope will have happened?

Level Two: Big Feelings

The depth and breadth of our emotional reaction to recent social and political events have reached toxic levels for many people. In the recent Stress in America™ survey conducted by the American Psychological Association, about two-thirds of adults report that the current social and political climate is a source of significant stress for them.

This finding is even more meaningful if you consider the impact of chronic continuous stress on your reactivity in a specific situation. In other words, if you are already feeling on edge, it won't take as much to push you over it.

Feelings matter, of course, especially when it comes to those painful rifts in the fabric of family relationships. Under the attributions and accusations that form your position on the topic of discussion, your strong feelings may get in the way of listening to anyone with a different viewpoint. But these big emotions are even more overwhelming because they inevitably involve both your ongoing distress about the topic *and* the specific challenge of trying to communicate with someone you love who feels so differently.

In the thick of it, someone might say things like "I can't believe you think that!" or "You have got to be kidding!" These sorts of reactions suggest disdain and anger but also, notably, an element of disbelief. Are *you* really saying this to *me*? The experience of betrayal is both primitive and real—and it will need to be contained for you to engage in productive difficult communications.

When we feel attacked, our stress response kicks into gear and we almost have to react. Once fearful feelings flood through our bodies, we have no choice. Unfortunately, the fight-flight response is also a problem for the one initiating a difficult conversation. Anticipating what might happen can itself be stressful. And when you begin to listen, already a little on edge, it will be all the harder to keep calm and carry on as your mind races and you don't feel quite so curious anymore.

Emotional flooding, frustrating though it is, makes good evolutionary sense—it's wise not to dither too much when you need to decide whether to fight or flee a saber-toothed tiger. Unfortunately, this level of emotional reactivity may be a bit much when facing Uncle Jim, who drove four hours for a family meal, or elderly Nana, who always makes her delicious eggplant parm with you in mind. Because human wiring hasn't kept up with the times, it takes some planning and self-awareness to keep your body from readying you for taking on tigers. You need to have a sense of how you'll handle emotional flooding *before* overwhelming feelings take over.

And, remember, a threat can feel real whether it is or not. We know well that people won't be able to speak clearly about things that matter deeply to them if they feel threatened. If you suddenly move into righteous argument mode—and this includes falling into those traps like being logical and patronizing, presenting evidence, sniping, name-calling, lecturing, and feigning curiosity—the person you are trying to reach will probably become emotionally flooded. Once her rational brain shuts down, she will have a diminished capacity to hear you, to think clearly about what you are saying, or to respond productively. And if she gets flooded, you are much more likely to join her there.

. . . .

Emotional flooding is contagious.

. . . .

Here Comes the Flood: Adrenaline! Cortisol! Action!

Not all who get so stressed that they feel emotionally flooded act the same way. Some people get aggressive, others withdraw—they may become silent or disengage completely. Some even smile and nod pleasantly even though, mentally, they are barely in the room at all.

How do you know you are getting emotionally flooded? Here are some of the physical signs that can let you know you are no longer thinking with your rational brain and the conversation will soon devolve—if it hasn't already:

Throbbing head	Sweaty palms
Shallow breathing	Trouble hearing
Clenched jaw	Feeling cornered
Feeling hot	Stomach in knots
Heart pounding	Headache
Dry mouth	Agitation
Speaking louder and faster	Angry thoughts
Confusion	Tension

You may experience some or many of these signs and symptoms and have little memory afterward of what happened, why it was such a big deal, or what either of you said. *What's most important to understand is that when you are emotionally flooded, nothing useful will come out of the conversation.* It's fine to have strong feelings about something that is compelling for you; however, no good will come when one or both people are emotionally overwhelmed.

. . . .

As you get more flooded, your cognitive ability declines.

. . . .

Manage your emotionality. Naturally, it would be best if you could go into the conversation with sufficient self-awareness and planning so that you can stay controlled and reasonable. You'd know the signs of emotional flooding and have some strategies for managing it before it swamps your cognitive ability. You can control some of the emotionality by setting intentions, establishing clear boundaries for yourself and the discussion, and having a plan to postpone responding until you are calmer. But don't forget that having to do all this preparation means you are anticipating stress—which is, itself, stressful.

. . . .

Once flooded with emotion, people don't hear each other.

. . . .

If you sense the tension rising but you are still not overwhelmed, you can try to stay reconnected by noticing what happened, validating the experience of the other person, taking responsibility for your role in the escalation, managing your tone of voice, and opening up space for the other person to try again. But, when anyone gets flooded with emotion, you'll need to stop and deal with the flooding as soon as possible. The issue may still be extremely important, but you won't really have won a debate if you've lost the relationship.

If you feel yourself getting emotionally flooded, try this brief grounding exercise to reorient and calm yourself:

- Notice five things that you can see.
- Notice four things that you can hear.
- Name three things that you can touch.
- Name two things that you can smell.

Take a few deep breaths, plant your feet on the ground, and be sure you feel calmer before trying to listen some more.

Level Three: Personal Identity

When we summon the courage to venture forth into a challenging discussion, we are putting more than our ideas and our feelings on the line; this crossing of the cultural and political divide is also about identity itself. Daring to engage in social and political conversations may be even more high risk, because they are actually deeply intimate exchanges that fundamentally reveal our core sense of who we are, what matters most to us, and what it means when someone we care about doesn't see the issue that way.

I'm not suggesting that your great-aunt Marnie poses an existential threat to you when she says that if you think there's global warming, you should come visit her in Wisconsin next winter—but if you now think of her with more than a little contempt, let's get curious about that. Why the inner turmoil? What just happened to you there?

Here are some questions that may suggest what's at stake for you in conversations across the cultural divide:

Am I smart enough? Political and cultural conflict affects our personal sense of competence. The less competent we feel, the more we may feel compelled to redouble our efforts to prove it, to hammer home that our conclusions are correct. Most of us (like Celeste) practice these passionate conversations in an echo chamber of information, sharing opinions with people who agree with us. So when our beliefs get challenged, it's possible that we don't feel as confident as we expected we'd be.

When someone you love and perhaps respect comes to opposing conclusions about the world, don't be surprised to find yourself wrestling not only with the person but also with your own self-doubt.

Am I good enough? When opinions diverge into two camps, it's almost inevitable that we then divide people into the good guys and the bad guys. If the conflict is with someone you care about, you may find yourself struggling to resolve this issue, perhaps by dismissing or marginalizing her. This act of polarization is fueled by identity politics. You can say that it doesn't matter what the other person thinks because he's _____ (a white male, a Democrat, a Fox news watcher, a homophobe, a millennial, an old fogey, or whatever). It doesn't actually work out that making someone else a bad person automatically confers goodness on you, but if you are understanding the conflict as a moral battle, it makes sense to want to be on the right side.

Am I lovable enough? It can be hard to stomach the idea that someone who matters to you doesn't value the principles you hold dearest. Intellectually, you might realize that people can both care for one another and disagree, but these primordial feelings of distress don't come from the intellect. We feel valued when our relatives give us comfort and support; when they tell us we are wrong, it hurts. The conflict can feel like rejection. To protect ourselves, we get angry and self-righteous. These feelings are miserable, so we project them onto others; *they* are the self-righteous ones.

People are hard to hate close up. Move in.
—Brené Brown

Adrian and Demetrius have an ongoing sibling conflict based on brotherly competition to be the one to care for their alcoholic mother, who is newly diagnosed with Alzheimer's disease. When they disagree (which is pretty much every time they try to have a conversation), one or the other will bring up issues from forty years ago, when they were in high school. They disagree about everything, from food preferences to charitable contributions.

But they also have a lot in common. In addition to their similar salt and pepper hair, they share excellent memories for injustices done. When Adrian called me for an appointment, he informed me that he and Deme had not spoken to each other for a couple of years over some rift he couldn't even remember the details of. He said that the lawyer helping them with their mother's long-term care intended for my office to be "Switzerland," a neutral place for the brothers to make plans on her behalf.

The emotion in the room our first meeting was, at first, hard to manage. After a couple of niceties and an awkward hug, all at once, as if by some ancient code, they began shouting at each other over years of pent-up anger. The torrent of accusations merged fear about their mother's illness, experience of rejection and loss from the other, and raw emotional upset into a tangled rehashing of the cause of the most recent rupture. Once they were flooded with emotion, the reasons for their upset lost relevance; they each felt betrayed.

Addressing the emotionality first, I thanked them for showing me how hard this all was for both of them. I acknowledged that they were undertaking a painful task planning for their mother's end of life. Then I took a deep breath and asked if we might start over. I had them put their feet on the ground and sit for a couple minutes in silent reflection. I asked them to breathe and rethink what they might be able to accomplish safely in the hour. We could not have any conversation at all if they didn't feel safe. Once their thinking brains were engaged again, I taught them a five-step strategy to develop the skills necessary to collaborate about their mother's estate.

Here are the five steps: Ask, Listen, Reflect, Agree, Share:

1. **Ask** open-ended, genuinely curious, nonjudgmental questions.
2. **Listen** to what the person you disagree with says and deepen your understanding with follow-up inquiries.

3. **Reflect** back that perspective by summarizing the person's answers and noting the underlying emotions.
4. **Agree** before disagreeing by naming ways in which you agree with the person's point of view.
5. **Share** stories by asking for personal narratives and offering your own reminiscences.

If you try this approach on your own, you will also want to pay special attention to the problem of emotional flooding. No referee will be there, so it will be up to you to stay reasonably calm throughout the conversation. Notice if you are triggering the other person; check in with him if you are unsure. Notice also if you are getting flooded yourself. If that happens, stop the conversation and try a strategy that works to calm you down. Give yourself permission to take time to get your rational brain back in charge before proceeding.

. . . .

To listen better during a hot-button conflict,
try paying attention to the storyteller instead of the story.

. . . .

Listening To and Telling Stories

We humans are storytelling creatures. When people have the chance to tell the stories of their lives, they are more apt to experience a sense of calm and connection instead of rage and rupture. Only when we are safe and certain there are no saber-toothed tigers in the room can we present our reflective selves. It's much more likely (though not a sure thing) that someone who feels heard this way will return the favor. You will usually have more of a chance to share your own perspectives *after* you have demonstrated curiosity and interest. Try to avoid the temptation to go first. You can generally start like this:

"Will you tell me your story? I'd love to know how you came to this point of view."

Then see what happens when you ask for more—another story or an experience that informs current feelings and belief. You could say something simple: "Tell me more."

Or you can ask more detailed questions that help you get to know the person better. Here are a few examples that engage conversation more specifically across political differences; the inquiry can easily be adapted to help you ask about any subject on which you hold a strong, opposing opinion.

"What experiences helped to shape your political views?"

"How have your political views changed over time?"

"What lessons learned from your parents show up in how you see the world now?"

"What is the most hurtful thing that people across the political divide say about people on your side?"

"Do you believe that there are some threads that bind us all together, even when it seems there is so much more that divides us? What do you think they are?"

"Can you think of any traits you admire in people on the other side of the political divide?"

"Was ever there a time when you felt doubt about your political beliefs?"

"What is it like for you to hear that I have such different experiences?"

"What is it about the current political climate that you don't like?"

"Do you feel misunderstood by people like me who have different beliefs than you do? How so?"

"Is there someone you disagree with but still respect? If so, why?"

"What scares you most when you think about the future?"

Learning to listen in difficult conversations without overreacting is an exercise in accepting that each of us is different and separate. You can even learn to enjoy the differences. Formerly "impossible," "disagreeable," or "obviously wrong" friends and relatives begin to soften perceptibly as soon as you let them be who they are and express authentic curiosity about their ideas and experiences.

Not all relationships can be sorted out when political and cultural differences become too polarized to accommodate. Releasing yourself from slavish and unrewarding obligations helps stem the energy drain from a few expendable relationships. But since most of our relationships—particularly with family—aren't expendable, the most important thing you can do to avoid getting caught up in emotionally reactive transactions is to stay calm and kind and be yourself. Staying open means honoring other people's individuality; being yourself means not denying your own. Remember that this act of thoughtful listening is not just good for you and the relationship with a loved one—although that is a great reason to give it a try. Your willingness to reach across and find common humanity, listening deeply at this divisive time, also has the potential to radiate outward, offering a rewarding and meaningful sense of connection, belonging, and engagement in your other relationships too.

EXERCISES

1. Think about a person with whom you would like to try to have a difficult conversation. Ahead of time, try to ground yourself by making a commitment to the relationship.

   Values: It is important to me in my relationships that I am _____.

   Gratitude: I'm thankful for _____ in my life because _____.

   Positive Memory: I recall one time when, together, this person and I _____.

   Intention: At the end of the conversation, a realistic expectation is that we will _____.

   Calming: When I start getting upset, I can do these three things to calm down:

   (a) _____

   (b) _____

   (c) _____

2. See if you can fill in this *empathy map* to develop some insight into the person with whom you disagree so strongly:

   What does _____ think and feel?

      What really matters to _____?

      What are _____'s major preoccupations?

      What are _____'s worries and aspirations?

   What does _____ hear?

      What do friends say?

      What are news sources?

      What are the attitudes of the people from work and the neighborhood?

   What does _____ see?

      Environment?

      Social media?

      The community?

   What does _____ say and do?

      Attitude in public?

      Appearances?

      Behavior toward others?

   Pain

      What are _____'s fears?

      What are _____'s frustrations?

      What are _____'s life obstacles too great to overcome?

   Gain

      What are _____'s wants/needs?

      What are _____'s measures of success?

      What are _____'s obstacles that have been overcome?

Epilogue

An epilogue is where the author can be expected to wax philosophical. Here, for example, I might tell you that better listening not only transforms personal and professional relationships (which it does) but can also bring understanding across the gender gap, the racial divide, between rich and poor, and even among nations. All that may be true, but if I'm going to indulge in the unearned right to preach, maybe I should confine myself to matters closer to home. After all, I'm a psychologist, not a philosopher.

Having read this far, you've probably been reminded of some things you already knew but perhaps also come to see that listening is even more important and difficult than people realize. The urge to be heard is so compelling that even when we do listen, it's usually not with the intent to understand but to reply. And, as if that didn't make listening hard enough, at times of heat and conflict it takes a real effort to overcome, or at least restrain, the reactive emotionalism that jolts us into anxiety and out of sympathy with each other.

Few things can do as much to bring mutual understanding to your relationships as responsive listening—hearing and acknowledging other people's thoughts and feelings before voicing your own. You can make responsive listening a habit but, like any new habit, it takes practice.

One of my least favorite remarks has come from certain individuals in therapy to improve their relationships. They've complained. I've listened sympathetically. Then I've suggested things they could do to start giving and getting the understanding they say they long for. Then comes The Comment: "Why does everything have to be so artificial? Why can't we just talk to each other?" I hate that! They *were* talking, and it wasn't working.

It's annoying when people say that it's unnatural to hold their response until they've acknowledged what the other person has to say, because this protest seems so stubborn and self-defeating. But the thing that really annoys me about this comment is that it's true: good listening *doesn't* come naturally.

> Listening is a skill, and like any skill it must be developed. But although listening can be looked at this way—as a performance—it can also be looked at another way, as a natural outgrowth of caring and concern for people.

• • •

Caring about people doesn't require a lot of thought; it's something you feel. Caring about others almost automatically impels you to act with consideration for them. This consideration isn't wholly unselfish, because caring about someone means that your well-being is tied up with theirs. When a bad thing happens to someone you love, something bad happens to you as well. But *showing* that you care, suspending your own interests and making yourself receptive, isn't always easy.

Listening a little harder—extending what we do automatically, extending ourselves a little more—is one of the best ways we can be good to each other. Attending a little harder to other people—enough to hear their feelings, enough to consider their point of view—this takes a little effort.

Caring enough to listen doesn't mean going around selflessly available to everyone you encounter. Rather, it means being alert to those situations in which someone you care about needs to be listened to.

• • •

Ironically, our ability to listen is often worst with the people closest to us. Conflict, habit, and the pressure of emotions makes us listen least well where listening is most needed. As we move outside the family circle to those we care about but don't live with, we tend to be more open, more receptive, and more flexible. It's not—as we're sometimes accused of—that we care more about our friends than about our family but that these relationships are less burdened with conflict and resentment.

You won't get far with your efforts to listen better without running into the problem of your own emotionality. Listening better requires not only a greater openness to others but also a greater awareness of yourself. Do you express yourself in a way that makes listeners anxious and defensive? If so, what can you do about it? (If the answer is nothing, then that's the improvement you can expect in the listening you get.) Under what circumstances do you become reactive and give advice or interrupt or make jokes instead of listening?

· · ·

Concern for other people is an instinctive expression of the best part of us. Unfortunately, frustrations at home and a sense of powerlessness in the wider world mean that we don't always act with generosity and concern.

· · ·

Everywhere around us we're encouraged to claim our victimhood and right to bitterness. This feeling of injured entitlement can be understood as a product of insufficient emotional nourishment. People who are hungry for attention are suffered, shunned, or shamed. Others let them know in some way that their need to be heard is excessive. And where does that leave them? Hungry for attention. And so the problem of listening, like all human problems, is circular: inadequate appreciation makes us insecure in ourselves and less open to others. The listening we don't get is the listening we don't pass on.

Our inability to get the attention we crave leaves us feeling powerless—a feeling reinforced by living in a world marked by economic decline, crime, pollution, and bureaucratic ineptitude. So it's not surprising that we've lost faith in our capacity to make a difference. Public disillusion and private disappointment deplete and discourage us. We feel put upon and let down, and so, naturally, we turn our resentment outward and our sympathy inward.

When you feel beleaguered and insecure, it's natural to think about looking out for number one. Unfortunately, self-absorption is self-defeating.

Trapped in self-consciousness, we become polarized and resentful. Sadly, anger and despair have fueled a decline in concern and a retreat to the dead end of preoccupation with ourselves.

You can't simply reverse the process of misunderstanding, but you can realize that relationship problems are circular, and circular patterns can be broken—if someone is willing to make the first move.

The great reward of making that move is that listening allows us to be open, generous, and connected; to touch others' lives and to enrich them and us in the process. Listening—empathic listening—promotes growth in the listener, the one listened to, and the relationship between them.

That better listening enhances our own well-being is the natural perspective of psychology, in which all human behavior is seen as motivated by the agendas of the self. But when you narrow down human relations to a collection of selves, and the self to the early conditioning of the child, what you have left is fixed characters, and you're stuck with them.

It's a dogma of American life that all actions are motivated by self-interest. But this dogma is false. The tendency to view our lives on the planet from the perspective of individualism obscures the larger view that we are part of systems within systems: the family, the extended family, the community, the nation—vast networks of associations. The truth is that looking inside ourselves can show us only part of the reason for feeling empty and unfulfilled.

Should the idea of self-interest include interest in others? Yes. Benevolent self-interest goes hand in hand with interest in others. But is it only a matter of enlightened self-interest to take an interest in other people?

Trade-offs have their place in the conduct of life. But it would leave too much out of the story of human affairs to give an account of relatedness to others only in terms of utilitarianism.

Caring about other people, which takes shape in political justice, the relief of suffering, and the love of family and friends, is fundamental to our sense of who we are and what makes our lives hang together. Pressures that block or obscure this impulse reduce, even damage us.

Respect for human dignity doesn't mean only feeling sympathy for others or doing for them. It means respecting them enough to listen to them, to hear and appreciate their voices—to view them as subjects, worthy of hearing, not just as objects of our needs.

Listening to others is an ethical good, part of what it means to have just and fair dealings with other people. Listening is part of our moral commitment to each other.

• • •

Listening better to those you're closest to is easier when you remember that we are separate selves. Openness and autonomy are correlated. If you are to have the courage to be yourself, to stand squarely on your own two feet, then you must accept that other people are entitled to their own point of view. The idea isn't to separate yourself from others but to let them be themselves while you continue to be yourself.

Learning to listen involves a paradox of self-control: controlling yourself and letting go of control over the relationship. It's like letting someone else drive. To listen, you have to let go.

Trying harder to understand another person's perspective takes effort, but it isn't just a skill to be studied and practiced. Hearing someone is an expression of caring enough to listen.

One of the things I've hoped to do in this book is to help restore a sense of balance to the way we think about relationships. First because seeing our relationships as mutually defined enables us to change what we get out of them by changing what we put into them. And second because recognizing that we live in a web of relationships, which give meaning and fullness to our lives, may inspire us to a little more generosity and concern for other people.

Does talk of rebalancing relationships and rediscovering concern sound a little pious? After all, you probably picked up this book to learn a little more about listening, not to read a sermon on benevolence. Sorry. But maybe the sympathy for other people that we're born with is something we have to remind ourselves to express from time to time.

We all believe in fairness and respect for the rights of others. We believe in compassion and justice and that everyone has a right to be heard. Of course these standards are regularly violated. It remains that they are valid standards. And they do from time to time galvanize us to action—as when we somehow manage to listen instead of arguing in the midst of a heated discussion or when we remember to take a little extra time to hear what's going on in someone's life.

The obligation to listen can be experienced as a burden, and we all sometimes feel it that way. But it is quite a different thing to be moved by a sense that the people in our lives are eminently *worth* listening to, a sense of their dignity and value. One thing we can all add a little more of is understanding—respect, compassion, and fairness, the fundamental values conveyed by listening.

• • •

As I said at the beginning of this book, the reason we long so much to be listened to is that we never outgrow the need to communicate what it's like to live in our separate, private worlds of experience. Unfortunately, there is no parallel need to listen. Maybe that's why listening sometimes seems in short supply. Listening isn't a need we have; it's a gift we give.

Notes

Chapter 1

Brodkey, H. (1991). *The runaway soul*. New York: Farrar, Straus & Giroux.

Fingerman, K., Huo, M., & Birditt, K. (2020). A decade of research on intergenerational ties: Technological, economic, political, and demographic changes. *Journal of Marriage and Family, 82*(1), 383–403.

Kohut, H. (1971). *The analysis of the self: A systematic approach to the psychoanalytic treatment of narcissistic personality disorders*. New York: International Universities Press.

Turkle, S. (2015). *Reclaiming conversation: The power of talk in a digital age*. New York: Penguin Books.

Chapter 2

Macfarlane, A. (1977). *The psychology of childbirth*. Cambridge, MA: Harvard University Press.

Stern, D. (1990). *Diary of a baby: What your child sees, feels, and experiences*. New York: Basic Books.

Sullivan, H. S. (1953). *The interpersonal theory of psychiatry*. New York: Norton.

Tronick, E., Adamson, L. B., Als, H., & Brazelton, T. B. (1975, April). *Infant emotions in normal and pertubated interactions*. Paper presented at the biennial meeting of the Society for Research in Child Development, Denver, CO.

Turkle, S. (2017). *Alone together: Why we expect more from technology and less from each other.* New York: Basic Books.

Chapter 3

Bateson, G. (1972). *Steps to an ecology of mind.* New York: Ballentine Books.

Chodorow, N. (1978). *The reproduction of mothering: Psychoanalysis and the sociology of gender.* Berkeley: University of California Press.

Gilligan, C. (1982). *In a different voice: Psychological theory and women's development.* Cambridge, MA: Harvard University Press.

Gottman, J., & Silver, N. (2012). *What makes love last?* New York: Simon & Schuster.

Gottman, J., & Silver, N. (2015). *The seven principles for making marriage work.* New York: Harmony Books.

Gray, J. (1992). *Men are from Mars, women are from Venus.* New York: Harper Collins.

Hyde, J. S. (2005). The gender similarities hypothesis. *American Psychologist, 60*(6), 581–592.

Miller, J. B. (1976). *Toward a new psychology of women.* Boston: Beacon Press.

Chapter 5

Arnett, J. (2014). *Emerging adulthood: The winding road from the late teens through the twenties* (2nd ed.). New York: Oxford University Press.

On the subject of subpersonalities:

According to Henry A. Murray, "A personality is a full congress of orators and pressure groups, of children, demagogues, Machiavellis . . . Caesars and Christs . . ."; "What should psychologists do about psychoanalysis?," *Journal of Abnormal and Social Psychology,* 1940, *35,* 160–161.

Eric Berne's transactional analysis personified Freud's superego, ego, and id as parent, adult, and child. *Transactional analysis in psychotherapy* (New York: Grove Press, 1961).

Although many people have used the metaphor of subpersonalities, I have found the internal family systems model of Richard Schwartz particularly useful.

Schwartz, R. C., & Sweezy, M. (2019). *Internal family systems therapy* (2nd ed.). New York: Guilford Press.

Settersten, R., & Ray, B. E. (2010). *Not quite adults: Why 20-somethings are choosing a slower path to adulthood, and why it's good for everyone.* New York: Bantam Books.

Chapter 6

Becker, W. J., Belkin, L. M., & Conroy, S. A. (2019). Killing me softly: Organizational e-mail monitoring expectations' impact on employee and significant other well-being. *Journal of Management*. [Epub ahead of print]

Fogarty, T. (1979). The distancer and the pursuer. *The Family, 7*, 11–16.

Johnson, S. (2008). *Hold me tight: Seven conversations for a lifetime of love.* New York: Little, Brown Spark.

Radicati Group. (2019). Email statistics report 2015–2019—Executive summary. Retrieved from *www.radicati.com.*

Chapter 9

Perelman, S. J. (1950). *The Swiss family Perelman* (pp. 4–5). New York: Simon & Schuster.

Chapter 10

Christensen, A., Doss, B. D., & Jacobson, N. S. (2014). *Reconcilable differences: Rebuild your relationship by rediscovering the partner you love—without losing yourself* (2nd ed.). New York: Guilford Press.

Nelson, T. (2012). Nagging: Is it killing your marriage? Retrieved from *www.huffpost.com/entry/nagging-is-it-killing-you_b_1245574.*

Chapter 11

Godfrey, N. (2017, June 11). Working millennial moms: Are you getting the support you need? Retrieved from *www.forbes.com/sites/nealegodfrey/2017/06/11/working-millennial-moms/#bd0d2433775.*

Minuchin, S., & Nichols, M. P. (1993). *Family healing: Strategies for hope and understanding.* New York: Free Press.

Walsh, F. (Ed.). (2011). *Normal family processes: Growing diversity and complexity* (4th ed.). New York: Guilford Press.

Chapter 13

Better Angels. (2018). *Fussing and fighting: How we don't get along and sometimes do: A primer on polarization and social conflict.* New York: Author.

Chen, M., & Rohla, R. (2018). The effect of partisanship and political advertising on close family ties. *Science, 360,* 1020–1024.

Isay, D. (2019). *The great Thanksgiving listen: Teacher toolkit 2019.* StoryCorps. *Thegreatlisten.org.*

Kim, A., & Prado, A. (2019). *It's time to talk (and listen): How to have constructive conversations about race, class, sexuality, ability, and gender in a polarized world.* Oakland, CA: New Harbinger.

Tamerius, K., & Campt, D. (2019, November 18). Your angry uncle wants to talk about politics. What do you do? *New York Times.* Retrieved from *www.nytimes. com/interactive/2019/11/26/opinion/family-holiday-talk-impeachment.html.*

Index

"Accepting influence," 75
Accommodation
    dynamics of polarization between
        parents and, 286–287
    in intimate partner relationships,
        250–254, 261–263
Acknowledgment, of the other person's
    viewpoint, 158–163, 330
Active listening, 102, 163
Adolescents
    giving advice to and the notion of
        subpersonalities, 119
    reactivity to parents, 115–116
    silent arguing, 134–135
Advice
    asking for, 118
    credibility of the advice giver and,
        108
    giving advice and not listening, 164
    giving advice that's not followed,
        98–99
    giving advice with emotional pressure,
        137–138
    giving unsolicited advice, 94–95
    how to ask for support without getting
        unwanted advice, 172–173
    notion of subpersonalities and,
        118–119
American Psychological Association,
    74–75, 334
Anger
    how to understand a speaker's anger,
        210–213
    importance of expressing without
        losing control, 229–230
    projection and, 287
    See also Arguments; Conflicts
Anticipation. See Assumptions;
    Expectations
Anxiety, emotional reactivity in one's self
    and, 224
Apologizing, 136–137
Appreciation
    as the opposite of nagging, 256
    of the other person's point of view,
        153–156

Arguments
  active listening and, 163
  apologizing, 136–137
  couples and, 135–137
  emotional reactivity and, 130–132
  how to complain without starting a
      fight, 257–263
  intimate partner relationships and, 263
  listening with a clenched mind, 134
  reasons for and ways to alleviate,
      132–133
  responsive listening and, 165–167
  silent arguing, 134–135
  See also Conflicts; Misunderstandings
Ask, Listen, Reflect, Agree, Share
    strategy, 339–340
Assumptions
  creating a climate of understanding
      and, 177–178
  cutting people off or talking out of
      turn and, 178–181
  effects on listening, 176–177
  how to move beyond assumptions to
      openness, 188–192
  preparing for tense encounters,
      209–210
  See also Expectations
Attachment
  listening and the emergent self, 34
  listening and the shaping of self-
      respect, 32
Attention
  expectations from prior experiences
      and, 112
  going through the motions of,
      100–103
  impact of cell phones on, 153
  impact of contemporary pressures on,
      1–2
  listening and, 2–3, 14, 151–153,
      164–165
  one's need for attention and its impact
      on listening, 347–348
  problem of parental disengagement,
      281–283

Attunement
  child's development of a core self and,
      37–39
  child's development of a personal self,
      41
Authority
  being a parent-in-charge and, 279–280
  forging a unified family leadership, 286
  of parents, 272
Autonomy
  enmeshed relationships and, 283
  openness and, 349
Avoidance, 47, 131

Bearing witness, 16–19
Being heard
  digital communication and, 24–27
  means being taken seriously, 19–24
  not being heard by the listener, 96–98
  why some are hard to listen to, 70–73
Being understood
  adult self-awareness and, 35–37
  importance to child development,
      32–43. *See also* Child development
  listening and the urge to be, 9–10
  repression and not being understood,
      46–48
  shaping of character and, 29–30
Beliefs, about people one disagrees with,
    327
Biases
  attitudes about the speaker, 106–109
  expectations from prior experiences
      and, 109–112
Bitterness, intimate partner relationships
    and, 263–265
Blended families, family leadership and,
    286
Boundaries
  enmeshed relationships in families
      and, 283–286
  friendships and, 302
  importance in families, 270
  judgment by friends as a boundary
      violation, 296

problem of parental disengagement and, 281–283

problems around blurred boundaries in families, 271–273

setting limits at the workplace, 319–321

Breathing exercise, 201

Caring about others, 346, 347, 348–350

Cell phones

digital communication and being heard, 24–27

impact on attention, 153

iPhones and thought bubbles, 18

listening and texting, 156–157. *See also* Texting

See also Digital communication

Character, shaping of, 29–30

Child development

emergent self, 33–37

importance of being listened to and, 30–33

self-assurance and the listened-to-child, 43–44

sense of a core self, 37–39

sense of a personal self, 39–41

sense of a verbal self, 41–43

Childishness, 115

Children

divorce and, 288–289

the parent's gift of empathy and, 182–184

responsive listening with, 167–168

See also Adolescents; Child development; Families; Infants; Parent–child relationship

Colleagues, listening at the workplace and, 317–319

Command, 64

Committed relationships. *See* Intimate partners

Communication

being heard means being taken seriously, 19–24

break downs in. *See* Communication break downs

child's development of a personal self, 39–41

child's development of a verbal self, 41–43

components of, 61

context of and its impact on listening, 66–70

developing self-reflective awareness and, 199–202

effective managers and, 312–314

implicit messages and the problem of multiple meanings, 63–66

importance of efforts in mutual understanding, 158–163

importance of expressing feelings without losing control, 228–230

keys to success in, 5

messages and the problem of indirectness, 62–63

rules of the listening game, 60–70

sharing expectations about how and when it should take place, 198–199

texting and listening, 156–157

See also Digital communication

Communication break downs

effects of, 50

listening as a two-person process, 50–53

misunderstandings, 53–60. *See also* Misunderstandings

notions of gender differences and, 73–78

why some are hard to listen to, 70–73

Communication styles, 200–201

Competence, 338

Complaints

about the boss in a workplace, 315–316

accommodation of differences and, 261–263

active listening and, 163

complementarity and, 238

confrontations from pent up complaints, 140–141

cross-complaining, 214

expressing at the office, 308–312

Complaints (*cont.*)
friendships and, 298–302
as hidden requests, 128
how to complain nicely, 129
how to complain without starting a fight, 257–263
See also Criticism
Complementarity, 237–239, 265
Compliant people, 155
Conflicts
notion of subpersonalities and, 119
from pent up complaints, 140–141
preparing for, 209–210
projection and, 287–288
resolving with friends, 298–302
See also Arguments; Misunderstandings
Control
being a parent-in-charge and, 279–280
importance of expressing feelings without losing control, 228–230
importance of relinquishing, 163–171, 349
self-control and the burden of listening, 87–91, 349
Conversational styles, 192–194
Conversations
balance between expression and recognition in, 29
emotional reactivity and arguments, 130–132 (*see also* Arguments)
misunderstandings and differences in conversational styles, 193–194
See also Difficult conversations
Core self, 37–39
Countertransference, 56–57
Couples. *See* Intimate partners
Courtship, 239–240
Credibility of speakers, 108–109
Criticism
complaints as hidden requests, 128
how to complain nicely, 129
how to complain without starting a fight, 257–263

how to listen to, 128
how to offer to friends, 303
how to take without overreacting, 213–216
overreaction to, 123–129
See also Complaints
Cross-complaining, 214
Curiosity, shifting from being right to, 333–340
Cutting people off, 178–181
Cyber bullying, 25

Defense analysis, 72
Defensiveness
how to avoid as a behavior, 206–209
preparing for tense encounters, 209–210
reasons for, 205
responding to with empathy, 204–205
Depression, 42
Differentiated individuals, 139–140
Difficult conversations
caring about the other person's opinions in, 329–330
challenges for personal identity and, 337–340
demonstrating an open mind in, 332–333
emotional reactivity and, 130–132, 334–337
listening to and telling stories, 340–342
listening when it feels impossible, 328–340
making the shift from being right to curiosity, 333–340
preparing for, 209–210
setting intentions for, 331–332
Digital communication
empathy and, 186–188
how to handle emotional reactivity in one's self, 223–224
listening and, 24–27
making time to listen to friends and, 306–308

problem of parental disengagement and, 281–283
responsive listening and, 170–171
See also Cell phones; Social media; Texting
Disagreements. *See* Arguments; Conflicts; Misunderstandings
Disengagement, 281–283
Dismissing the speaker, 96–98
Distancer–pursuer dynamic, 146–147, 247–250, 264
Distancing
disengagement and, 282–283
between intimate partners, 245–247
Divorce, 288–289
Dueling points of view, 161–162

Effective questions, 90–91
Email
empathy and communication, 186–188
how to handle emotional reactivity in one's self, 223–224
receiving criticism by, 128
responsive listening and, 170–171
See also Digital communication
Embarrassment, 96
Emergent self, 33–37
Emerging adulthood, 113–115, 116
Emoticons, 187
Emotional flooding, 335–337
Emotional intolerance, 197
Emotional reactivity
arguments and, 130–137. *See also* Arguments
challenges of difficult conversations and, 334–337
communication break downs and, 59–60
empathy turns defensiveness around, 204–205
getting to the root of, 217–220
giving advice with emotional pressure, 137–138
healing hurt feelings and broken connections, 143–145
how to avoid when provoked, 206–217
how to handle in one's self, 223–227
how to respond to recurring issues, 216–217
how to take criticism without overreacting, 213–216
how to understand a speaker's anger, 210–213
impact of the speaker's emotionality on listeners, 138–143, 347
importance of expressing feelings without losing control, 228–230
listening to hard-to-listen-to people and, 322–327
overreaction to criticism, 123–129
preparing for tense encounters, 209–210
reasons for increasing as relationships evolve, 220–223
ways to resolve, 227–228
See also Feelings; Overreacting
Emotional reticence. *See* Reticence
Emotional triangles
complaining about the boss in the workplace, 315–316
in families, 273–280
Emotional validation, 168–170
Emotional well-being, empathy and, 46
Empathic immersion, 183
Empathy
activities required in, 190
the burden of listening, 87–91
characteristics of, 94
conveying to another, 42–43
defined, 42
developing to become a better listener, 181–182
digital communication and, 186–188
distinguished from sympathy, 94
emotional validation and, 168–170
emotional well-being and, 46
escapism in the absence of, 26–27
friends and, 294–298
good listening and, 10, 15, 46, 84, 177, 348

Empathy *(cont.)*
impact of digital communication on, 26
intimate partner relationships and, 263
listening to your partner's repeated stories, 184–186
moving beyond assumptions to, 188–192
parents and, 182–184
reticence and the lack of empathic listening, 43
self-assurance and the listened-to-child, 43–44
turns defensiveness around, 204–205
understanding and, 189
Enmeshed relationships, 283–286
Escapism, 26–27
Excessive sympathy, 93–94
Expectations
hypersensitivity and, 109–112
preconceived notions, 58–59
sensitivity and, 192–199
transference and countertransference, 54–57
See also Assumptions
Expression
in balance with recognition, 29
self and the need for, 32

Faking attention, 100
Falling in love, 239–240
Families
contemporary family diversity and challenges for listening, 268–269
dangers of parents becoming polarized, 286–289
divorce and, 288–289
emotional triangles, 273–280
enmeshed relationships, 283–286
forging a unified family leadership, 286
importance of family pairs having time alone together, 270–271
parents and taking charge of children, 279–280
problems around blurred boundaries, 271–273

relationships and the creation of family structure, 268
rigid boundaries and the problem of parental disengagement, 281–283
subsystems and boundaries, 270
See also Adolescents; Children; Infants; Parent–child relationship
Family therapy, cotherapists and, 276
Favoritism, emotional triangles in families and, 277–279
Feelings
about people one disagrees with, 327
acknowledging and appreciating in others, 154, 160–161, 194, 205, 330
balancing with thinking, 190
blurring the distinction between facts and feelings, 63
challenges of difficult conversations and, 334–337
expressing and becoming better listeners, 57–58
expressing criticism and, 259–260
feeling embarrassed, 96
healing hurt feelings and broken connections, 143–145
importance of expressing without losing control, 228–230
questions to help the other person express, 155–156
resolving conflicts with friends and, 301–302
See also Emotional reactivity
Feminist psychologists, 74
Fight–flight response, 335
Friends
as the best listeners, 291–294
challenges of maintaining friendships through time, 303–305
digital communication and making time to listen to, 306–308
how to offer constructive criticism to, 303
as providers of judgment instead of empathy, 294–298
resolving conflicts with, 298–302

Gay relationships. *See* Same-sex relationships
Gender, communication and, 73–78
Gossip, 315–316

Hard-to-listen-to people
challenges and importance of listening and maintaining connections, 322–327
listening to and telling stories, 340–342
listening when it feels impossible, 328–340
reasons to get better at listening to, 325–326
why some people are hard to listen to, 70–73
Housework, women and, 255
How Good a Listener Are You? (questionnaire), 78–80
How Prepared Are You to Listen to Someone Who's Hard to Listen to? (exercise), 329
Hypersensitivity
expectations and the making of, 109–112
unresolved sensitivities from childhood and, 112–116

Identity, difficult conversations and, 337–340
Identity politics, 338
"I Don't Have a Minute to Catch My Breath" (breathing exercise), 201
Implicit messages, 63–66
Independence, balancing intimacy with, 243–247
Indirectness, 62–63
Ineffective questions, 90–91
Infants
need for listening and the emergent self, 33–37
the parent's gift of empathy and, 184
sense of a core self, 37–39
sense of a personal self, 39–41

sense of a verbal self, 41–43
See also Children
Inner experiences, development of a personal self and, 39–41
Inner voices, 197–198
Insecurity, emotional reactivity to criticism and, 127
Insensitivity, 195–197
Intentions
communication and, 53
setting for difficult conversations, 331–332
Internet, impact on our intimate lives, 244–245. *See also* Digital communication; Email; Social media
Interruptions
effects of interrupting the speaker, 99–100, 163–164
how to handle, 172–173
Intersubjectivity, 41
Intimacy
balancing with independence, 243–247
enmeshed relationships and, 283–286
Intimate partners
accommodating differences, 250–254, 261–263
arguments and, 135–137
balancing intimacy and independence, 243–247
challenges of very similar partners, 253–254
concept of complementarity and, 237–239, 265
divorce and, 288–289
dynamic of needs for space versus closeness in, 241–243
example of not listening to each other, 235–237
favoritism in families and, 278–279
getting beyond bitterness, 263–265
giving advice with emotional pressure, 137–138
how to complain without starting a fight, 257–263

Intimate partners *(cont.)*
impact of the emotional climate on the quality of understanding in, 140–143
importance of having time together in families, 270–271
importance of seeing the patterns of interaction in, 265–266
listening to a partner's repeated stories, 184–186
nagging and, 254–257
pursuer–distancer dynamic, 146–147, 247–250, 264
rhythms of change in committed relationships, 239–241
Intolerance, 129
iPhones, 18

Joking, 95–96
Judgment, 294–298

Leading questions, 165
Lesbian relationships. *See* Same-sex relationships
Limits, setting at the workplace, 319–321. *See also* Boundaries
Listeners
countertransference and, 56–57
good listening and suspending the self, 83–86. *See also* Suspending the self
impact of the speaker's emotionality on, 138–143
misunderstanding and the listener's own agenda, 57–58
transference and the speaker's expectations, 54–56, 57
Listening
appreciating the other person's point of view, 153–156
as bearing witness, 16–19
being heard means being taken seriously, 19–24
the burden of, 87–91
caring about others and, 346, 347, 348–350

consequences of losing the art of, 2
difficulty and importance of, 345–346
digital communication and, 24–27
elements in the process of, 61
empathy and good listening, 10, 15, 46, 84, 177, 348. *See also* Empathy
failures of understanding and, 3–4
going through the motions of, 100–103
guidelines for good listening, 171
to hard-to-listen-to people. *See* Hard-to-listen-to people
impact of contemporary pressures on, 1–2
impact of emotionally on, 132, 347. *See also* Emotional reactivity
impact of one's need for attention on, 347–348
importance of efforts in mutual understanding, 158–163
importance of relinquishing control, 163–171, 349
importance to child development and the shaping of self-respect, 30–43. *See also* Child development
importance to successful relationships, 10
mutual sharing and, 44–46
narcissism and, 20–21
paying attention and, 2–3, 14, 151–153, 164–165
resisting the temptation to turn away, 173–174
rules of the listening game, 60–70
sense of self and, 10–11
shaping of character and, 29–30
as a skill to be developed, 178, 346, 349
successful communication and, 5
suspending the self and, 83–91. *See also* Suspending the self
texting and, 156–157
as a two-person process, 50–53
types of failures in selfless listening, 92–100

the urge to be understood and, 9–10
when it feels impossible, 328–340
See also Active listening; Prejudiced
    listening; Responsive listening;
    Selfless listening

Managers
    getting one's point of view across with,
        308–312
    good managers as good listeners,
        312–314
    problems of not listening, 314–317
Marriage, modern "capstone" approach
    to, 240–241. *See also* Intimate
    partners
Meaning
    implicit messages and the problem of
        multiple meanings, 63–66
    levels of, 64
Memory, overreaction to criticism and,
    125–127
*Men Are from Mars, Women Are from
    Venus* (Gray), 73
Messages
    communication and, 53
    implicit messages and the problem of
        multiple meanings, 63–66
    the problem of indirectness and,
        62–63
Metacommunication, 64–66
"Me too," 93
#MeToo movement, 75–76
Mind reading, 39
Misunderstandings
    active listening and, 163
    attributing to other person's character,
        61
    blurring the distinction between facts
        and feelings, 63
    communication break downs and,
        53–54
    context of communication and,
        66–70
    differences in conversational styles
        and, 193–194

emotional reactivity, 59–60
    failures of listening and, 3–4
    failure to acknowledge what the other
        person says, 159–161
    implicit messages and the problem of
        multiple meanings, 63–66
    the listener's own agenda, 57–58
    listening with a clenched mind, 134
    messages and the problem of
        indirectness, 62–63
    preconceived notions, 58–59
    problem of linear thinking, 60–61
    suggestions for minimizing in digital
        communication, 187–188
    transference and countertransference,
        54–57
    See also Arguments
Mothers, enmeshed relationships and,
    284–285
Mutual sharing, 44–46
Mutual understanding, 158–163

Nagging
    in families, 272
    in intimate partner relationships,
        254–257
Narcissism, 20–21
Narratives, emergent self and, 34
Nonselves, 155
"Not me," 30
Nurture, being a parent-in-charge and,
    279–280

Oedipal conflict, 273–276
Openness
    autonomy and, 349
    demonstrating an open mind in
        difficult conversations, 332–333
    effective managers and, 312–313
    how to move beyond assumptions to,
        188–192
    questions that may help children open
        up, 90–91
    setting the intention for with difficult
        conversations, 331–332

Opinions, difficult conversations and, 329–330. *See also* Viewpoints
Overly sympathetic listeners, 93–94, 102–103
Overreacting
  to criticism, 123–129
  how to take criticism without overreacting, 213–216
  preparing for tense encounters, 209–210
  unresolved sensitivities from childhood and, 112–116
  See also Emotional reactivity

Parent–child relationship
  adolescents and silent arguing, 134–135
  being heard means being taken seriously, 20, 21–24
  child development and the importance of listening, 30–33 (*see also* Child development)
  digital communication and, 25
  divorce and, 288–289
  emotional reactivity in adult children and, 125–127, 217–220
  empathy and listening to children, 182–184
  questions that may help children open up, 90–91
  reactivity to parents during adolescence, 115–116
  unresolved issues and hypersensitivity in adult children, 112–116
  See also Adolescents; Children; Families; Infants
Passive listening, 155
Personal identity
  development of a sense of, 39–41
  difficult conversations and, 337–340
Peter Principle, 312
Phubbing, 100
Points of view. *See* Viewpoints
Polarization, and complementarity in parenting, 286–289

Political conversations
  questions to aid engaging in, 341
  shifting from being right to being curious, 333–340
  See also Difficult conversations
Preconceived notions, 58–59
Prejudiced listening
  attitudes about the speaker, 106–109
  expectations from prior experiences and, 109–112
  notion of subpersonalities and, 116–120
  unresolved issues in the parent–child relationship and, 112–116
Projection, 287–288
Pursuer–distancer dynamic, 146–147, 247–250, 264

Questions
  controlling listeners and, 165
  to demonstrate an open mind in difficult conversations, 332
  to engage in conversations across political differences, 341
  to help children open up, 90–91
  to help the other person express their feelings or thoughts, 155–156

Reacting, distinguished from responding, 182
Reassurance, 21
Recognition
  in balance with expression, 29
  self and the need for, 32
Recurring issues, how to respond to, 216–217
Relationships
  adult need for being understood and, 35–37
  challenges and importance of listening to hard-to-listen-to people, 322–327
  emotional reactivity and, 59–60, 220–223
  expectations from prior experiences and, 109–112

healing hurt feelings and broken
connections, 143–145

impact of the emotional climate on the
quality of understanding in, 139–143

importance of listening and being
listened to, 10, 29

listening and caring about others, 346,
347, 348–350

listening as a two-person process,
51–53

notion of subpersonalities and,
117–118, 119–120

pain of not being listened to, 11–15

preconceived notions and, 58–59

transference and countertransference
in, 54–57

See also Intimate partners; Parent–
child relationship

Repeated stories
how to respond to, 216–217
listening to, 99, 184–186

Repression, unshared thoughts and,
46–48

Reproduction of Mothering, The
(Chodorow), 74

Responding, distinguished from reacting,
182

Responsive listening
with children, 167–168
creating a climate of understanding
and, 177–178
description of, 165–167
with digital communication, 170–171
emotional validation and, 168–170
with hard-to-listen-to people, 328–330

Responsiveness, friendships and, 302

Responsive unavailability, 173–174

Reticence
characteristics of, 145–146
lack of empathic listening and, 43
pursuer–distancer dynamic, 146–147,
247–250, 264
questions that may help children open
up, 90–91
reasons for, 72

responding to, 72–73, 222–223

unshared thoughts and being
diminished, 46–48

Runaway Soul, The (Brodkey), 20

Sadness, not being listened and, 42

Same old story (SOS), 184–186

Same-sex relationships, pursuer–
distancer dynamic in, 249–250

Saying "no," 257

Secure self, 30–33

Self
the act of bearing witness and, 18–19
bad listening and focusing on one's
self, 103
how to handle emotional reactivity in
one's self, 223–227
impact of one's own emotionality on
listening, 347
intolerance and, 129
listening and the notion of
subpersonalities, 116–120
listening and the sense of self, 10–11
listening to one's self, 200–202
one's need for attention and its impact
on listening, 347–348
personal identity and the challenges of
difficult conversations, 337–340
suspending. *See* Suspending the self

Self-assurance
illusion of solitude and, 47
the listened-to-child and, 43–44

Self-awareness
adult need for being understood and,
35–37
developing self-reflective awareness,
199–202

Self-compassion, 129

Self-conscious listeners, 101

Self-control, the burden of listening and,
87–91, 349

Selfless listening
being a good listener and, 83–86
types of failures in, 92–100
the work of listening and, 87–91

Selfobjects, 18–19
Self-reflective awareness, 199–202
Self-respect
  bearing witness and the confirmation
    of, 16–18
  being listened to and the development
    of, 30–33
Self-righteousness, 338
Sensitivity
  being responsive to other people's
    feelings, 194
  developing self-reflective awareness,
    199–202
  insensitivity to those we love, 195–197
  to other people's conversational styles,
    192–194
  to other people's inner voices, 197–198
  sharing expectations about how and
    when to communicate, 198–199
  ways to show, 194–195
Setting, impact on communication and
    listening, 67–69
Shame, emotional reactivity to criticism
    and, 127
Shaming
  impact on a child, 228
  to provoke attention, 224–225
Sharing
  development of a personal self and,
    39–41
  listening and mutual sharing, 44–46
Silent arguing, 134–135
Single parents, 285
Smartphones, 68. *See also* Digital
    communication; Texting
Social media
  avoidant people and, 47
  bearing witness and, 16
  cyber bullying, 25
  digital communication and listening,
    24–27
  empathy and communication, 186–188
  friendship and, 293–294
  impact on our intimate lives, 244–245
  mutual sharing and, 44–45

narcissism and, 21
  See also Digital communication
Solitude, 47
Sons and Lovers (Lawrence), 275–276
SOS. *See* Same old story
Speakers
  attitudes about and biased listening,
    106–109
  being dismissed by the listener, 96–98
  credibility of, 108–109
  effects of interrupting, 99–100,
    163–164
  how to understand anger in, 210–213
  impact of emotionality on listeners,
    138–143, 347
  resisting the temptation to turn away
    from, 173–174
  See also Being heard; Being
    understood; Hard-to-listen-to people
Step-families, family leadership and, 286
Still-face response, 41
Storytelling
  emergent self and, 34
  listening to hard-to-listen-to people
    and, 340–342
Stress, emotional reactivity in difficult
    conversations and, 334–337
Stress in America™ survey, 334
Subpersonalities, 116–120, 198
Subsystems, 270–271
Support, how to ask for without getting
    advice, 172–173
Suspending the self
  to appreciate the other person's point
    of view, 153–156
  being a good listener and, 83–86
  moving beyond assumptions to
    empathy, 188–192
  overcoming assumptions about what
    someone is going to say, 180–181
  resisting the temptation to turn away
    from the speaker, 173–174
  types of failures in selfless listening,
    92–100
  the work of listening and, 87–91

Sympathy
  empathy distinguished from, 94
  overly sympathetic listeners, 102–103
  responding with excessive sympathy, 93–94
  therapists and, 85

Talking out of turn, 178–181
Technology. *See* Digital communication
Teenagers. *See* Adolescents
Tense encounters. *See* Difficult conversations
Texting
  empathy and communication, 186–188
  how to handle emotional reactivity in one's self, 223–224
  listening and, 156–157
  making time to listen to friends and, 306–308
  misunderstanding and the problem of metacommunication, 65
  receiving criticism by, 128
  resolving conflicts with friends and, 298–299
  responsive listening and, 170–171
  See also Digital communication
Thinking, balancing with feeling, 190
Thinking about the SOS (exercise), 186
Third parties, impact on communication and listening, 69–70
Thought bubbles, 18
Timing of communication, 66–67
Topics, difficult conversations and, 333–334
Transference, 54–56, 57
Triangulation. *See* Emotional triangles

Understanding
  acknowledgment of the other person's viewpoint, 158–163, 330
  authority of parents and, 272
  creating a climate of, 177–178
  empathy and, 189
  how to understand a speaker's anger, 210–213
  importance of efforts in mutual understanding, 158–163
  See also Being understood
Unshared thoughts, 46–48
Unsolicited advice, 94–95

Values, 331
Verbal self, 41–43
Viewpoints
  acknowledging in the other person, 158–163, 330
  appreciating in the other person, 153–156
  difficult conversations and, 329–330
  dueling points of view, 161–162
  listening to and telling stories with hard-to-listen-to people, 340–342

Workplace
  getting one's point of view across at, 308–312
  good managers as good listeners, 312–314
  listening to and getting listened by colleagues, 317–319
  problem of managers not listening, 314–317
  setting limits at, 319–321

"Yes, but . . . ," 273

Zero-sum games, 229

About the Authors

Michael P. Nichols, PhD, has been practicing and teaching family therapy since the 1970s. He is Professor of Psychology at the College of William and Mary. Dr. Nichols is the author of numerous books for general readers, professionals, and students.

Martha B. Straus, PhD, is Professor in the Department of Clinical Psychology at Antioch University New England in Keene, New Hampshire. Dr. Straus consults and trains internationally. The author of books including *Treating Trauma in Adolescents*, she maintains a small private practice in Vermont.